A Patient-Expert Walks You Through Everything You Need to Learn and Do™

CLAUDIA CRAIG MAREK is a medical assistant who has counseled fibromyalgia patients for more than a dozen years and the co-author of *What Your Doctor May Not Tell You About Fibromyalgia*.

THE COMPLETE FIRST YEAR™ SERIES

THE FIRST YEAR™

Fibromyalgia

An Essential Guide for the Newly Diagnosed

Claudia Craig Marek

Foreword by R. Paul St. Amand, M.D.

MARLOWE & COMPANY ■ NEW YORK

THE FIRST YEAR™—FIBROMYALGIA:
An Essential Guide for the Newly Diagnosed

Published by
Marlowe & Company
An Imprint of Avalon Publishing Group Incorporated
161 William Street, 16th Floor
New York, NY 10038

The First Year™ and A Patient-Expert Walks You Through
Everything You Need to Learn and Do™
are trademarks of the Avalon Publishing Group.

Library of Congress Cataloging-in-Publication Data
Marek, Claudia
    The first year—fibromyalgia: an essential guide for the-
newly diagnosed / Claudia Craig Marek.
        p. cm.
Includes bibliographical references and index.
    ISBN 1-56924-521-5 (trade paper)
    1. Fibromyalgia—Popular works. I. Title: Fibromyalgia.
II. Title.
RC927.3.M5786 2003
616.7'4—dc21   2002141445

9   8   7   6   5   4   3   2

*Designed by Pauline Neuwirth,
Neuwirth and Associates, Inc.*

Printed in the United States of America

Distributed by Publishers Group West

FOR MY PARENTS, AND FOR EVERYONE WHO
SUFFERS WITH FIBROMYALGIA AND THE
WONDERFUL PEOPLE WHO LOVE
AND SUPPORT THEM

"YOU'RE BRAVER THAN YOU BELIEVE,
AND STRONGER THAN YOU SEEM,
AND SMARTER THAN YOU THINK."

—CHRISTOPHER ROBIN

Contents

CONTENTS

Foreword

by R. Paul St. Amand, M.D.

THE FIRST time I met her, Claudia Marek had an impressive presence and there was no doubt about her persona. I saw enough during our brief encounters during the course of our workdays to try and lure her into coming to work with me. She had been raised in a world inhabited by super scientists, some of them Nobel laureates. Was that experience sufficiently overbearing to explain her initial reluctance to join me? I don't know, but finally, during our first real interview something seemed to change and her earlier refusal became an almost eager acceptance. She was soon my medical assistant—kudos to us for our mutual decision!

She was immediately immersed in the daily pool of my fibromyalgic patients. Within a few weeks she described one sister who lived in the strange realm of all too familiar complaints. Before long she began speaking about her own two boys, her beloved "puppies," one brown and the other white. The six-year-old darker one shared some of auntie's symptoms. We wouldn't have to wait too many years for the blond one's company.

Then one day she asked, almost commanded me, albeit sheepishly to "check me." As I swept my hands over her muscles and sinews she began her own litany of symptoms. There seemed to be one to match every lump and bump I found.

When I completed my examination and she her recital, there was no doubt: Claudia also had fibromyalgia.

The early weeks working together provided me daily surprises. Whatever is the genetic code that creates medical talent I could see its expression emerging in this brilliant woman. It seemed like a silent explosion if such is possible. It wasn't long before we were working at comparable levels. Within a few years, she had assimilated my life's work and many times since I have wondered which of us is leading the other.

I have worked with Claudia for nearly fifteen years. Together, we've listened to patients, examined them, gloated over our successes and despaired with our early-on failures. We moved forward in large part because of her. She sometimes heard what I had not. She often surmised facts intellectually and sometimes had to drag me along until I grasped her concepts. I amazingly found myself alongside a colleague in every sense. When I have to yield to her better perceptions I save my waning ego by reminding her that I hold the license!

Claudia has pored over countless e-mails, oftentimes screening literally from fifty to sixty a day, seven days a week, 365 days a year. She has collected data from incessant phone calls, letters, and technical information as this book well reflects. She has continuously interfaced with thousands of patients in our practice including over six hundred new ones each year. Her eyes see and she has trained herself to hear not only what's said but to interpret within the memory gaps so common in fibromyalgic patients. Empathy and intuition are always added to her tactile skills to validate patient complaints. She has lived the tired and achy life in its depths and has emerged whole.

I am happy to report that her sister is well and teaching at the university level. Malcolm, the brown puppy, is now a tanned, strapping twenty-one-year-old who interjects his computer talents in Month 12 of this book. The white puppy is six feet tall, pure brawn, and is turning seventeen while dreaming of his future career in law enforcement. These are Claudia's most cherished fibromyalgics, who now lead healthy lives unimpeded.

You are fortunate to have chosen this book. You will learn from an expert in the field. She is co-author of two other books with me. No position papers leave our office without her editorial touches and embellishments. We write, instruct, and lecture almost interchangeably. Claudia Marek is analytical about her personal experiences while painting her word pictures about fibromyalgia. In these pages she combines science and her prodigious memory to let you study what she has learned. She writes as a fellow sufferer, not some disinterested author. You will understand what she is telling you since both you and she have been there.

This is not simply another book about coping. It's a structured, factual recitation of I've-been-there experiences accumulated from patients and author. This is a compendium for diagnosis, understanding, and overcoming a miserable, badly understood disease. Claudia will adeptly walk you through your first year with fibromyalgia.

Once upon a time, I faltered in my frustration from years of working with a nameless disease. There was no acceptance for what I was doing. There was usually open sneering when I tried to promote the concept of a new entity. I hesitated and withdrew within the confines of my practice and expounded the diagnosis and my treatment protocol only to my own patients. Then came the empowerment of the Claudia years. She simply would not allow less than worldwide dissemination of our cumulative experience and physical findings. It seems to me that just about the time when I cried "uncle" I was lucky to have her answer "niece" and now, through her spirit, the job will somehow get done.

R. PAUL ST. AMAND, M.D., has been on the teaching staff at the Los Angeles Harbor/UCLA Hospital, Department of Endocrinology for over forty-five years and is co-author of *What Your Doctor May Not Tell You About Fibromyalgia*. Amand lives in Los Angeles.

Introduction

FIBROMYALGIA IS a confusing word and an even more confusing illness. The name means muscle pain, but muscle pain is only the tip of the iceberg when it comes to the symptoms you will encounter. If you're like most of us, getting a diagnosis meant that while you were relieved to finally learn that something "real" is wrong with you, you still don't really know exactly what that something is. You know that fibromyalgia is responsible for your pain and fatigue, but what else it means, why you have it, and what caused it is a mystery to you. Let's face it, you're probably feeling stunned, lost, and unsure of what your next step should be.

What happened to me

In 1987, I was thirty-six years old and the single mother of two small boys. I was working full-time, battling fatigue, headaches, back pain, constant pelvic pain, and one bladder infection after another. My gynecologist, desperate for some explanation for my symptoms, wanted to do exploratory surgery. Heavy-duty antibiotics were making me queasy, dizzy, and even more miserable. A friend looked at me and said, "I don't understand. The doctors don't know what's wrong with you, but they give you medication, and *you're taking it!*" Her words struck home: I was letting the doctors treat me for symptoms they didn't understand with medications that were not helping. I stopped the medications, canceled my appointments, and concentrated on getting through each day the best way I could, propped up on coffee, sugar, Tylenol, and all the extra sleep I could muster. I was weary of doctors anyway, having wasted much of my life, from childhood on, looking to them for answers that they simply did not have.

Fibromyalgia hasn't been around very long

It was only about fifteen years ago that an eminent rheumatologist, Frederick Wolfe, M.D., brought together a group of twenty-plus physicians and scientists—all of whom were observing an array of similar symptoms in their patients. They came from all over the United States and Canada and gathered at his home in Wichita, Kansas. Their goal was to develop criteria—a basis from which they could begin to study this condition. Dr. Wolfe's purpose, he declared, was not to name an illness (it already had a name, albeit a woefully inaccurate one, "fibrositis"), but to put into place a standard so that they could start to unravel the mystery. They all knew the history of the condition they were observing: it had been noted in medical literature since the early 1800s. An approach needed to be devised before they could initiate research into the perplexing cluster of symptoms they were looking at: widespread pain, deadening fatigue, disturbed and non-restorative sleep, irritable bowel and bladder, painful menstrual cycles, mood swings, anxiety, and depression.

The odd combination of the mental (depression, anxiety, nervousness, irritability, cognitive deficits) and the physical (headaches, backaches, leg cramps, shoulder pain, neck pain) begged the question: Which came first, the chicken or the egg? Were patients in pain because they were depressed, or depressed because they were in pain? Did the lack of sleep cause the pain, or did the pain cause the lack of sleep? Why were women predominately affected? Was this an inherited condition or a by-product of the stress of the modern world? Are certain personalities at risk to develop these woes? They did not know the answers; they did not even know all the questions. But, as Dr. Wolfe reminds us today, the purpose of this meeting was to voice questions, not to find answers. The collection of symptoms they were studying was given a new name, *fibromyalgia syndrome,* which simply means pain in muscles and fibers, and with this an unexpected phenomenon began.

Fibromyalgia is born

Though Dr. Wolfe insists he did not mean to define a disease, that's exactly what happened. Physicians started to use the criteria and the name in their practices; patients suddenly had an explanation for all their pesky complaints. They were validated: There was something wrong with them and it wasn't all in their heads; they were really sick. And, in 1991, when the World Health Organization accepted the criteria, almost word for word, it became official. Modern fibromyalgia was born, and almost simultaneously I was finally diagnosed. "I'm not crazy, I'm sick," I said aloud, slowly and almost carefully. And most wonderful of all, "Other people have what I have. I am not alone." Working in a medical office I saw the magic of that moment then, and I still do today. I know how they feel. I never forget how I felt. I am achingly aware of how much easier their lives, and my early life, would have been if any doctor had ever said, "I have other patients like you. They hurt all over just like you do, and I don't know why." I wouldn't have cared if my illness had a name. I wouldn't have minded that there was no cure. I would have been comforted just to know that there was someone else like me, someone who had strange symptoms no one could explain. There were times when I was hanging on by the skin of my teeth when a gesture *that simple* would have made all the difference in my world.

In 1992 there were no books about fibromyalgia, no Internet groups, no support groups—nothing but a few vague pamphlets by the Arthritis Foundation assuring us that our fibromyalgia wouldn't get worse, and all we needed to do was exercise and learn to relax. Coasting on the high of getting a diagnosis, most of us didn't even notice there was no substance to what we were being told. But in 1996, that changed. There was a site on the Internet where fibromyalgics would meet to chat and compare notes, and one of us rose up. Fibromyalgics were given a new voice by Devin Starlanyl, whose groundbreaking book, *Fibromyalgia and Chronic Myofascial Pain Syndrome,* has now sold a million or so copies. Offering ideas and detailed explanation, teaching empowerment, and daring to question authority, Devin blazed a trail for all of us. Alternative treatments were proposed, advocacy encouraged, conventional wisdom challenged. There was no going back; fibromyalgia and we fibromyalgics would never be the same. A diagnosis was no longer enough; the revolution had begun.

Fibromyalgia is still controversial

Meanwhile, back in Wichita, Dr. Frederick Wolfe was having doubts. He saw an army of patients armed with journals and pain charts for writing down their symptoms and feelings, with motorized scooters and handicapped placards, and carrying copies of preprinted demands for narcotic pain medication. He recoiled, and stated, "By receiving this diagnosis and taking medications, these people become card-carrying members of the fibromyalgia club." In *The Journal of Rheumatology,* looking like a distinguished elder statesman with a neatly trimmed gray beard, Dr. Wolfe renounced the work that had won him fame. Like Alfred Nobel, he looked at the fruits of his well-intentioned labor and hung his head. "For a moment in time we thought we had discovered a new physical disease. But it was the emperor's new clothes. When we started out in the '80s we saw patients going from doctor to doctor with pain. We believed that by telling them they had fibromyalgia, we reduced stress and reduced medical utilization. This idea, this great humane idea . . . didn't turn out that way. My view now is that we are creating an illness rather than curing one."

His colleagues did not share his torment. Drs. Russell, Goldenberg, Pellegrino, Wallace, and others have written books of their own about fibromyalgia in the wake of Devin Starlanyl's success. They never mention her book or her dominant presence on the World Wide Web. Instead, they cheerfully tout exercise and antidepressants, and listening to your doctor, of course. Good posture helps, and prescription drugs in personalized combinations, and, of course, de-stressing your life. They refer and defer to each other, as if no one will notice that the best known voice of fibromyalgia and all that she stands for is missing from their work. Yet still, they inadvertently do us all a favor: They let us know that most fibromyalgics continue to be productive, to work, and to live full lives, that they under- rather than over-medicate, and actually try to steer clear of doctors.

I will not prescribe

I am not a doctor; I will not prescribe for you. I will not tell you which treatment I think is best or what you should take and what you should try. Luckily for all of us, research is ongoing both in fibromyalgia and in its related syndromes such as irritable bowel syndrome. New medications and supplements hit the market weekly, each with its own advocate and cheering section. New breakthroughs appear often on the nightly news, or in magazines and even published books. I hope to give you the basic information, and, in the end, the tools to evaluate new information as it comes to you, as well as how to find it. You and your doctors should always decide what is best for you and what is safe. Weighing the risks and possible benefits is something you will both need to do. No practicing physician has time to keep track of all the new information that comes out. It will be up to you, by and large, to find this information and learn about how it might help you. This book is meant to be an introduction to lifelong learning about and living with fibromyalgia.

• • •

Where the focus is

In 1998, Dr. R. Paul St. Amand and I were approached about writing a book called *What Your Doctor May Not Tell You About Fibromyalgia*. The urgent reason was to get his protocol into the hands of patients, but we also sought to share our firsthand knowledge, both as members of the medical field and fibromyalgics, with our readers. We wanted to interweave both voices.

What is left to do? Why did I write this book? I wrote this book for you: the newly diagnosed. I want to tell you what I've learned and what I wish someone could have told me back when I was given a word I could barely spell and was left wondering what it would mean to me. This is not a manual for being sick; it is not a treatise to defend you for doing nothing because you feel so lousy. This is a book about learning what you need to know, and then getting on with it. There is a lot to learn about how to handle your symptoms, and what your options are. I have tried to keep the explanations simple and the format easy to follow. Words in **boldface** can be found in the glossary in the back, and there are reference and resource sections for those of you who want to learn more. I have tried to weave a combined message from all the expert voices for those of us who inhabit the middle world, who live in sickness and in health. My goal is to show you how to be a person with fibromyalgia, not a fibromyalgic who happens to be a person. I agree with Dr. Wolfe that a preoccupation with your symptoms isn't healthy, but I disagree with the rest of what he says. My diagnosis made me powerful, and it led me here and gave me an important purpose for my life. It did not isolate me from the world; it brought me back into it.

Where a diagnosis of fibromyalgia leaves you

Fibromyalgia is a chronic disease for which today there is no known cause and no known cure. The good news is that you can still lead a full life and control most of your symptoms at least most of the time. You can take this opportunity and use it to turn your health around. Now more than ever you should commit yourself to getting into the best possible shape that you can and take good care of yourself each and every day. If you do this, and you take charge of your fibromyalgia, you have the opportunity to feel better than you have in years. Managing stress, eating properly, and exercising—these are keys to more than controlling your illness, they are keys to improve the quality of your life. And remember: you are not alone. There are large groups of fibromyalgics (also known as *fibromites*) who suffer as you do from what we call *this DD,* or darn disease. They understand you. I am sorry you have joined us, but I welcome you to our community. I hope that when you read this book you will decide that you are in good company.

> Though nothing can bring back the hour
> Of splendour in the grass, of glory in the flower;
> We will grieve not, rather find
> Strength in what remains behind
> In the primal sympathy
> Which having been must ever be;
> In the soothing thoughts that spring
> Out of human suffering;
> In the faith that looks through death,
> In years that bring the philosophic mind.

—WILLIAM WORDSWORTH

Getting the Right Doctor to Diagnose You

BEFORE WE get into a long discussion about fibromyalgia, it's important for us all to be on the same wavelength. If you've picked up this book because someone's told you that you might have fibromyalgia, or if you've read about it and think it sounds like you, the next paragraph is for you.

The first thing to do if you think you may have fibromyalgia is to get a diagnosis. This sounds obvious and even silly, but it is important. It's dangerous to treat yourself or to assume that all your symptoms are from fibromyalgia. So if you have not yet been diagnosed, then make an appointment with your doctor. If you don't have a doctor, then it's time to find one.

This is not as easy as it sounds. The fact is, if you do not have a supportive physician, or you don't choose one wisely, you may be walking out of the doctor's office without a definitive diagnosis. So here's the most important bit of wisdom to heed—and one that will serve you well on your road to recovery—the sooner you learn to act as your own personal health advocate, the sooner you will get results.

Find a believer

Your first task when you call to set up your appointment is to be sure to mention that you suspect you have fibromyalgia.

Let's face an unpleasant fact right now: Not every doctor believes fibromyalgia is a real illness. Some firmly believe it's what's called a "wastebasket diagnosis"—a sort of trash bin into which they throw neurotic hypochondriacs who complain a lot. It once had a name to match this philosophy, "the tender lady syndrome," and there are still some people who think fibromyalgia is a name that sympathetic doctors give to patients to shut them up. Luckily for all of us, things are changing. You won't encounter this school of thought now as often as you would have a few years ago, but it's still out there, so be prepared.

Even if you're lucky enough not to ever come across a doctor who thinks this way, I promise you'll encounter this mind-set eventually when you discuss your illness with family and friends. As you know, there's no test for fibromyalgia, no black-and-white proof that this illness exists. And for some medical professionals, if your illness doesn't meet a certain fixed set of symptoms, with a blood test to confirm it, then there's nothing really wrong with you. But, as FMS researcher Jon Russell, M.D., Ph.D., points out, "Twenty years ago rheumatoid arthritis was considered a psychological illness, its symptoms exacerbated by stress and life changes. Today we know that stress has nothing to do with it. Fibromyalgia is undergoing the same transition."

The wrong physician can cost you more than money

Don't skip the very important step of getting a diagnosis, but don't waste your time and money on a dead end. This is why it's crucial to take a moment when you make contact with a prospective doctor's office to discuss fibromyalgia and find out if the physician you're going to be seeing will set aside time for you and take your concerns and your illness seriously. The average patient spends thousands of dollars before ever receiving an accurate diagnosis, and many of us are acutely aware that our mothers and grandmothers went unheeded and unaided before us. Too many fibromyalgics have had unnecessary surgeries and have endured too many dissertations from physicians who could not help us, or did not listen to us. The bottom line here is that if your physician believes that your symptoms are largely imaginary, you are not going to get the help you need.

If the doctor you have called doesn't believe fibromyalgia exists, *do not* make an appointment. Instead, call a different doctor. This may seem harsh, but because the road to recovery is a difficult one, you need to have a doctor you can work with. The best doctor is one who is willing to partner with you in your journey back to good health. Save your strength for getting better, and don't waste it trying to convince some doctor that you're really sick or really in pain. Find a doctor with a proven track record of listening to and caring about patients.

Finding the right doctor

If you need help finding a doctor, there are several things you can try. First of all, ask your friends. If one of them has a doctor they describe as a good listener or open-minded, this is a good place to start. If they happen to mention that their doctor spends time with them when they go in, you've probably found a good doctor. You do not need a specialist to make the diagnosis of fibromyalgia.

Another possibility for finding a doctor is to call local fibromyalgia support groups. Online newsgroups and Web sites may also have lists of doctors. Even though you may be in a hurry to get in to see a doctor, take your time with this step. Get several names and get a feel for each of their offices. When you get a good feeling from one of them, make your appointment. And remember: the American College of Rheumatology, the World Health Organization, the National Institutes of Health, and the American Medical Association all accept fibromyalgia as a real medical entity. You don't need to put up with people who don't believe it's real, whether they have "M.D." after their names or not.

What to expect from your doctor's visit

Once you are face-to-face with a doctor you should expect a few things. First of all, the doctor should listen to your complaints, and be interested in how long you've had them. This information is important because you want to make sure nothing is missed. Most fibromyalgics have learned not to tell a doctor all of their symptoms because they have so many and, in the past, physicians have been impatient with them because of this. It's hard not to feel crazy when you look at your own long list of symptoms, so it will help if you put your complaints in a logical order, with the most important symptoms first. If you do a little homework and speak in a clear, logical way, it will help your doctor and it will make you feel a little less stressed or panicked that you've forgotten something. Fibromyalgia is confusing enough to most doctors because of the sheer number of symptoms it creates, not to mention the fact that symptoms can fluctuate wildly from day to day.

You may be sent for blood tests

If you haven't had recent blood tests, your new physician should order them. Since there's no blood test for fibromyalgia, it's a diagnosis of exclusion, meaning your doctor must rule out all other possible reasons for your symptoms. Only then can he or she settle on a fibromyalgia diagnosis with a clean conscience.

Blood tests you can expect to have

A basic workup will include a blood count to rule out anemia or other blood-borne illnesses that can cause fatigue or muscle pain. You can also expect a thyroid panel including a test known as a **TSH-HS**. An underactive thyroid can cause fatigue, so your doctor will want to make sure your gland is functioning normally. Fasting blood sugar should also be measured. High (**diabetes**) or low blood sugar can also cause fatigue and muscle pain. Liver tests should be performed to rule out hepatitis, and you can expect an arthritis panel to rule out other conditions. **Rheumatoid arthritis**, polymyalgia rheumatica, **lupus**, and **gout** all have specific tests that your doctor will ask for if there's any suspicion at all that you may have something else. Having one of these conditions doesn't mean you can't have fibromyalgia as well, but it's important that they be treated aggressively and appropriately.

The hands-on evaluation

After your doctor is satisfied that your symptoms and history suggest fibromyalgia, a physical examination will be conducted. One of the important diagnostic criteria for fibromyalgia is the presence of **tender points**. Your doctor will palpate eighteen predetermined sites looking to see if you experience pain when they're pressed on. There's some controversy about how useful these points are, and we'll talk about that in Day 7, but this examination is standard for making the diagnosis so you should expect to have it. There are some new concepts on the tender points that have recently come to light, which you'll learn about in Day 3, but right now you should just know that most doctors and patients do understand that these points do not adequately describe the pain that people with fibromyalgia feel. We all know that we have pain throughout our entire bodies. Medical articles usually advise physicians that if they have a patient that hurts *all* over, they should think fibromyalgia. But keep in mind that no doctor can make a diagnosis of fibromyalgia without physically examining you.

Things to Look for in a Physician if You Suspect Fibromyalgia (FM)

○ Believes FM is a legitimate medical condition
○ Believes that treatments exist and that there are specific steps that can be taken to improve the quality of your life. (You don't want a doctor who is going to write you a prescription for an antidepressant and tell you to exercise and leave it at that.)
○ Listens well and answers questions
○ Addresses your concerns, takes your concerns seriously
○ Is willing to read information that you bring to the office about fibromyalgia and will consider treating you with things that may be "outside the box" but that will not harm you
○ Permits and encourages your family members to accompany you if you feel that you need support and validation

IN A SENTENCE:

You need to find an understanding physician you can work with to make sure that fibromyalgia is the correct diagnosis for you.

learning

Relaying Your Symptoms to Your Doctor

TO DATE there is no single accepted theory about the cause of FM or what is causing your symptoms, but through the course of this next year, we'll touch on some of the theories. For now, the best thing that you can do for your visit to the doctor is to make a list of your symptoms, how long you've had each one, and the severity.

So what is this illness really?

In making your list, it's extremely helpful to understand the accepted medical definition of fibromyalgia. Fibromyalgia **syndrome** (FMS) is a painful condition that primarily affects muscles, tendons, and ligaments. Tender points must be present—which by official criteria means that a patient must have pain in eleven out of eighteen predetermined locations. Pain must have been present for at least three months with no other explanation for its cause. Other symptoms that are officially recognized as part of fibromyalgia are: deadening fatigue, headaches, irritable bladder, painful menstrual cycles, intolerance to cold, restless legs, numbness and tingling, exercise intolerance, and poor stamina. It's recognized that there are psychological symptoms, which include depression, anxiety, and cognitive deficits. It's also accepted that some patients may have fewer areas of pain, but if they

Symptoms of Fibromyalgia

CENTRAL NERVOUS SYSTEM SYMPTOMS

- O Dragging fatigue that gets worse as the day goes on
- O Exhaustion at the end of the day
- O Irritability, nervousness, and anxiety
- O Depression, apathy
- O Impaired memory and concentration (this is also known as *fibrofog*)
- O Dizziness
- O Headaches (often called migraines when they are sufficiently intense)
- O Insomnia (difficulty falling asleep, staying asleep, or falling back asleep)
- O Nonrestorative sleep (waking up unrefreshed)
- O Sensitivity to light, smell, and sounds (which can cause headaches and nausea)
- O Chemical sensitivities

MUSCULOSKELETAL SYMPTOMS

- O Pain most often in the back (upper and lower including neck, shoulders, and buttocks), in the arms (wrists, elbows, shoulders), hips, legs, thighs, knees, ankles, feet, and chest wall
- O Pain described as throbbing, burning, stabbing, stinging, grabbing, with intensity that varies from hour to hour and can increase with cold or damp weather, anxiety, stress, and activity
- O Being able to predict a change of weather by an increase in certain symptoms
- O Muscle spasms and cramps
- O Widespread stiffness in muscles, tendons, and ligaments
- O Pain typically worse in the morning and may improve somewhat during the day, but then will return in the evening
- O Numbness of the extremities or face
- O Diffuse pelvic pain
- O Chest wall pain (chostocondritis)
- O Temporomandibular joint pain, facial, and head pain originating in the neck area
- O Feelings like electrical impulses in their muscles
- O Restless legs
- O A feeling of general weakness often described as "poor stamina"

GASTROINTESTINAL SYMPTOMS
- Irritable bowel syndrome
- Gas, pain, bloating, and constipation
- Diarrhea
- Nausea
- Hyperacidity
- Crampy abdominal pain that can be intense and unpredictable

GENITOURINARY
- Vulvodynia
- Vulvar vestibulitis
- Vaginal spasms or cramps
- Burning discharge
- Increased menstrual and uterine cramps
- Dyspareunia, or painful intercourse
- Bladder pain
- Recurrent bladder infections
- Interstitial cystitis
- Dark, pungent urine that burns

DERMAL
- Crawling feelings
- Itching, scaly patches
- Rashes (many varieties) in strange patches
- Small areas of pimples occur
- Perspiration that is pungent and irritates the skin
- Sensitive allergic skin
- Dermatographia is fairly common.
- Raynaud's phenomena

MISCELLANEOUS
- Excessive nasal congestion and mucus or postnasal drip
- Brittle nails, inferior hair quality
- Scalded or metallic mouth sensations
- Bitter (sometimes even salty) taste in the mouth
- Eye irritation or blurring, burning eyes
- Ringing in the ears or popping sounds
- Vertigo

have enough of the other symptoms they can also be acceptably diagnosed with fibromyalgia.

By and large, symptoms can be grouped into the following categories: cerebral, musculoskeletal, gastrointestinal, dermal, and genitourinary. These are discussed in more detail in the following chapters, but they're outlined here to assist you in making a symptom list. There are a few other isolated problems that do not fit easily into any classification-and they'll be covered later, too. Never forget that symptoms are what define fibromyalgia. Nothing you feel is too trivial to list, nothing that bothers you is too unimportant to make a note of. Controlling all your symptoms is what you are striving to do, and therefore, you must list them and pay attention to how much they bother you.

Bear in mind that very few people have all the complaints listed. Not every symptom is listed on the chart above, only the most common complaints, and as you learn more about your condition you will discover more.

The most important thing to remember is that your symptoms may not match those you've heard of, or those of your colleague with fibromyalgia, or those of the woman who works at the library. Part of the reason fibromyalgia is so often misdiagnosed and undertreated is just this: Everyone is different.

IN A SENTENCE:

> *Your best hope for dealing with fibromyalgia is an early, accurate diagnosis combined with active patient involvement—you are your own best advocate.*

DAY **2**

living

What Fibromyalgia Is—And Isn't

SO, WHO gets fibromyalgia? The answer to this question is: Anyone can. The typical fibromyalgia patient is a woman between the ages of twenty and fifty, but men and children get it as well. Roughly 85 percent of patients are women, although some people (myself included) feel that while it is certainly more common in women, fewer men are represented in the statistics because they are more hesitant to go to doctors. I also believe more doctors are apt to diagnose men with **chronic fatigue syndrome (CFS)** simply because of a sexual stereotype—namely that fibromyalgia is a women's complaint. It occurs in all races and ethnicities, and appears to be equally common in little girls and little boys[1]. I know fibromyalgics as young as two and as old as seventy-two. I've seen three and four generations in families with the illness, and I've watched my own sons struggle with it as children.

What fibromyalgia is not

Fibromyalgia is not a life-threatening disorder. Medically, it is a syndrome, meaning that it is a collection of symptoms that can vary from one person to another in type and severity. Fibromyalgia is not an **autoimmune illness,** like **Hashimoto's thyroiditis** is, for example. There is no tissue destruction in

Conditions with Symptoms That Mimic FM but Are Not Related:

Degenerative disc disease	Rheumatoid arthritis
Sjogren's syndrome	Carpal tunnel syndrome
Lyme disease	Polymyalgia rhematica
Lupus (connective tissue disease)	Polymyositis
Hypothyroidism	Gastric or duodenal ulcers
Spondyloarthropathy	Reiter's syndrome
Parkinson's disease	Multiple sclerosis
Myasthenia gravis	Gout and pseudogout

fibromyalgia, which is how an illness is categorized as autoimmune in nature. Autoimmune illnesses are easily diagnosed by the presence of antibodies in the bloodstream. In fibromyalgia there are no antibodies and no toxins. (One small footnote here: It has been documented that it is common to see a positive test for **antinuclear antibodies [ANA]**, although such tests usually turn up weakly positive (or speckled) and will fluctuate back to negative on occasion.)

Fibromyalgia is not infectious. There are physicians who believe that fibromyalgia is caused by an infection, but no **virus** or **bacterium** has yet been identified, and the body does not mount an **antibody** response as it does when a person is exposed to a virus.

THE HISTORY of fibromyalgia is rather fascinating. The name we use today only dates from around 1990, which means we have to be detectives to learn more. Like Americans whose family names were changed at Ellis Island when they disembarked, it takes persistence, imagination, and luck to find out what occurred before.

If we look back through medical history we can find many references to our illness and see that only the name *fibromyalgia* is new. Some physicians have even found passages in the Bible that sound as if they're describing fibromyalgia. The condition really began to come under scrutiny in the 1880s, when both German and British physicians were studying a perplexing form of what was then called "rheumatism." This was a period of huge strides forward in medical research, when physicians typically studied the entire body, and made notes and drawings of their findings. They did not have fancy machines, or even blood tests, so they relied upon their senses, including touch, to learn about the human condition.

One of these was Robert Froriep, a German physician who noted in the mid-1880s a type of **rheumatism** in which he would palpate what he called "muskelschwiele"—muscle calluses, or welts. In nineteenth-century Germany, this condition was called Weichteilrheumatismus, or soft tissue rheumatism.

In England in the early 1900s the physician Sir William Gowers studied his own **lumbago** and became interested in back pain that did not have a mechanical nature. He noted a complex of symptoms that occurred in "ladies of blameless habits and abstemious clergymen" (unlike, I suppose gout, which was considered a consequence of rich living). Dr. Gowers also observed that his patients were exhausted, unable to sleep, and that their illness was "so painful it would make a strong man cry out." He tried everything he could think of in an attempt to relieve this pain, and like his modern counterparts, found that nothing worked very well. He chronicled a list of failed therapies, including salicylates (the newly discovered aspirin) and noted a few things that seemed to help, such as gentle manipulation and cocaine injections. Eventually, after deciding the illness he was studying was more than lumbago, he named it **fibrositis**. Gowers chose this name carefully, supposing there was some sort of inflammation he couldn't measure that was causing the pain. Eighty years later, when physicians confirmed that this was not the case, fibrositis was discarded in favor of fibromyalgia, a name that is only slightly more accurate.

In the interest of time, let's now skip ahead past the studies of Civil War and World War I soldiers with fibrositis (perhaps an early form of Gulf War syndrome!) to 1960, when Canadian Dr. Hugh Smythe wrote an article about fibrositis that appeared in a textbook. He is thus credited with being the man who brought our illness into the modern spotlight. It was his interest and tenacity that began the avalanche of research and study that commenced in the 1970s.

In 1990, Dr. Smythe, along with Drs. Yunus, Wolfe, Bennett, Goldenberg, and Bombardier, carefully detailed the location of eighteen tender points symmetrically located around the human body for the American College of Rheumatology's Criteria for Classification of Fibromyalgia. After much serious debate, the presence of at least eleven out of eighteen became the standard for making a fibromyalgia diagnosis, along with pain in all four quadrants of the body for at least three months' duration. These spots have been poked, prodded, biopsied, and scanned. What's more, they are commonly measured on a scale from 1 to 10 with a special contraption called a dolorimeter, a spring-loaded device designed to provide a numerical measurement for the point at which the patient cries out or flinches.

IN A SENTENCE:

Although the cause of fibromyalgia is unknown, it is not a new fad disease, but rather a condition that has been well researched over the last century.

learning

Coming to Terms
with a Complex Illness

BY NOW you've heard the words from your doctor that
you've been expecting but dreading, hoping for but also not
wanting to hear: "You have fibromyalgia." This is a strange and
difficult moment, one that I am used to sharing with people.
It always brings back the moment that I heard the words
myself. Relieved in one breath that I wasn't crazy, vindicated
that I had an illness and that the illness had a name, but in the
same moment terrified and sobered by what I had learned. But
it isn't entirely bad news, is it? You don't have cancer, or need
surgery. You don't have terminal leukemia that is causing your
fatigue and weakness. But what does this diagnosis mean? One
search is over—you have a reason for your suffering. You know
that you are no longer alone, that there are other patients like
you. Now what?

You may feel a little lost at first

It's normal to feel alone in the beginning. But this loneliness
will send you on a quest. It will make you want to learn about
your illness, which is exactly what you're going to do over the
course of this first week. At the end of these first seven days,
you will have a clear picture of what fibromyalgia is and the
symptoms involved, what to tell your friends and family, and

how to understand and be kind to yourself, and how to start to help yourself with your symptoms.

If you've come this far, you already know what a challenging illness fibromyalgia is. It is certainly overwhelming in the sheer magnitude of complaints, and its unpredictable nature makes things worse. By now, you're probably used to people telling you: "You don't look sick. You look fine, why don't you feel fine?" Or perhaps you feel like you're complaining all the time, so you stop saying you don't feel well, which makes it even harder for people to realize or remember that you're sick.

It's human nature to question and to second-guess things. We all play devil's advocate with ourselves. It's also normal to wonder if your diagnosis is really correct. It's common even at second and third doctor's visits for patients to ask again, "You're sure this is what I have?" I understand. During some of my own down times I've asked the same questions. I've gone to labs and had my blood tests repeated. I've told myself, "This can't just be fibromyalgia. Something else is wrong." But in the end I realized it was true. I really *do* have fibromyalgia. And so do you. You are not alone.

Learning acceptance

The first step is to accept that you have a **chronic illness** for which there are treatments, but there is no cure. There is no chronic illness that doesn't require lifestyle changes, whether it is diabetes, heart disease, high blood pressure, arthritis, or kidney disease. A chronic illness changes your life in ways you will spend the rest of your life learning about, and it will take time to come to terms with this. Your doctor can be your partner and your adviser, but can't do the work you need to do. Fibromyalgia is high maintenance, and you have to work on it every single day. You may get guidance, but the path you take will still be your own.

Acceptance is difficult, but you must get to that point. Get over your feelings of denial and turn your mind to learning about your illness. It will help you with your second problem: the isolation you feel in being different from everyone around you. This is a frightening time, and you must accept that and be kind to yourself.

Your new affirmation: You are not alone

Some experts believe that as many as twenty million Americans have fibromyalgia to some degree. (Everyone else agrees that at least 5 percent of the population does.) As you learn about how fibromyalgia affects you, you will meet other sufferers who will underscore the truth that you are now part of a big club. You will meet people who are better off than you are,

---

I've often wondered

I'VE OFTEN wondered what the world would be like if we all had fibromyalgia

You wouldn't be seen as a slacker if you didn't work overtime.

People would spend more time at home with their families and cherish time spent with friends instead of overscheduling themselves.

Everyone would take the time to stop and smell the roses. Heck, even sit among them for an afternoon and watch them grow.

Nap time would be a given time every day, and we'd shut off our phones, computers, pagers, etc., for a couple of hours.

We'd be more thankful for what we have, rather than caring about how many toys we own or how big our houses are.

Maybe we'd all cut each other a little more slack and forgive people for making mistakes and not being everything we want them to be.

Nobody would discriminate against you for your illness, and there would be no need to decide what to tell an employer.

Then again, would you want heavily fibrofogged people designing and building bridges and other things that would cause disaster if they didn't work right the first time?

OK, so maybe the best route is to take the things this disease has taught us, and try to infect the rest of the world with a sense of balance and permission to slow down the frenetic pace our culture idealizes.

—*Amy Harth*

---

and some who are worse off. From their stories you will learn much about yourself.

Handling your emotions

It's very normal to feel angry that you have an illness. "It's not fair" and "Why me?" are the hallmarks of this emotion. It's hard not to feel sorry for yourself, especially when you're constantly around people who aren't sick. Two things in my own past experience stand out. One is the memory of being a sick child when a big new living room was added onto our house.

I was having a severe bout of what they now call irritable bowel, but what was then mysterious diarrhea. My sisters and the neighborhood kids were jumping from beam to beam on the structure and I was watching from the window. I was different: the only kid who could not go outside. No one knew what was wrong with me, I didn't know what was wrong with me, and there I was watching the other kids wistfully from behind glass.

But that first memory doesn't hurt the way my other one does. I remember being a young mother at the park with first one little son, and then two of them. I used to drag my exhausted butt to the park to get them out of the house, where the noise they made would drive me nuts, and collapse on a blanket. The boys would run around and beg me to push them on swings and watch them go down slides. I could hardly move. I had to force myself to stand up and put one foot in front of the other to do things with them. I begged them to swing by themselves. I promised I would get up in a minute. All around me I could see moms running with their kids, playing ball with them, holding jump ropes. I didn't know what was wrong with me then. But I knew I would never be one of those moms and my boys would never have me to play tag with them in the park. I would look at my sons and my heart would ache for what I could not give them.

It's OK to be angry

Which leads us to the next normal emotion—anger. It's normal to rail against your body, which has defeated you, imprisoned you, and keeps you from doing what you want. There's turning the anger inward, but there's also the outward kind. Believe me, it's very easy to become a martyr with this illness, very easy and very awful. You can punish people because you don't feel well or lose it when they don't do enough to help you, or when they don't understand what your limitations are. It's so easy to torture people who care about you and are trying to help you because your life isn't going the way you want. Remember, I see fibromyalgics every day as part of my job, and I am one. There have been times when I played the victim, and nothing anyone did was ever right. I would sigh and struggle to do things the right way for myself because no one could do them the way I needed them done. Or I would be angry because nothing was right, nothing was enough, it wasn't fair that I had to do everything myself when I wasn't feeling well. I have also felt abandoned, miserable, and as if everyone was having a great old time except for me.

Eventually, though, you have to let your anger out. You can't keep it inside. The key, of course, is to channel it into a productive emotion. Focus your mind on getting better. Be determined to get control of yourself and your illness. Educate those you come in contact with, write letters to the doctors who misdiagnosed you.

Depression is also normal in the beginning

The good thing about big emotions like anger and fear is that they fade. They just take too much energy to maintain. The problem is that they often leave behind depression. Yes, after anger comes depression.

I'm not saying it's not normal to be depressed, or to mourn for the things you can't have and won't have. When I had my second son, despite the joy I had from my beautiful child, I mourned the fact that I would never have a daughter. If you can mourn at happy times like that, and it's normal, think how normal it is to be sad when you've had to deal with the loss of a whole lot of your cherished dreams. You'll never be like other people. Maybe you will on the outside, maybe for a few hours, maybe for days at a time. But you'll always have this illness as a companion, taking over when you least expect it or want it. Your life isn't just yours anymore. Things are out of control. To gain back control you have to accept that you may have this condition for the rest of your life and it won't go away. You're not going to wake up one morning and find out that this was all some awful nightmare. I promise you that it won't happen. Only acceptance of your condition will help you overcome your depression

Your life isn't over. And you can, as Walt Whitman wrote, find "joy in the things that remain behind." You can cut out a lot of nonessential things, and you can reestablish your priorities. This book will help you learn how to do it. You may have fewer friendships, but the ones you have will be deeper, stronger, and truer. A door has closed, but another door has opened. It may sound trite, but things become more precious when you've suffered. You know all those quotes about not being able to see a rainbow unless it's raining? Well, there's truth to them. You can be a better person, help others, love more deeply, and be more open when you've come to terms with and embraced your own limitations, whatever they are. You've got to get real about your situation and stop resenting things and wasting your precious energy looking for miracle cures. It's not all a mistake, and there isn't going to be an easy answer, or even one simple set of steps to follow. When and if a miracle cure comes along, you will certainly hear about it.

You are in charge of your life

The surest way to improve the quality of your life when you have a chronic illness is to develop a sense of control over it. The most frustrating things about fibromyalgia are the flare-ups and constantly changing symptoms that make it impossible to make plans and to predict how well you'll be able to function. The scary, maddening, and infuriating thing is not knowing what to expect, how to manage, or how to trust your own body. So it makes sense that you should learn as much as you can about your illness, what's available to help you, and what has and hasn't helped others. The more you know, the more you'll understand and the more you'll be in control.

Fibromyalgia affects everyone differently

Like most disorders, the impact of fibromyalgia differs from person to person. Some are able to lead relatively normal lives. Others become home-bound and some become completely debilitated. Many fibromyalgics feel relatively fine until some traumatic event occurs, such as a car accident or an emotional setback. Then they begin to notice symptoms that don't go away. Some fibromyalgics live with their symptoms for years, until finally they succumb to excruciating pain.

In addition to the physical complaints, many people also have difficulties with memory and concentration—cognitive difficulties that are nicknamed "fibrofog." These symptoms take as much of a toll on you as do the physical disturbances. Diminished mental clarity and fatigue can have a profound effect on your life. Most everyone I've talked to with fibromyalgia confirms exactly what I've always said: If I had only pain I wouldn't bother to complain. I could deal with the pain somehow. It's the other symptoms that do me in, that keep me from being myself, keep me from being the person I was. I really don't care about the pain most of the time. If I could just be the person I was before I got sick, I'd stop complaining about the pain.

Dealing with your personal issues about fibromyalgia

If you're anything like me, discovering that there is, in fact, a diagnosis for the many things that ail you was probably a huge relief. They say that the average patient goes five years looking for a diagnosis, and has spent—well, you can imagine what's been spent, and maybe you've spent it yourself. So take that deep breath now. You know what you have. You'll need the ammunition of that satisfaction to battle through the journey ahead.

Thankfully, fibromyalgia doesn't carry with it the helplessness or stigma that it did merely a few years ago. Yet today, that won't make your body feel any better or your mind any clearer. The saying "Anything that's worth having is worth working for" never resonated more clearly to me than when I was struggling to reclaim my life.

You have the power to make things better

If it's any consolation, I understand the combination of shock, confusion, and fear you're feeling. Not only do you have to come to grips with the concept that you have an incurable, chronic condition, but no one can predict the course your illness will take or how you will feel tomorrow. I've had people who have survived cancer tell me that fibromyalgia is worse. They've told me that with cancer treatments they were told what to expect, and how long things would last, and given facts and figures, and black and white. Fibromyalgia isn't like that. It's a gray area, and changing shades of gray at that. But if you learn, as I have, to take care of yourself, to listen to your body, and to take charge of your life, you will absolutely have a better life despite your illness. Fibromyalgia can be your excuse to get into the best shape that you can, to eat well, to sleep enough, to get strong, and to learn about what makes you feel good about yourself. But the most important thing to understand now is that you are not alone and that there are things you can do about your illness. I know because I've done them. And we'll work through all of this together.

IN A SENTENCE:

> *Fibromyalgia can be successfully managed by educating yourself about your condition and getting the support you need.*

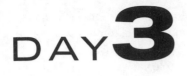

DAY 3

living

Musculoskeletal Symptoms: Mapping Your Pain

THE REASON we're turning our attention to the musculoskeletal symptoms, or pain, first is because tender points are crucial to the official diagnosis of fibromyalgia. It is these spots and the pain around them that made fibromyalgia the province of rheumatologists, who now, almost by default, are the main physicians involved in research and treatment of our illness. Though pain may not be your primary concern, today you will learn about what might cause it, what might help it, and what we know about it.

Pain is a daily reality

Nearly all fibromyalgics have daily pain, which is thus chronic, and most have debilitating pain at least some of the time. There are a few fortunate people who complain only of stiffness or occasional joint pain, but they make up only about one percent of patients. These are the same people who may have been told that they have chronic fatigue syndrome simply because their primary complaint is fatigue. Most physicians now admit that this is not a separate illness but a complex of

Musculoskeletal Symptoms
of Fibromyalgia

○ Widespread, aching pain

○ Stiffness in muscles, tendons, and ligaments—worse upon awakening

○ Stiffness and pain that can get worse as the day wears on

○ Pains that burn, sting, stab, and pull and are both changeable and variable

○ Numbness and tingling usually of extremities but anywhere on the body

○ Temporomandibular joint pain (TMJ), with difficulty chewing, and excruciating facial and head pain

○ Headaches, often migraine intensity, and duller tension headaches that arise from points on the back of the neck

○ Muscles that can often actually be seen twitching

○ Restless leg syndrome

○ Leg and foot cramps, often in the evenings or in bed at night

○ Feelings like electrical impulses in the muscles

○ General weakness

○ Exercise intolerance and poor stamina that get worse when you are inactive

○ Joint pain not from the joints themselves but from tendon insertions above and around the joints themselves

symptoms that falls under the umbrella of fibromyalgia syndrome. (Remember that a syndrome merely means a collection of symptoms.)

Despite the fact that almost all fibromyalgics have pain, many of us don't regard it as our worst symptom. Most of us think we could deal with our illness if all we had to worry about was pain. Pain without exhaustion, anxiety, depression, pain without irritable bowel syndrome, pain without compromised memory and concentration seems like a vacation to us. That's not to say that when we're in one of our pain cycles we don't go to doctors begging for respite, and that at times we don't feel like we can't deal with any more pain. It's just that pain is simply one of our many concerns. But since we have to start somewhere, let's start with the musculoskeletal symptoms.

What are tender points?

We know these areas exist, but what causes them? Books and articles focus on their location, but don't offer any explanation for what they actually might be, other than painful. The reason for this is that so much is still

Tender Points

TENDER POINTS are bilaterally symmetrical:

- ◯ Located at the base of the skull directly below the hairline
- ◯ Above the shoulder blades near where the neck and shoulder join
- ◯ Between the shoulder blades
- ◯ On the front of the neck above the collar bone
- ◯ Chest at the second and third costochondral junction (second rib)
- ◯ Below the elbows
- ◯ In the lower back right below the waist
- ◯ On the hips right under the hip bones
- ◯ Behind the knees

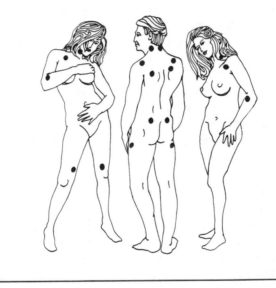

unknown. Tender points are areas of contracted muscle, and we know from biopsy reports and electromagnetic scanning technology that they are areas where energy production is markedly decreased. This has been determined by measurements showing that these areas have less **ATP,** the now measurable currency of energy. Early muscle biopsies that point to this conclusion have been reported in Scandinavian journals and have now been corroborated by more modern methods. But why these spots occur where they do, and how they come to exist, is still a mystery.

What we do know is that muscles are made up of different types of muscle fibers. The exact location of different fibers varies to some degree from person to person depending on how they use their muscles. Muscles are fast twitch or slow twitch, striated or striped. It appears that certain types of these fibers, bundled together, may be more prone to the contractions that cause the hard spots where we feel pain.

If we know where the pain is, what's the problem?

To make things complicated, not every physician agrees with the tender point measurements. Many physicians have never liked them, and consider them to be arbitrary. Others, like R. Paul St. Amand, M.D., have pointed out that tenderness has more to do with pain thresholds than anything else. Also, as he is fond of remarking, "On a bad day, every inch of your body hurts. On a good day, you can tolerate a lot more. Even in the same person pain thresholds vary tremendously."

And what about the patient who may have, say, ten, but not eleven tender points? "Many of us feel that if you've excluded any other disease or explanation for the symptoms, and the patient describes pain and has the other frequently associated problems like sleep disorder, migraine headaches, and so on, then regardless of whether they have the prescribed number of tender points, the diagnosis is likely to be FMS," says David S. Caldwell, M.D., a rheumatologist at Duke Medical Center in Durham, North Carolina. This was the consensus of the physicians who devised the tender point criteria, but much of their original comments have been lost, as doctors preferred to focus on the black and white, the yes or no, of tender point counts.

Pain thresholds are different in different people

Another problem is that while these predetermined areas can be exquisitely tender in fibromyalgics, it is clear that most of the rest of the body can be tender as well. Some people are so hugely tolerant to pain they can have teeth pulled without anesthesia. Others are not so lucky. Chronic pain may also create some sort of pain amplification, and research has been done showing that there is some of this in fibromyalgia. As a result, many doctors believe tender point measurements should be disbanded. Others have suggested adding to their number, suggesting up to sixty additional sites! Helpful as this is, it has added to the confusion about fibromyalgia, and given those who don't believe in it ammunition. To them, if the physicians who first defined it can't even agree on the importance and location of tender points, then the whole concept of fibromyalgia is even more cockeyed.

For those of us with the illness, I believe it's best to steer away from these preordained sites and concentrate on our entire bodies. There's no

---

Known Laboratory Abnormalities in Fibromyalgia

○ Elevated substance P
○ Elevated prolactin
○ Elevated angiotensin converting enzyme
○ Elevated pyruvate
○ Elevated inorganic phosphate/adenosine diphosphate
○ Elevated melatonin (nocturnal)
○ Elevated nerve growth factor
○ Elevated antinuclear antibodies
○ Elevated rheumatoid factor
○ Elevated calcitonin related peptide
○ Decreased human growth hormone
○ Decreased insulin-like growth factor 1
○ Decrease of 7 amino acids in the blood
○ Decrease of cortisol on 24-hour urine test
○ Decreased ionized calcium
○ Decreased serum lactate
○ Decreased adenosine triphosphate (ATP)
○ Decreased serotonin
○ Decreased neuropeptide

---

reason to spend hours tracing the patterns of pain caused by pressure on a nerve. Tender points will continue to rear their ugly heads, but their only real use is as diagnostic criteria to ensure we're all talking about the same illness, or for research purposes, which is the reason they were initially defined. In terms of healing ourselves, we have more important things to think about. You know where you hurt.

Fibromyalgics may have a systemwide sensitivity to pain

In the early days, when Dr. Gowers initially palpated tender points, he didn't have sophisticated tests to look at possible system-wide defects. He and other physicians like him could only write about what they could examine and observe—their hands and other senses were their primary diagnostic tools. In the ensuing years many other abnormalities have been found, and as our tests become more sophisticated, still others will certainly be found. Many studies today are focusing on fibromyalgia as a pain amplification syndrome, but this hardly explains why there are palpable hard areas in the muscles, or why certain patients experience very little pain.

I know that when I have a lot of pain, my body becomes oversensitive to pain. Sometimes when I'm feeling lousy I do something like stub my toe, and even though this is a minor injury, the pain seems excruciating. I tell myself I'm being silly, but at the same time I know it hurts horribly. I say this here because I can't help but wonder if there isn't some chemical change in my body from the overabundance of pain I'm experiencing that is like a circuit overload. I don't think this means that fibromyalgia is caused by a defect making me more sensitive to pain, but just that my pain causes me greater intolerance to pain.

Why is this important?

The purpose of the preceding list is not to send you running off to your doctors for more tests, because as we've repeatedly seen, there are no abnormalities that are diagnostic of fibromyalgia. Some of these abnormalities have been found on tests too expensive and too invasive to serve as useful markers, and others are only marginally elevated or decreased, and occur in only a majority of tested subjects. And because we don't know what causes the abnormalities listed or the concrete abnormalities we can palpate, there is little consensus among researchers. It's just important for you to remember that while you'll read a lot about abnormalities in fibromyalgia, they are, like the symptoms you have, just a loose collection of data.

The bottom line is that we don't really know why fibromyalgics have so much pain. It may be that pain sensitivity is increased because the pain is continuous. There may be biochemical reasons—many physicians feel we have a defect that causes us to perceive pain where it may not exist. It is believed that we may have a reduction in pain threshold. But it is also true that fibromyalgics have all sorts of different tolerance levels to pain. We are not all the same. Then there is the psychological aspect—the fact that we are depressed and beaten down by the pain. It is abundantly clear that pain is not just in our heads, it is all over our bodies, and the proof of this lies in physical findings in our muscles, tendons, and ligaments that can be easily felt by a simple examination.

IN SENTENCE:

> *Fibromyalgia causes many different kinds of muscle pains, but usually in specific areas.*

learning

Taking a Closer
Look at Your Pain

IT'S EASY enough to see what causes most of your pain.
Hard swollen areas in the muscles, tendons, and ligaments
cause pressure on the **nerves** underneath. Where these nerves
branch and radiate, so does the pain. Thus, when you have a
headache, poking around at the hairline on the back of your
neck will usually reveal a spot that is "exquisitely painful."
When you press harder on the spot you've found, you'll notice
your headache is more intense. If your headache is on the right
side, the spot will be there. If your headache is all over your
head, look in the middle.

Pain in the back, legs, shoulders, arms, and chest are the
pains we live with every day. I used to poke around and find the
spots and try to push them out. It's one of those pains that hurts
so bad, it's good. If anyone who doesn't have fibromyalgia is
reading this chapter, that last sentence won't make any sense to
you. But trust me, those of us who suffer with it will tell you
that it makes perfect sense to us. My younger sister once put
it succinctly: "You can diagnose fibromyalgia just by asking people if they've had fantasies about doing awful things to their
bodies." She used to think about sticking an ice pick into her
eye when she had a horrible headache. When my back hurt, I
used to fantasize about lying on one of those beds of nails the
fakirs have in India. I figured the nails would actually feel good

in comparison to the pain I was feeling. Other people visualize hacking off body parts, or bashing themselves with a hammer.

Part of my job is to examine patients manually and make notations of **muscle calluses.** It's a system called mapping that some doctors use instead of tender point examinations. Patients are often amazed at how easily and quickly I can find the spots that hurt them. I laugh and tell them it's easy. I know exactly where they are because I used to find them on my own body. You hurt all over and you have these spots all over. You know where they are but don't know how to get rid of them. It's that simple and that difficult.

Local therapy might help your pain

Some doctors do trigger point, or tender point injections. A little synthetic **cortisone** and something like the Novocain they give you for dental surgery is injected into the area that hurts. This may sound like it would work well, and it does, but it has limitations. First of all, if you hurt all over as most of us do, you'd need to have fifty of these injections before you'd feel better. Secondly, of course, we all know that Novocain wears off in a few hours' time. There's also a limit to how many injections it's safe to have, especially if you're also injected with cortisone. I used to tell my doctor that the only thing accomplished by an injection was that my second-worst pain became my worst pain, meaning remove the main one and another takes its place. It stands to reason that these injections are the most useful when you have only one or two areas that hurt.

Some work has been done with "dry" needles, or needles that don't contain anything. This therapy is based on the idea that the injections cause inflammation at the site of the injury and the body's response to inflammation may make the area feel better. This technique is known as **prolotherapy.** Some people swear by this therapy, but I'm not a big fan of needles.

Acupuncture, or Chinese needle therapy, has been recognized as having some benefits for fibromyalgia in recent studies. Some insurance companies will even cover it, and some medical doctors endorse it. You may want to investigate this, especially if you can get it done without too much expense.

Other local therapies that might help

Local heat and cold therapies can also bring you relief. They have the benefit of not being intrusive, or, like medications, systemic. Hot showers are especially useful in the morning to ease morning stiffness. A warm bath in the evening may relax your muscles enough to help you fall asleep.

At other times, it's a matter of personal preference as to whether or not you prefer heat or cold compresses. I'm a big fan of heat, so old-fashioned hot water bottles are one of the things I've grown to depend on. They're portable, and don't need to be plugged in or microwaved, so you can use them in the car. You can use them at night and don't have to be afraid that you'll burn yourself as you might on a heating pad. I honestly don't know how I would have survived without my faithful hot water bottle. My sons are involved in sports and music so I've had to sit through countless concerts and games. My hot water bottle behind my back made those events tolerable on my bad days.

For a headache, though, ice or cold packs can do wonders. Cold, of course is a sort of anesthesia all by itself. So sometimes you can try ice packs for certain kinds of pain. A cold compress or pack should be used when you have itching or skin irritation because heat will make those symptoms worse. Remember to wrap a cold pack in a towel just as you would something hot. Cold things can burn your skin, too, especially if you're hypersensitive.

Compounds you can apply for skin pain

For certain skin pain, you may find a topical cream helpful. The most common are topical **salicylates** such as menthol, methyl salicylate, and peppermint oil. If you can't use salicylates, there are also ammonia compounds on the market. Pharmacists often make and sell topical anti-inflammatory creams, most commonly **ketoprofen** cream or gel. You may also find these helpful for joint pain and even for headaches when applied on the temple.

Chronic pain is different from other pain

The problem with our pain is that technically it isn't really pain. Pain is caused, the dictionary tells us, by the destruction of tissue. A burn hurts because you've destroyed something. Pain is the message that your body sends out to tell you to pull your hand away from a hot stove. When oxygen is cut off to the heart because the artery is occluded or closed, there's a crushing pain. The pain of a heart attack is caused by the destruction of tissue—dying because it has no oxygen.

All this is to simply explain why pain medication doesn't work very well in fibromyalgia. In fibromyalgia, there's no tissue destruction whatsoever. There's no **inflammation** as in **osteoarthritis,** when the cartilage in your joints is being worn away. If you've ever had surgery, or dental work, or had a severe sprain, you might recall amazement at how well the medication they gave you worked. Once when I was on a trip in Italy I walked too far in the wrong pair of shoes. My lower legs ached terribly. I took some ibuprofen because that's what people take for sprains. I was amazed at the fact that it took my pain away. No matter how many I took, ibuprofen had never done anything for my fibromyalgia.

Pain medications are available

Still, pain medication is prescribed for fibromyalgia, and the list is long. People typically switch around and try every new thing that comes out only to be disappointed that nothing works completely. Over time, you will learn through experience that nothing works very well for your pain. You can take a huge amount of something, or a cocktail combination of many things, but the end result isn't very satisfying, and there are always trade-offs. Stronger medications make you groggy, or hazy, when you're already tired and not thinking clearly. Doctors get nervous prescribing a lot of drugs, and get even more nervous when you need constant refills. A lot of prescriptions are expensive and insurance companies are notoriously stingy with the quantity and quality of their coverage.

Try simple things first

A combination of acetaminophen (Tylenol) and ibuprofen (Motril, Advil) may relieve pain as well as narcotics without the side effects or the issue of habituation or dependence. Usually you can get by, at least some of the time, with something purchased over the counter. On the other hand, when the pain is intractable, mild narcotics can restore functioning. Studies show that tramodol (Ultram) or antidepressant medications may also help you function despite your pain. These last two have side effects, but they are not generally as severe as those of narcotics like codeine. Headache patients have many new options and can now avoid the curse of the older medications that contained caffeine: the rebound headache. We'll explore some of the medications you may be familiar with in Month 4. For now, just remember that the less you use pain medication, the better it will work for you. Does this mean you should do without it? Of course not. It just means that you should treat it with respect and be careful about how much and how often you put medications into your body. It's easy to build up a tolerance and then the medication will no longer work at all.

Medication is not the only option

Relaxation and meditation techniques can be extremely helpful. Some people practice yoga and swear by it. Stretching and deep breathing are also wonderful tools if you learn to use them properly. In the For Further Information section at the end of this book you'll find a list of some tapes that might help you. The importance of setting aside this time for yourself and focusing on getting control over your body should not be undervalued. When you read about endorphins a bit later, in Month 3, remember that any form of relaxation will help you release them. Slowing down, you'll find, is a healing activity.

Body work and physical therapy are also helpful if you can afford them. Unfortunately, many insurance polices won't cover them for extended periods. However, if you're at your wits' end and can find practitioners who are well versed in fibromyalgia, you may benefit from their help.

Why your pain is so hard to control

We've all read stories of people who heroically cut off one of their own body parts to save themselves, or who walk miles on a broken leg. Women lift up cars to rescue their husbands, people dive into freezing water to save a child. It's natural when you hear these stories to wonder why you have so little tolerance for pain. Sometimes you might even think you're weak and it's your own fault that you can't just suck it up like other people do. Well, that just isn't the case. I can tell you honestly that fibromyalgics are among the bravest people I know. There are lots of other people who could never put up with the pain we do on a daily basis. It's easy to think of yourself as a hypochondriac, or a baby, but you're not.

Chronic pain is different from episodic pain, and it's a whole lot more difficult to treat for a variety of reasons. Fibromyalgics have pain somewhere in their body every single day. They have no rest or respite. Something always hurts, and this wears us down. In addition, there are physiological differences between chronic pain and, say, the pain caused by an accident. One of the things we know about chronic pain is that, after a time, the message system in the body reverses. Instead of the body sending a message to the brain about injury, the brain actually begins to send messages to the body telling it has pain. This is why researchers are looking at fibromyalgia pain closely. But the major difference between chronic and episodic pain is found in our hormones. For example, a surge of mighty **adrenaline** gives us the strength for supernatural feats like lifting cars in an emergency. But adrenaline isn't triggered by chronic pain.

Harnessing your natural painkillers

Trauma, both physical and emotional, causes the release of **endorphins**, our bodies' own natural painkillers. A cascade of physical responses over which we have no control begins in the **hypothalamus** and **pituitary** when our bodies are threatened. Other glands, including the **adrenals**, respond as well. The resulting chemicals, endorphins, spurt out into the body to blunt the body's sensation of pain. Nature has good reasons for this: When we are in less pain we can better protect ourselves.

The word *endorphin* is abbreviated from "endogenous morphine," which means a **morphine** produced naturally in the body. What they do is block the signal of pain to the nervous system. Endorphins, like narcotic pain medications, bind to pain receptors in the body. In fact, the term **opioid** is used for all endorphins and morphine-like chemicals. By occupying the pathways used by the pain signal, endorphins blunt our perception of pain, and even produce the same semi-euphoric, detached feeling associated with opiates. Unfortunately for those in chronic pain, endorphins cannot work for a long time because our body also makes enzymes called **endorphinase**, which chew up the endorphins. And, in time, our body accepts the chronic pain as normal and no longer produces endorphins.

Endorphins were only discovered in 1975. Medical research is now being done that will tell us more about the nature of pain, and how we might better harness our body's own resources to help us. There is certainly the possibility of relief on the horizon for various kinds of pain, among them; hopefully, the chronic kind fibromyalgics must endure.

Neurotransmitters and pain

Many of the medications used for fibromyalgia work in the part of our bodies known as **neurotransmitters.** Though we often think of the nervous system like a telephone line, it's not exactly an accurate analogy. In the body, the nerves are not one continuous cable, but rather a series of small ones, a long string of cells arranged end to end. There's an area between the cables where a message must jump from one to the other—and this is the province of neurotransmitters. These are simply chemicals excreted by the nerve cells that enable a signal to jump from one cable to another. Neurotransmitters have receptor sites to plug into, and this is where opioid medications fit. Here they can enhance or block messages, including pain. Opioids plug into receptors so pain signals cannot get through. And, as you now know, opioids enter your body via medication or are produced there naturally.

Can we make more endorphins?

You're probably thinking how great it would be if we could make our bodies release more endorphins. And, actually, there's a simple way to do this that doesn't cost anything or require a physician's help. One of the greatest ways to produce high levels of endorphins is through daily aerobic exercise lasting at least thirty minutes. This has a potent effect on endorphin production, more than laughing, meditation, or even eating. Aerobic exercises that seem to contribute the most to increased endorphin production include cycling, running, weight training, swimming, and brisk walking, although these are not the only exercises that have such an effect. Remember that you have to convince your body you're in distress to produce endorphins. This means you need to exercise at around 76 percent of your maximum heart rate to get the endorphin release going. Anything less won't do it.

It has also been noted that you are more likely to experience an endorphin high if the exercise performed is one that is familiar to you and your body. By following an exercise program on a regular basis, your body will produce a greater level of endorphins. This is why exercise staves off the blues, makes you less hungry, and helps with pain. As you'll soon learn, exercise will work to combat depression and many symptoms of fibromyalgia. This is why doctors keep telling you to do it.

Managing your pain—A constant challenge

To manage chronic pain successfully means you'll have to work at it in various ways, getting a certain percentage of relief from different things. For example, you could experience some relief from medication, some more from exercise, and a bit more from meditation or from relaxation exercises. Finding the right balance will take time and may require periodic changes, but any break from your pain will help you tremendously, both physically and mentally.

Pain has changed your life and the only way to control it is to make lifestyle changes to compensate. By learning all you can, and by making permanent changes based on what you've learned, you can take steps to regain your former self. Chronic pain is not just pain that has lasted a long time. It is a separate condition and you have to work to achieve control of it. And then you have to work some more to stay in control.

By the way, there are other things that stimulate the release of endorphins. Pleasant thoughts, laughter, happy memories, sexual pleasure—these also do the trick. So you can see that all of this leads to the same conclusion—you must get control of your body and your life. Being well begets well-being. Fear, stress, and inactivity are your enemies. You will not vanquish pain until you vanquish them.

IN A SENTENCE:

> *Researchers are looking more deeply into a systemwide cause for fibromyalgia pain—though they remain divided on what the defect may be and how best to treat it, there are certainly things you can do to help ease your pain.*

Some of It *Is* in Your Head: The Central Nervous System

IT'S A difficult call, but I believe that the central nervous system (CNS) symptoms of fibromyalgia are really the most awful and the most difficult to live with. It's common to suffer from the sensation of a scattered mind, waves of depression, exhaustion, irritability, poor short-term memory, difficulty with concentration, apathy, insomnia, nonrestorative sleep, nervousness, and a vague sensation that the brain is not connected to the body. These symptoms are hideous enough, but they're often made worse because no one but another fibromyalgic can understand them. You'll find that saying "I'm tired" doesn't come close to describing your numbing fatigue, and saying "I don't feel like doing that right now" doesn't do justice to your apathy. Just try to explain that you can't read a book because you can't comprehend the words on the page, or try to explain why you're still tired when you've slept twelve hours straight—it can't be done satisfactorily. Or maybe you sleep and wake up in cycles. My husband used to ask, "Why were you up and down all night?" I couldn't explain it, especially when I didn't remember getting up at all.

Brain cycles: A very real problem

Physicians who treat fibromyalgics know that almost every patient has said at one time or another, "I can stand the pain, but I need my brain." Bless my friend Devin Starlanyl for introducing the now-famous word **fibrofog**. (I'm not sure if she made it up, but she surely made it famous.) All I can say is if people think London fog is thick, they ought to spend a day with a fibromyalgic who is having a brain cycle!

(By the way, though there is no doubt whatsoever for those who have the disease that **brain cycles** exist in fibromyalgia, the mechanism that causes them remains obscure. Brain cycles coincide with pain cycles and can last for a few hours, a few weeks, or for months.)

The cerebral, or brain cycles, of fibromyalgia entered medical literature somewhat late in the game, and mostly through the back door. As you read in the last chapter, fibromyalgia was viewed in the beginning as a physical pain syndrome, or a rheumatic disorder, despite the fact that early researchers had mentioned other symptoms. Even Dr. Gowers stated in a paper dating back to 1904 that he was describing a "very terrible malady" and that the term "muscular rheumatism was inadequate." The medical papers written in the 1970s and '80s by experts trying to define fibromyalgia did discuss sleep disturbances, but they hardly mentioned the mental dullness and were mostly devoted to tender points and other painful syndromes such as irritable bowel, bladder, and painful menstrual cycles. This approach helped to create the criteria for diagnosing the illness, which led to its recognition as a distinct medical syndrome, but it is hardly descriptive for those of us who suffer from it.

This new classification left out the brain symptoms, the ones that for too many years had been the reason why women were diagnosed with hysteria. The emotional overlay, the mood swings, depression, and cognitive problems were left on the cutting room floor. Oddly enough, during the 1950s and '60s, when fibromyalgia was generally considered a manifestation of hysteria, no studies were actually done to support this idea. When these emotional symptoms were finally studied beginning in 1982, fibromyalgic patients fared about the same as other chronic pain patients on standard tests of emotional well-being. This discovery actually led to an important change. It became evident that standard psychiatric tests needed to be reevaluated and rescaled for patients who were in chronic physical distress.

• • •

Diminished cognitive skills

Today, it is common for fibromyalgics to talk about the toll the disease has taken on their cognitive abilities. To many it is the most disabling part of the whole illness, and the most difficult to explain (and prove) to employers and insurance companies. There is no way to measure this ever-changing galaxy of symptoms. I know. I've tried.

Researchers still don't know much about the relationship between pain and depression, sleep deprivation, and cognitive abilities. Some believe that pain, or pain sensitivity, is the cause of all our symptoms; others believe that if we could only sleep we would heal. We certainly do know that pain and depression occupy many of the same receptors in the body. Yet underneath all this lies the simple truth: Fibromyalgics can barely make enough energy just to cope. That above all is the fundamental problem we face.

Central Nervous System Symptoms of Fibromyalgia:

- ○ Insomnia and nonrestorative sleep
- ○ Irritability, nervousness, anxiousness
- ○ Mood swings
- ○ Depression
- ○ Apathy, listlessness
- ○ Impaired memory and concentration ("fibrofog")

Fatigue is a huge problem

Fatigue is the number one complaint of fibromyalgics. According to the latest statistics, 100 percent of fibromyalgics have pain, 98 percent fatigue, and an overwhelming number have a mixture of both. While that may be true, I absolutely believe I can speak for all of us when I say that fatigue is our most serious problem. We wake up tired, and by the afternoon we're exhausted. On a bad day, just taking a shower can seem daunting, and it's not an exaggeration to say that after taking a bath you may have to lie down and rest. One woman put it even more succinctly when she told me: "I feel like I have to lie down when I'm already lying down." Deadening fatigue, exhaustion, lack of stamina, and apathy are just the grueling icing on an already bitter cake. It really is the most extreme form of chronic torture. Most fibromyalgics don't feel guilty about their pain, they just deal with it.

But they feel horribly guilty about their fatigue, the things they can't do, the person they can't be.

There isn't enough energy to go around

Fibromyalgia is caused by a systemwide energy deficit. Fatigue and malaise are constant. I think the best description of the situation is to say that our bodies are operating in a brownout or under energy rationing. Just in case you're not familiar with that term, it's when a system of energy ration is imposed by a power company when need exceeds production. In the hottest days of summer, for example, when everyone is running air conditioners and appliances and there isn't enough energy to go around, energy keeps flowing, but at a lower level than normal. Lights aren't as bright as usual; the air conditioner doesn't work at high. In our fibromyalgic bodies, it's the same thing. Energy isn't cut off, we're not dead, power is running through our lines, but at a lower level. Every part of our body is fatigued, running at 50 percent power or less, and that's exactly what it feels like. If you try to do more than you feel up to, you'll find that the next step after a brownout is a power blackout. You'll know the moment you've overdone it, and the price you pay will be bed rest for days.

Insomnia and nonrestorative sleep

Even in healthy people lack of sleep causes impaired mental function and a lowered pain threshold. In fibromyalgia, fatigue and pain are made worse by insomnia and nonrestorative sleep. It's one of the most basic malfunctions in the illness, one that every doctor will ask you about. Fibromyalgics cannot sleep well and awaken frequently throughout the night, especially during their pain cycles. We suffer from a lack of deep restorative sleep, no matter how many hours we stay in bed. To most people, sleep seems like a simple act. You lie down in bed, close your eyes, and it happens. But it's not simple at all when you have fibromyalgia. Sleep is actually a complex function orchestrated by our brains where nerve cells in our hypothalamus control our sleep/wake cycles. Deep sleep, the kind that's hard to fall into when you hurt—when your bladder wakes you up, when your legs are restless—is the time when the body repairs itself. This is known as Stage IV sleep, and it's the kind of sleep you need to physically function at a normal level. It's the time when **serotonin** is produced, as well as other hormones, and the time when your body repairs itself down to each individual cell. When you aren't making demands on your body by walking around and engaging in other physical activities, your body is making demands on itself. In that quiet time, your body works hard, preparing itself for the coming day. More than one study has shown that even one sleepless night has an effect on hormone production, particularly growth hormone, serotonin, and the adrenal hormones—which unfortunately are the hormones that have the most effect on stress levels. Not enough restorative sleep also depresses the immune system. Lack of sleep, like too much sleep, can deepen depression.

REM sleep, the earlier "dreaming" stage of sleep, is important to your body as well. It appears that what Stage IV sleep does for your body, dreaming sleep does for your mind. All of the natural sleep stages serve essential restorative functions and, to function at your optimum level, you must experience all of them.

So what's the sleep-fibromyalgia connection?

After years of sleep studies and muscle biopsies, scans and other tests, no conclusive evidence has emerged that explains the relationship between fibromyalgia and poor sleep patterns. It does appear evident that there is some central abnormality. Yet nonspecific abnormalities in skeletal muscle are unlikely to explain most of our symptoms. Besides, overwhelming new evidence demonstrates that there is a disturbance in pain perception that extends beyond muscles and tendons. Poor sleep is a common complaint, but while it is clear that sleep deprivation may amplify existing symptoms, it's also unlikely that disturbed sleep alone is the cause of our illness.

Irritability and mood swings

A normal but horrifying part of brain cycles are mood swings. The horrifying part is that you are acutely aware of your mood swings but feel powerless to control them. For fibromyalgics, anger, frustration, fear, depression, and self-pity can come and go in the matter of minutes and with great intensity. We cry easily, become frustrated at the drop of a hat, and get unreasonably angry at the slightest provocation. But the real curse is the heightened sensation that somewhere inside you know you are wrong, or overreacting, yet can't admit it, let alone stop it.

The reason for these mood swings, again, is unclear. Some doctors have speculated that it's due to fluctuating or abnormal hormone levels; others believe the fault may lie somehow with the neurotransmitters that relay messages of emotion and pain. Overstimulation, understimulation—right now it's anybody's guess. It's certainly true that it feels like something has gone awry at a fundamental level.

• • •

Don't do too much when you don't feel up to it

An article called "Witch or Martyr?" once caught my eye on the Internet. I stopped dead in my mental tracks when I saw it because it summed up in only two words my emotional gamut when I'm having my fibromyalgia mood swings. When I'm tired and feel overwhelmed I get frantic and try to do too much. This exhausts and then frustrates me, and I become consumed with guilt, and then I start feeling sorry for myself. I force myself to struggle on, when it's obvious to everyone but me that I should just stop and let things be. This is my martyr cycle: I have to do it because no one else can or will. Can't anyone else see the pile of laundry, the trash that needs emptying, or the dirty handprints on the door?

Being a martyr sets up the witch cycle because I can't quite identify with being a martyr. I start to get angry because no one else feels as sorry for me as I do. Why can't anyone else see the extra work they're creating by their lack of assistance? Why can't anyone stop and see how awful I feel and understand me? I am angry at whatever vexes me at the moment and the truth is I don't really know why. The closest I can come to describing it is to say that it's because people don't see everything exactly as I do.

Battling your mood swings

After anger rolls in the sadness, despair, anxiety—or does anxiety start the cascade of emotional symptoms? It's one of those things that spirals to a point and finally explodes like the other symptoms of fibromyalgia. I don't know what sets me off, but I think exhaustion plays some role in it. I know that when I'm in a cycle I can't be reasonable, though when someone tells me to be reasonable I insist that I am. In our office I've heard Dr. St. Amand tell patients, "I used to come into the office some days spoiling for a fight. In my heart I knew that someone that day was going to get it." It's an emotional edginess you can feel, but you can't admit.

Back in the 1980s, Dr. Hugh Smythe penned one of my favorite definitions of fibromyalgia. When I first read it, it struck me as a perfect description of my illness, and I've never changed my mind. "The irritable everything" syndrome. Sound familiar?

Heightened sensitivities and senses

During brain cycles, we become oversensitive to noise, bright lights, smells, and other external stimuli. These are more severe in women whose senses are more acute. Ordinary sounds from television can drive you straight up a wall. On a bad day even the noise from fluorescent lights is intolerable.

Children's voices and other noises get on your nerves, you can hear the barking dog down the street that doesn't bother anyone else, and the neighbor's gardener makes you scream out loud. When you're sensitive to sounds sleep can be impossible, even when you put your head under your pillow and hold it down with your arm, even when the bedroom door is closed.

Bright lights or certain kinds of ungentle light (like florescent) can't be tolerated and you need to wear dark glasses to protect yourself in a house or in an airport terminal. The glare from sunlight on cars is blinding and can cause frontal headaches and your eyes to tear, burn, and ache. Headaches and nausea are commonly caused by flickering light sources.

Most fibromyalgics describe sensitivity to smells to some degree. These smells can cause nausea, headaches, and increased pain. Doctors will tell you that you're chemically sensitive, though natural smells like meat cooking or certain flowers will do exactly the same thing. These various stimuli will usually increase your mental symptoms and add to your anxiety and frustration. It is not surprising that these symptom combinations have led some doctors to think of fibromyalgia as a sensitivity syndrome that is caused by exposure to contaminants in the environment. For doctors who believe that fibromyalgia is a pain amplification syndrome, the next logical step in their thinking is that other senses are amplified as well.

Depression, apathy, listlessness

Many, many studies have been done on fibromyalgics and depression. Are we in pain because we are depressed? Or are we depressed because we're in pain? This dilemma always makes me think of the chicken-and-egg conundrum—and I don't think science has solved that one either!

You have good reasons to be depressed

If you're living in constant or almost constant pain and you don't have enough energy to get up and get out of the house, or even to get dressed on some days, is it any wonder you're depressed? If you can't be the kind of mother you want to be, or the kind of man you think you should be, shouldn't you be depressed? Who wouldn't be with all the symptoms we have to deal with? It's normal to be depressed when bad things happen. Depression, the abnormal kind—is what people experience when nothing's wrong. Most fibromyalgics have what's called situational depression. After all, there are plenty of bad things happening in our body at any given moment.

• • •

There's no simple answer for depression and apathy

The problem is that fibromyalgics aren't going to "get over" what's causing their depression. It's not the kind of a loss that grows distant over time and eventually you think about it less and less. There's always some new disappointment, some new source of guilt or sadness. Fibromyalgia is a loss that never goes away. And to top it off, you never really feel well. It's not like you can jump up and get out to new surroundings to cheer yourself up. It takes energy to be happy. It takes energy to step outside yourself and find things to do that will brighten your outlook.

It's normal to feel depressed—for a little while

In the beginning, after you've just been diagnosed with FM, it's normal to be a little depressed. It's normal to want some time to yourself to come to terms with the changes in your life. But, if this lasts—if you feel like the world is a bad place and you feel you are worthless and that life is worthless—think about getting help for your depression. Especially if you begin to isolate yourself—doing things like not answering the phone anymore—you must examine the situation. If you can't bring yourself to do anything, if you just want to sleep, or feel like ending your life, you need to talk to your doctor right away. There are things that can be done to help you. If you have severe depression, you need help. It may be a product of your fibromyalgia, the side effect of a medication, or another condition entirely. It's just like fibromyalgia itself. A car accident can't give you fibromyalgia. Getting pneumonia can't make you catch fibromyalgia. But both of those things drain your energy and when your body is under siege that's when bad genetic traits rear their ugly heads. It's the same thing with depression. If you are prone to clinical depression, for example, fibromyalgia might tip the scale and you could slide into it. So don't take depression lightly. If you feel like you're losing control or need help, get it. We're lucky that the stigma of depression isn't what it used to be. There's no shame in asking for help.

Apathy and listlessness are the little brothers of depression. That's not to say that they're not powerful, though. I've endured heavy apathy that was really overwhelming. I remember once talking to a patient, a young girl. She told me that she wasn't taking her medication at night; she just couldn't get up to get it. Her mother said to her, "Just get up and take it." I understood perfectly what this girl was saying because I can remember lying in bed at night and knowing the lights were on in the living room and I had to get up to turn them off and wash my face and brush my teeth. I would just lie there, too. I couldn't force myself to get up and get moving. It's almost more

---

Warning Signs of Depression

○   Feeling of emptiness, loss of interest in everything

○   Lack of pleasure in things that you used to enjoy

○   Feelings of guilt

○   Feeling isolated and overwhelmed

○   Taking no joy in anything good that happens around you

○   A feeling that life is not worth living, suicidal thoughts

○   Loss of appetite, weight loss

○   Inability to get out of bed, the desire to sleep twenty-four hours a day

○   Not wanting to socialize at all, or answer the phone when it rings

---

of a physical apathy than a mental one, though there's that, too. It's hard to rouse yourself to move, or care, or to get up and close the door!

Listlessness just means a lack of energy. It's sort of just there, and you can't get a spark going. Everything seems kind of gray, and everything you need to do just doesn't seem worth the effort of doing it.

Fibrofog: Impaired memory and concentration

It's hard to know where to start when describing fibrofog. It would be easiest to say: you know what it is, you have it. You may even have better war stories than I do! But here goes: Your short-term memory is very short or nonexistent. Often you can't remember things you've just been told or recall why you just walked into a room. Your sense of direction is disrupted, you get lost even in places you know very well. Suddenly on the freeway you've gone miles past your exit. You can forget what you are doing or saying in the middle of a conversation or task. Reasoning and deduction range from difficult to impossible, depending on the severity of a cycle. In severe cycles, you cannot even read because you can't follow a plot, or remember the names of characters from one chapter to the next. It's really hard to follow a television show if it's one of those detective stories with plot twists and turns. It's also common to misspell words, or not recognize how they are written incorrectly. If you're lucky, you may have the vague sense that they look wrong. However, this usually doesn't help because you have no idea how to make them correct. When fibrofog is bad, using a dictionary is impossible because you can't even string together the sequence of letters to look a word up.

• • •

The inconveniences of fibrofog go on and on

You'll have no idea where you left things, and be unable to "see things" even when you are looking directly at them, that is, if you are lucky enough to remember what you are looking for. Unless you put your keys in the same place every day or have someone to help you, you'll literally never find them. Somewhere in my house I have lost bank ATM cards, keys, lipsticks, hair clips, and many other assorted items. I have no idea where they are, except to say they must be in unusual places because I've never stumbled across them. I can't tell you how many times I've had to go through garbage Dumpsters, wastebaskets, and trash cans because I've absentmindedly thrown things away that I need. You'll completely forget appointments, conversations, things you have said or have agreed to do, and wake up at night wondering whether or not you have paid your bills this month or any month. Serious frustration is caused by this inability to count on your own brain. It's demoralizing and it can dramatically increase your irritability, nervousness, anxiety, and sense of isolation.

You can laugh at fibrofog, but it isn't always funny

Sometimes it's easy to laugh when you find the milk in the pantry with the cereal or your purse still in the car or on the back porch. Other times it's scary because your hot water has boiled out of the kettle and nearly started a fire. For reasons of sheer self-defense, I'd never buy an iron or a curling iron without an automatic shutoff.

Many people have had to go on disability and leave careers they love because their cognitive skills are so undependable and generally absent. This is especially true of high-pressure jobs, because with fatigue combined with bad cognitive days, there's no chance they can catch up.

It's nearly impossible and completely demeaning for these people to try to prove or explain what makes them disabled when physically they look fine and don't work demanding physical jobs. Most employers recognize that fibromyalgia has something to do with pain and chronic fatigue that makes you tired. Now try to explain why you can't do a job where your only physical activity is typing on a computer, or even doing dictation, and you can see the problem.

Brain symptoms make your whole life more difficult

This same problem translates into our personal lives as well. When your brain isn't working, it's practically impossible to express your problems clearly and eloquently. Most fibromyalgics have a problem finding the right words for a simple sentence, so it's out of the question to try to explain something abstract, changeable, and not generally accepted or easily understood. It's easy to say that if people care for you, they'll understand. But that's way too simplistic. When they care for you, they want to understand, and to be told how to help you. And that's where the frustration gets really bad. The most disruptive aspect of these symptoms is often the fact that people can't identify with them. Nearly everyone has had the flu or a toothache. But forgetting how to tie a shoe? Not likely.

Your brain cells use a huge amount of power. They have the most mitochondria, or power stations, of any cells in the body. If we apply the same brownout analogy to brain cells and circuits, it's easy enough to see what the problem is. Obviously you can still think to some degree, but in the systemwide energy rationing, each and every brain cell is working at diminished capacity.

IN A SENTENCE:

> Fatigue, fibrofog, low energy, and lack of sleep are among the most difficult symptoms of fibromyalgia to endure.

learning

Coping Strategies for CNS Symptoms

THE WORST thing about the fatigue of fibromyalgia is that you can't make it go away by resting. No matter how much rest you get, your fatigue won't go away for long. You can push yourself, but then you'll collapse and, believe me, the net result will be the same as if you paced yourself from the beginning. I've learned this lesson many times the hard way. And I still have to convince myself it's true. If you're like me—hang up a sign: More than anything else, pacing yourself is the key to surviving with fibromyalgia.

Where to start

Other than resting and taking breaks, what can you do when you're exhausted? Prioritize and pace yourself. Every day decide what the most important task is that you have and do that first. Decide what isn't important, and forget about it. Really. *Forget about it*. It's important to really forget about what you can't do. Thinking about what you don't have the strength to do will just stress you out and wear you out even more. Stress will wear you down faster than anything except running a marathon and it's a pretty good bet that you're not going to be trying that.

You really do have to learn to put things out of your mind. If you delegate something or hire someone to do something for you, (like housework or gardening) let them do it and accept the way they go about it. This may not be the easiest thing to do, especially if you're a control freak like me, but practice. And practice some more.

If you're a woman, think of it this way: it's practice at being graceful. Take help when it's offered and let the help *help* you. If you're a man—it's good practice, too. Men also need to know when to sit back and let things happen. I just think men are better at compartmentalizing than women are. I've learned a lot about this from watching my husband. For some reason, it's a lot easier for them to really put things out of their minds.

Plan, plan, plan

Planning is crucial. It's not a bad idea to make one day a week your planning day. I do my planning on Sunday afternoon. Maybe a dry erase board or a worksheet for the week is a good idea for you. If you plan ahead and group your tasks, you'll end up saving energy. So the time spent planning will pay off in extra energy when you need it.

First, make a list on a piece of scratch paper of the things you have to do. Group your tasks together so that you can do, for example, two errands at the same end of town on the same day. If you have to pick up your kids, write down what you have to do that is in the same region or neighborhood. If you have to go shopping, find a large store that carries groceries as well as the other things you need so you'll only have one place to go. You'll only have to get out of the car, walk into a store, and load and unload the car once. You might have to drive a little farther to get there, but the energy you'll save only waiting in line once will make it worth it. Some people have computer programs that create shopping lists with items organized by the aisle in the supermarket. I've never been organized enough to use one of those, but I can see how they would be a remarkable help especially if your mind is extra foggy on shopping day. I have to admit that I usually do have to double back a few times in the market to get everything I need.

Other shortcuts to remember

Another tip that's one of my favorites is to shop at small places when you only need one thing. If you're like me, shopping at a mall is an overwhelming and exhausting experience. You have to walk long distances and deal with jarring lighting as well the crowds and noise. You won't save energy, because distances are always farther than you think, and it may take going into many stores to find what you're looking for. I've found a whole network of smaller stores where I can park easily and shop quickly in a softer, less frenetic and hectic atmosphere.

If you have lots of occasions in your life, start a gift cupboard. I buy things like pretty picture frames, candles, books, pens, and stationery when I see them on sale and keep them in a special drawer at home. When I need a gift, or one of my kids needs something for a friend or a teacher, we don't have to run out that minute and get something. When you're sick it's stressful to have to muster the strength to run out and do something unexpected, especially on a really bad day. If you force yourself to do it, you'll pay for it for days afterward.

Experiment until you find an organizer or system that suits you. Keep it handy, and don't deviate from it. I know when I'm exhausted I flounder—everything seems insurmountable and impossible and impulsively I try to rearrange things. I'm always sorry when I do. Plan carefully and look at your plan carefully. Make your plans at the beginning of the week when you're rested and stick with the plans you have made. If you are really in bad shape, cross out tasks you don't really have to do right now. Some people bunch their tasks so that each day they have some that are essential and some things they could forgo if they aren't feeling up to it.

Get rid of clutter

Before we leave the topic of organization, I need to tell you one more thing. It's something that's really hard for me to do, but I know I'm right. One thing that will help you feel better and will also help with depression is to get rid of clutter. Get rid of all the clothes that will fit you "someday," the papers you're going to read, the projects you'll do if and when you feel up to it. If you can't bear to throw something away, put it away in a box in your attic or shed, where you can't see it. Free your living space of clutter. Clutter is depressing. It is a silent reproach of all the things you can't do. It's a mountain of things waiting for your time and your attention. Make a vow to only work on one project at a time. If you have a huge stack of magazines and things you want to read, tear out just the articles you'd like to read and keep them in a folder. To most people, clutter is just things. But to fibromyalgics, it can be a pile of guilt.

Consider learning to use a computer

Of course computers have made shopping (and everything else) much less of a problem. You can do banking and shopping online now. Groceries and books can be delivered to your door as well as prescription medications and other sundries. If you make lists and do a little planning you can shop at online stores that charge a nominal delivery fee or no fee at all if your charges are over a certain amount. That's another way that being organized will pay off.

The best investment I ever made was buying my laptop computer. I don't have to sit rigidly at my desk or stay in one room. I can lean back on the couch or sit in bed propped up on pillows to make my lists. If you get a long cord, you can plug in to phone jacks in whichever room you are working to get online.

If you're not computer literate, I promise you that it's easier than you think it will be to learn. Remember that you probably will only be doing a few things; you won't be doing fractals or computing the square root of pi. You don't have to put a man on the moon. All you want to learn to do is simplify your life. More than anything I can think of, computers have changed the face of having fibromyalgia. You can participate in support groups, do your shopping, write to your friends, and help your children with their homework without even having to get dressed, let alone get in the car and go somewhere. No more hysterics when one of your children has a report due tomorrow and you just can't take him to the library. You'll have the Internet and reference books right at your fingertips.

There are many ways to learn

There are lots of easy ways to learn what you need to know about computers, including teachers who give private instruction and classes at community colleges. I recommend the latter because that is where I learned the things that I couldn't figure out myself. I found that the classes were small and my fellow students were all "of a certain age" like I am. No smart-aleck kids, just people working at a pleasant pace to learn something new. Computer classes and other classes are also offered on-line or you can purchase tutorial CDs. Both of those approaches allow you to work at your own pace. Give it a try: Computers really can help you to restore many parts of life that you've lost.

Medications are tools, not solutions to fatigue

There are medications called stimulants that many fibromyalgics take, and you will certainly meet people who swear by them. These stimulants come in various forms—from caffeine and over-the-counter pep pills to prescription drugs. These should all be used very cautiously. By taking these drugs you are, in essence, whipping your body to keep it moving. This will certainly work for a while. But it should be obvious that what goes up must come down. You can't force your body to make energy: Eventually it becomes like beating a dead horse and it will take you a long time to recover. It's best to learn to understand your body, learn when you can do one more thing without harming yourself, and when you need to stop and take a short nap or take on an easier task.

Your thyroid usually isn't the problem

Don't allow yourself to be convinced you have thyroid problems if you don't. You're tired because you have fibromyalgia, and fibromyalgia isn't caused by a thyroid deficiency. (If it were, we could just take thyroid medication and be well!) If you're concerned, see a reputable **endocrinologist** and have your thyroid tested with a blood test called a TSH. If this test is normal, then your thyroid is functioning normally. An incorrect diagnosis of thyroid disorder can be a real problem because too much thyroid is dangerous for your heart and your bones. If your doctor wants you to try a little to see if it will give you more energy, insist on being tested two months after you start. If your TSH is still normal, then you're doing yourself no harm. (You may just be suppressing your own gland a little, but no harm is being done.)

Dealing with insomnia and nonrestorative sleep

There's no easy solution to the sleep problems of fibromyalgia, I'm sorry to say. Exercise and regular bedtimes are always helpful, of course. Being tired when you go to bed certainly at least helps you to fall asleep. Warm showers or baths before bed will help your muscles relax so you can get comfortable. Reading in bed, a warm decaffeinated beverage, and meditation can also be relaxing. Relaxation and soothing audiotapes can also serve a purpose, and popular versions are available in most music and bookstores. Heavy meals in the late evening can cause blood sugar to fall during the night, which may cause you to have nightmares, even more restless sleep, or waking panic attacks. It's best, if you're going to eat in the evening, to have protein and fat, not heavy starches or sugars. Keep your meals small in the evening, too, because feeling stuffed makes it very difficult to sleep. If your bladder wakes you up at night it's important to limit your fluid intake in the late afternoon and evening.

Assess your surroundings

Obvious mechanical things also shouldn't be ignored. Make sure your bed is comfortable and everything you might need is in reach. Curtains and shades will make your room quiet and dark and a fan can also be calming and even muffle outside noise a bit. Extra pillows, a heating pad, an electric blanket, or a hot water bottle can also help make you comfortable, especially if you turn them on before you go to bed so your bed will feel warm and comforting when you climb in. You really do have to be comfortable to sleep, so make sure the clothes you sleep in are the right weight and loose enough.

Some supplements might help

You'll hear people touting **5-HTP (5hydroxytrytophan)** and **melatonin.** These are the most natural and least habit-forming sleep aids. 5-HTP is a breakdown product of L-tryptophan, an amino acid present in protein foods. (Every Thanksgiving you can read about this—it's supposedly the reason that turkey makes you sleepy.) It increases serotonin in the blood, so similar to prescription antidepressants, it can help you sleep. For this reason, if you are taking an SSRI anti-depressant (especially Zoloft and Welbutrin), you should not take 5 HTP. In studies it has been shown to be helpful with relatively few side effects.

Melatonin is a hormone normally secreted from the pineal gland, a tiny gland deep inside the brain behind the forehead. (The pineal gland converts tryptophan to melatonin) It is produced only at night, and as we age, we produce less of it. It also has several studies behind its success, and is not implicated in rebound fatigue the following day. It is available over the counter or in health food stores. The usual dose is around 2 mg a night and it should not be used in adolescents because their natural melatonin levels are already high. One thing to bear in mind is that melatonin works better if used regularly, and since it is a natural hormone you can't develop a tolerance to it. Melatonin can, in some fibromyalgics, cause or worsen existing depression. Stop taking it right away if this happens to you. You do not have to wean off it.

There are compounds available to you if you don't have to restrict salicylates. Calms Forte, which contains magnesium, may help with restless legs or muscle cramps (as would a plain magnesium supplement). Valerian is another herb often used to help sleep. Though you might consider herbal medications natural and safe, newer studies show that a fair number of them are not. If you are taking prescription medications of any kind it would be wise not to use herbs because drug interactions can occur, and most herb/drug combinations have not been studied.

Other sleep aids

Benadryl (or **diphenhydramine**) is another over-the-counter option. It's the active ingredient in most over-the-counter sleep aids, many of which come in tablet form so you can chop them up with a knife and take as little as you think you'll need on any given night. It has a great safety record, but doesn't work for everyone. It has been proven safe for children and even pregnant women. Over the counter pills come in 25 to 50 mg. I often get by with an even smaller dose of 12.5 mg. Benadryl can cause excitability in some people, in which case you should not take it for sleep.

The next step up is prescription medication. **Ambien,** or Zolpidem, is the most common, followed by antidepressants (such as **Elavil** and **Desyrel—amitriptyline** and trazodone), muscle relaxants (**Soma** and **Flexeril, carisoprodol** and cyclobenzapreine), and other assortments of medications including doxepin, temazepam, lorazepam, and clonazepam. A newer pill, **Sonata,** or zalepron, is quite short acting and can be helpful if your problem is early-morning awakenings. Your doctor will help you decide which is best for you. Prescription medications will help you sleep, but you shouldn't take them every night because they can be addictive.

Remember that sleep medications will make you tired

They all, each and every one of them, will depress your energy level the next day, and some have more severe effects than others. Some cause increased morning somnolence; others have a rebound effect twelve hours later. You can build up a tolerance over time to many of them. Like all medications, they have a place in the treatment of your symptoms but should be used as an adjunct to exercise, relaxation techniques, and a good bedtime routine. Sleep medications can help you fall asleep, or stay asleep, or go back to sleep in a pinch, but they don't really help you get the deep sleep that you need. Use them carefully, respect their powers, and they will be useful assistants when you need them.

Managing your irritability and mood swings

The best coping strategy I can muster for these difficult symptoms is to take the time to explain them to the people around you. Next time you're having a cycle of better days, or feel more relaxed, write a letter to your family. Explain that these emotional symptoms are part of your illness, and ask them to understand and try to be patient. Ask for help. Explain that when you're in one of these cycles, it's extraordinarily difficult for you to be reasonable.

Communication with others is absolutely essential for coping with your invisible illness. Most of the time it's pretty easy to see how to help someone. If you come across someone who is visually impaired, or using a cane, you can instantly assess the challenges facing them. In contrast, to live around fibromyalgics isn't straightforward, and you need to remind yourself of that fact. When you feel better, be sure to show your gratitude to your friends and family. This simple fact alone will help them to understand that the other "you" isn't really you, but part of an illness neither you nor they can see.

Learning to recognize your mood swings and irritability can also help you better cope with them. Sometimes you can identify a feeling of restlessness and an uncomfortable manic energy surge that signals their onset. When these symptoms start it's essential to decrease your stress levels, as stress will certainly trigger huge emotional swings. Sometimes it helps to withdraw away from harsh external stimuli. Take a long bath or shower, or a quiet walk. Eat a simple meal on a tray in bed, and try to relax. This is an important time to take things off the table and simplify your life.

Simple solutions for nervousness and anxiety

Anxiety and nervousness, like other emotional symptoms, come and go. Take to heart the suggestions above about coping with mood swings, because nervousness and anxiety are closely related to them. The difference lies in how you handle them—you need to get out and be active, and keep your mind busy.

The best solution is exercise and meditation. Simple stretching exercises done to classical music or a gentle videotape can help get rid of nervous energy and focus your mind elsewhere. Taking a long walk can really take the edge off these unproductive emotions by burning some of the energy they churn up.

There are a variety of relaxation techniques that can be employed, practiced, or studied by you or in a class setting. Water **aerobics** and low-impact exercise classes have sprung up at centers like YMCAs, local parks, and extension classes. There are also many available tapes that can bring those classes right into your own living room.

Coping with depression, apathy, and listlessness

To pull yourself out of the normal depression that comes with a chronic illness and that crops up periodically when you're feeling sorry for yourself because you can't get things done the way you want is not impossible. What you have to do is retrain your thinking. For example, when you find yourself dwelling on all that you can't do, consciously turn your mind to how strong you are to still be functioning so well. Every time you think something negative, stop, think again, and this time think of something positive that you have accomplished. Think about good and rewarding experiences. Turn your mind away from yourself and what you can't do, and go do something you know you'll enjoy. Treat yourself to crossing one of the tasks off your to-do list, or do something just for you. Concentrate on things that you do well. This is not a time to be harsh on yourself, or make yourself feel worse with frustration that you can't accomplish what you set out to do. If you have a hobby, or activities that make you feel better, this is a time to devote what energy you have to these occupations.

Exercise helps in more than one way

Take a walk, or sit outdoors and take your mind off everything. Ten minutes of exercise will cause your body to release endorphins. When you come back and your mind is clearer for a moment, look around yourself and see things differently. Remember that exercise coupled with happy memories and laughter will release even more endorphins. Personally, I like the satisfaction of working in my garden, so even when I couldn't do a lot, I found that when I just did something little I could still get a great deal of satisfaction. Even planting a few pots of flowers, tending to them, and enjoying their blooms can boost my spirits. When you don't feel well, keep your tasks simple: Watering might be one day's job, for example. If you keep your tasks down to a reasonable size, you'll be able to accomplish them and enjoy the satisfaction of getting something done. That may sound silly, but I can remember so many days being depressed because I hadn't done even one thing. So pick your one thing wisely!

Keeping your mind busy

Gardening, walking, and exercising have something else in common. They're mindless activities—you don't have to think to do them and they take your attention away from the things that are pressing on you. This works the same way as meditation; it clears your mind and slows down the pace of life. Slowing down is very healing, and if you share this with your healthier friends, you'll be teaching them something important. Even healthy people can find that relaxation and meditation are also wonderful ways to fight depression, pain, or a simple case of the blues.

If you're physically exhausted, try watching a simple movie. Don't get something loud or violent. If you have children, some of their movies are perfect. You'll be surprised at how much fun and escapism you can experience by watching something simple and sweet with them. Lots of fibromyalgics have tried and true movies for certain days like this. For me, *An American in Paris,* with its beautiful music and sweet love story, is a real escape.

Don't be afraid to ask for help

If none of these measures help you, please don't try to tough it out. Overcoming depression is not proof of manhood or even womanhood, and actually women are much more likely to be depressed. When you're ill (and even if you're not), if something is overwhelming, it's time to ask for help. Depression is, after all, treatable. There are many antidepressant medications, and therapy or group therapy are other viable options. Be sure to confer with your physician, and be honest with him or her. Be clear that you have tried to control your emotions by yourself and now you need assistance. Antidepressant medications do have side effects, although there are many newer ones and you will have options. These medications have the added benefit of helping with sleep and cutting your pain perception. Remember that depression is a treatable illness and you have nothing to be ashamed of.

Life strategies for fibrofog

You need to recognize that all these cognitive impairments and emotional overreactions are a normal part of fibromyalgia, experienced to some degree by all of us who have this disease. This way, you can learn to be patient and understanding with yourself. Remember to laugh when your fibrofog has caused you to do something funny. There is a funny side to almost everything.

It is important to use all of your coping skills when dealing with fibrofog. The less "fibro frustration" you experience, the less stress will wear down your body. The underlying fear of forgetting something important, of not being able to count on your memory, are two huge looming stresses that will amplify all your other symptoms.

Repetition and simplicity are key

Practice being methodical, so that many of your tasks become second nature. This is the single most important thing that you can do to help yourself deal with fibrofog when it rolls in. The less complicated you can make things, the better you will cope. Train yourself to put things in the same place every time, and no matter how exhausted you are, don't cut yourself any slack on this one. Force yourself to put your things where they go before you collapse. For example, always keep your keys in the same place. Hang them by the door, or put them in a dish on your dresser. But never, ever put them down any other place. If you always put them there, eventually you will do it without thinking about it. It will become a habit. Do the same with your eyeglasses (especially sunglasses, because you probably use them less) and your purse or wallet. Think about it this way: You don't lose your toothbrush because you don't take it out of the bathroom.

Make a special drawer for your bills and your checks. Twice a month, once for the bills due the first and once for the bills due the fifteenth, schedule a time to attend to this. When my bills come in, I tear off all the extra stuff, throw away the advertisements, and put the payment stub in the envelope. On the back in large numbers I write the due date of the bill. That way, when it's time to pay them, I can easily check to see if I have paid what's due. If you write checks around town, for goodness sake, get the kind that have carbon paper and duplicates. If your bank lets you check your balance and transactions online, you can do that before you write out your batch of checks just to make sure you haven't forgotten to make a deposit. Also, if you can put your phone bill, cable bill, and other monthly fees on your credit card, you'll have fewer checks to write, and the credit card detail will have recorded all your payments for you.

Write it down

THIS IS the most important tip I can give you for dealing with fibrofog. Keep a small pad and a pen near the phone and make sure you leave them there. Don't walk off with them. When you take a message, write it down. Sometimes when the fog is very bad you may want to make notes while you are talking. You may even need to do this as you go along to remember who you are talking to and the purpose of the call. Insist that your family members and children write down phone messages. Again, if they tell you about who called when you're doing something else there's an excellent chance you'll have absolutely no recollection of the incident.

Post notes if you have to. Lots of us can't imagine what we did before Post-its, those little papers with a sticky part. These come in handy because sometimes you will want to post notes in other places, like on the dashboard of your car. If you are going somewhere in your car and you're foggy, take an extra minute to write out directions. If you have a computer, print out a map from MapQuest.com. When you're driving keep the radio off so you will have fewer distractions.

Make lists to take to your appointments. If you have a meeting with your child's teacher, your boss, repairmen, or a client, make a list of pertinent things. Make one to take with you when you go to the doctor. There is nothing more frustrating for the doctor and patient when a patient walks out of the appointment room and suddenly remembers a question she forgot to ask. You can also make brief notes of things you need to remember when you're meeting with other people. Keep them brief, so you don't slow things down trying to read them and ask and answer questions at the same time.

Lists are your safety net and your map

Put a shopping list pad on your refrigerator door, and tie a pen or pencil to it. When you run out of something write it down the minute you notice it. Have your family members do the same, because if they tell you when you're tired or doing something else you'll never remember it.

Keep a calendar and write down every appointment the minute you make it. Every morning and every night check this calendar. Do it at two specific times, like just before you go to bed and first thing in the morning, or pick other logical times and work these into your routine. You can put your calendar by your telephone, next to your bed, or on your computer. If you're afraid you'll forget something during the day, hang a note up where you are sure to see it. Never leave the house without checking your list of things to do. When you go out, take a copy with you if you have a habit of forgetting one of your errands.

Some people will tell you that if you're in a severe fibrofog, you shouldn't drive. This unfortunately isn't very realistic for most of us, but you can certainly limit your driving time. Run one errand at a time. Save complicated ones for when you are feeling better. Teach your children not to distract you if you have to drive with them. This is another good lesson, by the way, for children. They need to learn that cars are dangerous and drivers need to keep their concentration on the road and not be distracted.

Limit your sensory input

Another thing that will help is to decrease your sensory input. Fibromyalgics in general have a problem with noise, especially loud background noise. I'm not sure why this is, but I especially notice that I am unable to tune them out or keep them in the background. For example, I need to plug my other ear when I'm talking on the phone. If you're like this, turn off music when you need to concentrate. Even classical or soothing music can make you feel overloaded in a cycle. Filter out noise by closing the doors and windows. If you need to, run a small fan to make white noise. Too much light can also make it difficult to concentrate, and glare can make it impossible. Your ability to absorb information is impaired, so remember to keep things as simple, uncluttered and quiet as possible. This will help you function.

• • •

Just keep it simple and organized

To help your cognitive and central nervous systems function as effectively as they can, it all comes down to this: simplify and organize. Simplifying includes delegating work and turning down jobs or engagements you know you aren't up to. Being organized means keeping things accessible and checking and double-checking your plans. Being organized will keep your pace reasonable and help you conserve what energy and mental functions you do have. It will reduce stress and enable you to enjoy all the benefits that simple change will give you.

IN A SENTENCE:

> *The fatigue and cognitive challenges of fibromyalgia can be managed only by adjusting your routines to accommodate your symptoms and by simplifying and organizing your daily routines and chores.*

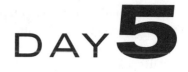

Understanding IBS and How It Affects Your Life

IRRITABLE BOWEL syndrome (IBS) is a syndrome by name, so like fibromyalgia; it's a collection of symptoms that occur together. Unfortunately, one of fibromyalgia's symptoms is usually irritable bowel syndrome. To make an IBS diagnosis, your doctor will have to rule out diseases that have overlapping symptoms. When all your test results are negative (again!), you'll be told that you have irritable bowel syndrome, and be given the "comforting" news that there is no cure for your condition, and that the cause of it is unknown.

IBS is common in fibromyalgia

Irritable bowel syndrome is common in fibromyalgics and upward of 70 percent of patients have at least some of the common complaints. Very often, it's the earliest symptom you may recall, or see in your children. Irritable bowel has a whole spectrum of severity and symptoms, just like fibromyalgia itself. For example, there are patients who complain of a dull but steady aching in some part of the abdomen and tenderness when that area is examined by hand or palpated. Others have nausea without actual vomiting, and still others have long periods of constipation (less than three bowel movements a week). At the other end of the spectrum are patients with severe diarrhea (more than three loose bowel movements a day) that occurs with little warning and disrupts their lives. When IBS is severe enough, patients are incapacitated by out-of-control symptoms and are often largely housebound.

Get ready for some serious testing

Irritable bowel syndrome is usually diagnosed like this: You go to your doctor complaining of digestive problems, cramping or pain, and alternating bouts of constipation and diarrhea. In response, your physician does a basic workup consisting of a rectal examination, X rays, and blood tests including a **sedimentation rate** and maybe a **CA-125 test** to look for ovarian cancer. Your doctor will probably also check for **celiac disease** and **lactose intolerance**.

When all your tests are normal but you're still complaining, your doctor will refer you to a **gastroenterologist**. This specialist has to call in bigger guns, because your case is complicated by the fact that nothing obvious is wrong with you. You'll probably have an abdominal ultrasound first to check your liver, spleen, and gallbladder. When those organs are found normal but you're still complaining, the saga will continue. **Endoscopy** of the esophagus, stomach, and upper part of the small intestine might be next on the list, or a **colonoscopy** to look down through your entire digestive system if you're over forty. If you're under forty you'll more likely be given a **sigmoidoscopy,** an examination of the last part of your digestive tract where polyps and malignancies most often occur. There are also tests such as **barium enemas** that, depending on your symptoms, you may be urged to take. This testing will continue because all your symptoms are caused by fibromyalgia, and we already know that fibromyalgia doesn't show up on tests. However, though these tests may be unpleasant and even embarrassing, they are important and necessary to rule out other possibilities.

Diarrhea reported to a doctor will often lead to stool testing for **candida** (yeast) or **ova** and **parasites**. If you have this testing done, make sure that your specimen is sent to a reputable laboratory such as a local hospital or university. Make sure that your results come from standardized testing by a specialist. If your specimen is sent halfway across the country to some specialty lab or ordered by someone other than a gastroenterologist, be suspicious. It is difficult to avoid errors because a certain amount of yeast is normal in stool specimens. Make sure that you really have a problem before submitting to treatment. There are many varieties of herbal purgings, colonic cleansings, or heavy cathartic "washouts" or "detoxings" done in the vain attempt to clean out something that was never there. Be careful of antifungal (yeast) medications such as **mycostatin,** nystatin, or fluconazole, because those will also kill off all the normal bacteria in your body. They should be used very cautiously and never without blood tests to check your liver function.

Another problem is that your symptoms may convince your doctor that you have food allergies. To prove or disprove this hypothesis you will have to submit to a battery of skin allergy tests. Unfortunately, many fibromyalgics test positive because our mast cells are already malfunctioning, and then you'll be told you have multiple food sensitivities. The next unpleasant step is to confirm these skin findings with a series of very expensive blood tests. Be sure to bear in mind that if your food sensitivities come and go they may be just symptoms of your fibromyalgia and nothing that needs an expensive treatment.

When your doctor finishes with testing, you will be informed that no serious problem was found. So now, by process of elimination, you will be given the official diagnosis of irritable bowel syndrome. If you've leveled with your specialist about your other symptoms, and if you make it clear that you have fibromyalgia, your specialist may tell you that it's secondary to your other illness. Of course, specialists by definition specialize and may not be interested in a part of medicine outside their area of expertise. If you try to discuss your fibromyalgia in general, you may run up against a brick wall, or just get the simple comment that a lot of people seem to have both conditions.

The real scoop

Let's get the good news out of the way first. IBS is not the same as **ulcerative colitis**, which is a serious condition. IBS does not progress to a more serious disease or cancer. As in all other facets of fibromyalgia, women are affected by IBS in far greater numbers than men, and their symptoms are much worse premenstrually. In fact, many women suffer from mild bouts of IBS at that time but are not overly bothered by it during the rest of their cycle. They may have increased gas production, and loose stools, and cramping. Just like with fibromyalgia, stress makes irritable bowel worse but does not cause it.

Again like fibromyalgia, IBS was originally thought to be a psychosomatic illness, and from time to time you'll encounter people in the medical profession who still believe this. Ignore them, and the help they offer, because they clearly do not have an understanding of what is actually wrong (or not wrong) with you. There are no cures for IBS, but some lifestyle changes will control it marvelously well.

Symptoms of Irritable Bowel Syndrome

○ Nausea, in repetitive waves (without vomiting)
○ Indigestion, acid stomach
○ Gas and bloating
○ Sharp jabbing pains in the abdomen
○ Knotted feeling in the stomach
○ Cramps (and a cramping feeling like you need to move your bowels but you can't)
○ Urgency (rushing to a bowel movement)
○ Diarrhea, often with mucous in the stool

You may not have all the symptoms of IBS

While the majority of fibromyalgics have some gastrointestinal symptoms, few of us have every symptom. You may, for example, notice an intermittent difficulty in swallowing. You may experience **gastroesophageal reflux** (GERD) where stomach acid can reflux back up the esophagus from the stomach. GERD can cause heartburn, which can take the form of an acid taste or a slight burning sensation. If the condition is bad enough, this can become an actual chemical burn. This acid irritation may cause esophageal spasms and produce chest pain that can closely mimic cardiac pain.

It's common for waves of nausea to appear and disappear out of nowhere. They can last for hours or for only a few seconds and come in frequent, repetitive waves. Sometimes you'll blame vitamin pills or the medication you take only to find that the nausea is the same when you forget to take them. It will baffle you completely if you're trying to pinpoint the cause.

You may have gas and bloating

Gas and bloating are among the most common complaints. Gas pains can be incredibly intense at times and send you flying to the doctor. The gas bubble is normally located on your left side, right under the lower edge of your rib cage. Gas, as you know, rises, and that's the highest point of the intestine. When the bubble is trapped there you can have an intense, almost claustrophobic sensation. I remember once having such intense gas pains that I was covered with sweat and writhing in pain. I prodded my abdomen testing for appendicitis. Everywhere I pushed, it hurt. I was sure that I had appendicitis but I didn't want to go to the hospital for fear it was

WARNING: IRRITABLE BOWEL SYNDROME AND FIBROMYALGIA DO NOT CAUSE HIGH FEVERS OR A SEVERE PAIN THAT IS PERSISTENT. YOU WILL NOT EXPERIENCE A DRAMATIC WEIGHT LOSS, OR SEE SIGNIFI-CANT BLEEDING. IF YOU ARE EXPERIENCING THESE SYMPTOMS, WITH OR WITHOUT NAUSEA, DIARRHEA, OR CONSTIPATION, SEE A DOCTOR IMMEDIATELY TO RULE OUT MORE DANGEROUS CONDITIONS SUCH AS APPENDICITIS OR DIVERTICULITIS.

just gas. Then I was terrified that it was appendicitis and that my appendix would rupture and I'd really be sick for not taking my complaints seriously. This went on for hours, all night, in fact, until my symptoms subsided finally, leaving me exhausted but relieved.

It's common for constipation and diarrhea to alternate

Constipation and diarrhea come and go in cycles. They're unpredictable and very debilitating for that reason. One day you have the uncomfortable feeling of being constipated, and the next day you wake up with diarrhea and are housebound in the morning until medication can take effect. If you're lucky these sudden bursts of diarrhea happen when you're at home. Too often they happen when you're traveling or when you're out shopping. These are just some of the nightmares of irritable bowel.

Understanding IBS

Let's look at the gastrointestinal system for a moment to better understand what happens in Irritable Bowel Syndrome. Essentially what we're looking at is a very long tube (of vastly changing dimensions) that begins at your mouth and ends at your **anus.** Altogether it's about thirty feet long. **Enzymes** and **digestive juices** enter this system from your salivary glands, your pancreas, your liver, and the cells that line your small intestine.

The function of the GI tract is essentially that of a high-tech conveyer belt in a factory. It takes the food you eat, processes it, nourishes the body with it, and transports the waste out the other end. Muscle contractions, called **peristalsis,** move the contents along. Peristalsis is best described as a wavelike motion that pushes the contents of the digestive tract slowly down the conveyer belt from beginning to end. In a normal person who eats properly, the transit time can be anywhere from twelve to twenty-four hours. People who don't eat enough fiber see a dramatic increase in the time, up to seventy-two hours. Imagine the difference now in a constipated fibromyalgic. Unfortunately, we've already seen how well muscles fare in fibromyalgia. And with IBS it's worse.

Hormones excreted from the adrenals and enzymes and juices from the pancreas and liver also do their chemical work, and again, we can assume that these are not quite up to par. **Digestion** is the process of breaking food down into units that your body can use for energy. The fact that your body isn't doing it efficiently is part of the fundamental problem of fibromyalgia.

In the **colon**, your body stores the waste products that are the undigested part of your food, including any fiber you may have consumed. The colon is also where water and some electrolytes are reabsorbed into your body. If your stool is moving too slowly, too much water is lost and the stool becomes hard, causing constipation. On the other hand, if the stool is moved along too quickly, when your fibromyalgic nerves can't get it quite right, your stool is liquid, causing diarrhea.

First Drugs Approved for Irritable Bowel Syndrome

ON JUNE 24, 2002, the FDA approved the first drug specifically for constipation-predominant IBS. It's called Zelnorm. It's usually taken twice a day for bloating and constipation. The catch is that it's only been tested on women. Safety and efficacy have not been proven in men. Transient diarrhea was the most common side effect.

Lotonex (alosetron hydrochloride) was the first medication to be approved for diarrhea predominant IBS, in February 2000. It was voluntarily withdrawn from the market by its manufacturer in November because of serious side effects. In January 2003, Lotonex was returned to the market but can only be prescribed for cases where the need is so strong that it outweighs the risks, which include constipation so serious it requires hospitalization and ischemic colitis.

A bad comedy of errors

As you can see, irritable bowel syndrome is really a cascade of sequential problems. They begin in the stomach, but include irritation of the rectum and internal or external **hemorrhoids** and small rectal **fissures**.

When you're constipated your lower bowel will form more mucus because the colon responds with mucus the same way your nose does when it's irritated by a cold. In the case of the colon, the irritant is a bowel movement that has hardened during the long wait to exit. This hard stool can press against the wall of the lower (sigmoid) colon, where it can cause both pain and spasms that can be felt in the lower, left side of the abdomen, To complete this comedy of errors, when the beginning part of the stool is really hard, or has food particles in it, the lining of your rectum can get scratched. This is the most likely cause of bright red blood seen on the toilet paper when you are constipated. But there's more. The discomfort of constipation can cause you to strain to try to push out the irritating stool. When the hard stool pushes a rectal vein ahead of it, this causes the rectal protrusion we call a hemorrhoid, which is really a **varicosed vein**. When the soft tissue is ripped by a hard stool, bleeding also occurs, and this is known as a rectal fissure.

Why you get gas pains

As much as 20 percent of the carbohydrates that a healthy person eats reach the large intestine undigested. These carbohydrates are the main source of nutrition for these bacteria. In fibromyalgics, with our not-up-to-standard digestion and our carbohydrate cravings, even more carbohydrate reaches the large intestine. Unfortunately, they greatly add to our gas because this sugar and starch residue actually ferments, especially when transit time is slow. It is this gas that causes the short-term, repetitive, sharp stabs of pain you may feel in your small intestine. The gas moves along easily and is quickly expelled into the much larger area of the colon, where it distends the area where it accumulates. Pockets collect in certain areas, and as pressure builds in that area, the gas is driven to the upper right abdomen, at the edge of the liver. This is what causes the pain in the left upper abdomen, the highest point in the colon just under the heart, because, of course, the hot air (gas) rises. When it is distended, shooting pains can travel up into the chest. Then the intestinal muscles contract and the results are a bit like grabbing a long, sausage-like balloon in the middle. The gas squeezes in both directions but, as soon as one end lets go, it gushes back to the center site. This causes shifting gas pains, especially when the colon is spastic.

Excessive gas contributes to constipation

Gas adds to the problem in another way. Stool inside the collecting area of the colon is not only deprived of too much water when the transit time is slow, but it is also exposed to gas, which has the same drying effect as hot air. Constipation is made worse, and the hard stool plugs up the rectal area and acts like a dam against the elimination of gas, and as a result more bloating and drying occur. This in turn causes even more discomfort and the result is often waves of nausea.

Another source of various abdominal pains is the muscles of the abdominal wall. The internal pain of IBS, which is due to cramping or gas pressure, is different from pains caused by areas of spasm. These muscle contractions are no different from the ones that occur throughout the rest of the body. Pain from these areas can mimic appendicitis, ovarian cysts, or radiate down a leg, or up along the side of your body. These more external pains will respond to heat or change of position, unlike the deeper pains from the intestinal tract.

Pain also originates from the inguinal ligaments. These double parallel cords on each side of the groin run from the pelvic bone in front of the hip to the pubic bone. When swollen, they create a steady pull on the attached muscles and cause them to spasm. This can cause radiating pain on the underside of the rib margins, where the muscles attach. This pain is not related to irritable bowel syndrome, though it causes pain in the same general area, and may occur in a flareup of your fibromyalgia just as your irritable bowel symptoms tend to.

IBS symptoms have a lot in common with the other fibromyalgia symptoms

Your digestive system has the same problem as your central nervous system and your musculoskeletal symptoms. The interactions between your brain and the rest of your body are not functioning properly. Heightened pain sensitivity is very real, and irregular GI muscle contractions make it worse. Things just don't work quite right.

GRETCHEN'S STORY

Most of my life has been regulated by my belly. Even as a schoolgirl our annual trip to the circus started anticipatory butterflies for days ahead of time. The big day was always punctuated with dashes to the bathroom. While I was still in elementary school I developed gripping chest pain that came on suddenly and disappeared just as suddenly. Years later I was told the cause was hiatal hernia and reflux. Beginning with college, every time there was either a stressful or exciting event I was able to mark it with cramps and the green apple shuffle. My honeymoon was some trip. My poor new husband was initiated with a wild drive in a blinding storm as his new wife lay in cramping pain near fainting and battling diarrhea. Not romantic. The decade following a hysterectomy everything worsened. Each day began to be marked by those mad dashes with cramping that twisted and grabbed my gut until I was doubled over. IBS slowly robbed me of my freedom; I had to be near a bathroom at all times. My energy was sapped and it whittled away at my ability to enjoy my children's lives or to work. I finally had to quit my job. I constantly begged off helping with the children's activities or social events. It was too embarrassing being with other people, having the sort of intestinal gas eruptions I created.

In the past thirty years I have had multiple sigmoidoscopies, barium X rays, and a multitude of treatments. The 1970s were the phenobarbital years; the 1980s brought on sulfa drugs. During the 1990s things started ratcheting up and I was treated for colon helicobacter pylori infection and food allergies and given ridiculous treatments for environmental illness (this treatment alone could fill a book). My life continued to nosedive. There was an ambulance trip to the ER for heart irregularities. Insomnia became unrelenting. If I could sleep for two hours at a time it was a lot. Many nights were punctuated with nightmares and a pounding heart. Just rolling over in bed would send it galloping accompanied by terrifying chest pain. I hated to go to bed because the nights seemed endless. I hated to get up because the pain and anxiety were unrelenting. During the day my heart would skip beats many times in a minute. I had grinding chest pain and could not catch my breath. I was convinced I was next in a long familial line of cardiac patients, but a full cardiac workup proved my heart to be wonderfully fit. I was puzzled.

Everything I ate went straight through my system. I lost weight and got so thin my daughter refers to that time as my Ethiopian days. For two years a physician tried to put weight on my emaciated frame by encouraging a high carbohydrate diet. The IBS worsened and I developed panic and anxiety attacks. I became paranoid. I didn't leave the house alone. I was terrified to drive the car for fear my heart would go wild and I could not get home. I was convinced that Halle-Bopp comet was going to collide with earth and we were all going to die. I read the obituaries daily, jealous of the people listed there. I daydreamed about tying a cement block around my leg and jumping in the lake or driving my five-speed V-8 into the biggest tree I could find. My days revolved around getting to my chair or bed. Walking across the room was exhausting. By midafternoon every day I was drenched in sweat. My life was not worth living and I told my husband of thirty years to please leave me so he could have a life. God bless him, he refused.

People ask how I can stick so religiously to a low-carb diet. Had they lived my nightmare existence for just a day they would know *how simple it really is. For me one small bite of chocolate cake means the difference between prison and freedom. The choice is so simple it makes me smile.*

IN A SENTENCE:

> *Irritable bowel syndrome is a common part of fibromyalgia and causes gas, bloating, constipation, and diarrhea.*

learning

Strategies for Living with IBS

THE FIRST thing you'll have to do to control your irritable bowel is change the way you eat. Though this may seem difficult, and you may be even more unhappy when you see the list of things you'll have to avoid, there's some good news. The good news is that if you eat correctly you'll find that you can control your symptoms and feel better in just a few weeks. I understand that you don't feel well, that you're miserable; I know how awful irritable bowel can be. (If you need proof, I'll take you for the drive I used to make every morning taking two sons to two different schools. On the way I'll point out every bathroom that's open at that time of the morning and tell you what they're like. I'll tell you about the beginning of the year when schools were changed, and how I had to map out a new emergency route, trying to drive with gut-wrenching cramping.) I know that when you don't feel well it seems hard to change the way you eat, and awful to think about giving up the comfort foods you're used to. Still, I urge you try the dietary measures that follow.

The treatment plan

The first things you'll need to avoid are the carbohydrates because they feed the bacteria in your intestine. This will eliminate the gas buildup, and once the gas is gone, your pain will

FOODS TO STRICTLY AVOID:

1. Caffeine: (a stimulant)

    Withdrawal from caffeine may take a couple of days. Headache and fatigue are common symptoms. (Be sure to do this over a weekend.) Drink plenty of water and comfort yourself with a soothing tea such as chamomile if this withdrawal makes you jittery. Discontinuing caffeine may also help you sleep, and if you have an irritable bladder it will help that as well. Unfortunately, if you love coffee, you may not fare any better with the decaf kind. Coffee contains a potent enzyme that can irritate your GI tract.

2. Sugar in any form: dextrose, maltose, sucrose, glucose, fructose, honey, brown rice syrup, corn syrup, or starch

3. Legumes: lentils, garbanzo beans (chickpeas), black-eyed peas, lima beans, baked beans, refried beans, pinto beans, black beans

4. Potatoes

5. Corn

6. Rice, except brown or wild rice

7. Barley

8. Bananas, or any dried fruit

9. Pasta

10. Mexican food such as tamales that contain corn meal; corn tortillas only

11. Fruit juice—especially apple and grape—contain a lot of fructose, which can cause gas, bloating, and diarrhea

12. Fruit is limited to one piece every four hours

13. Bread must be sugar-free and is limited to three slices a day (or can be replaced with sugar-free flatbread or corn tortillas)

14. Cereal and dairy products must have no sugar added

usually disappear as well. Begin with the elimination of sugars and complex carbohydrates. Try following these guidelines strictly for a month. This will give things time to settle down. Once you feel better, you can try a little of the forbidden foods and see how you fare. If your bowel problems flare up, you'll need to back off until things settle down again. You'll eventually come up with a diet that controls your symptoms and that you can live with. A food diary can help you keep track of which foods you've experimented with.

What about fiber?

Fiber has many health benefits. It helps to regulate blood sugar and lower cholesterol levels. Fiber may also help prevent heart attacks, other

MISCELLANEOUS THINGS TO AVOID:

Chocolate: I am extremely sorry to say that this is a problem for most people with irritable bowel because of chemicals it contains as well as the caffeine. Carob is OK.

White flour: use soy, gluten, or a low-carbohydrate bake mix. You can use wheat germ.

Sweet wines, champagne, sweet liquors (such as Irish Cream and Amaretto), and fruit brandy. Some people find alcohol except that used in cooking will cause attacks. Others find that moderate consumption has only a minimal effect

Carbonation in soda beverages causes bloating and cramps in some people.

Sugar alcohols (such as sorbitol and mannitol) and artificial sweeteners cause diarrhea as well as bloating and cramping in most people. Sucralose or Splenda is a better choice.

Artificial fats (Olestra) cause unpleasant bowel symptoms even in healthy people.

IF YOU ARE LACTOSE INTOLERANT AVOID: milk, buttermilk, yogurt, and cottage cheese. You can have heavy cream, sour cream, and natural cheeses (the kind you slice yourself).

The key to this diet is to avoid the above and to read all labels before you eat anything. I promise you will be astounded, when you start to read labels, at all the hidden grams of sugar we consume in a day. You can have cereals such as oatmeal that are sugar-free. You can have bread that does not contain sugar, cold cuts that do not contain sugar, salad dressings that don't contain dextrose, and so on. You can have a serving of peanut butter, but, yes, check it for sugar. There are many excellent sugar-free products on the market now for people on low-carbohydrate diet.

heart problems, and colon cancer. While it's true that legumes are an excellent source of fiber, and that meat and dairy products are not, it's absolutely possible for you to get enough on this diet. The daily recommended amount of fiber is 35 grams. You know you need fiber to help bulk your stools and move them along and avoid constipation. You can eat plenty of vegetables, and several pieces of fruit a day will help. Broccoli, green beans, plums, pears, apples, greens (spinach, collard, mustard, lettuce, chard), and Brussels sprouts are on the list of the foods highest in fiber. If you have oatmeal for breakfast, each cup contains 7 grams of fiber. A baked apple has about 5 grams. A raw apple and a pear contain about 4 grams. If you have a cup of broccoli for dinner you'll have 8 grams, and a cup of brown rice weighs in at 5.5 grams. A cup of cooked spinach has 7 grams.

In addition, you can always use sugar-free fiber supplements in powder or chewable form. Fiber supplements should be added very gradually to your routine because they may cause more gas and bloating if you move too fast. Remember to drink plenty of water as well.

Medications and remedies for irritable bowel syndrome

There are also medications to help when your condition flares. You should save these for occasional use, relying on your dietary restrictions to control your problems most of the time. You can build up a tolerance to, or become dependent on, most of them.

- For gas you'll find many effective over-the-counter medications, including Phazyme and Gas-X.
- For an acidy stomach there are calcium carbonate antacids such as Mylanta, Rolaids, and Maalox. If your stomach acid is severe, you can also use blockers such as Pepcid. Newer medications will work on the valve at the top of the stomach and can prevent acid from escaping upward and causing acid reflux.
- Diarrhea and cramping can be helped by Lomotil or Immodium. These work by enhancing intestinal water absorption, so should be taken with plenty of fluids. Lomotil is chemically related to narcotics and can be habit forming and so it is available by prescription. Immodium, by contrast, is over the counter.
- **Anti-spasmodics** such as Donnatol or Levsin can be prescribed for cramping and pain. Librax should be used with more caution as it has more side effects and can be habit forming. These drugs are by prescription only.
- For constipation, when it's painful, and exercise and increased fluids don't help, there are mild laxatives and stool softeners or glycerin suppositories. Remember that laxatives should be used as infrequently as possible because your body will come to rely on them. Chemical laxatives such as Ex-Lax or Milk of Magnesia are too strong—they work by irritating the bowel, which is the last thing you need. Soluble fiber supplements such as Fibercon or Metamucil are probably the best treatment. Again, you'll need plenty of water and exercise to help them work.
- **Tricylic** antidepressants in low doses can be prescribed for pain, diarrhea, depression, and other uncomfortable symptoms. Side effects can include weight gain, sedation, and, unfortunately, constipation.

○ Digestive enzymes: Some people find these helpful especially when they eat more fat than usual. The most common of these are papain and bromelain, which are available in pharmacies or health food stores.

○ Acidophilus can help maintain healthy flora in the digestive tract. Be sure to take this if you've been given an antibiotic for any reason. Make sure the label says "live cultures." Health food stores usually have the best selection.

○ Calcium helps control diarrhea. Caltrate is known for having good results. Take about 1500 mgs a day. Calcium should be taken with meals and will help your fibromyalgia also.

○ Magnesium helps some patients with constipation and cramping and is easy to find in the vitamin section of any store.

Medications can have good and bad effects on your bowels

It's worth mentioning here that many of the medications you take for other symptoms can contribute to constipation. This is especially true of pain medications that contain codeine (which can also cause nausea and even vomiting). Antidepressants such as Elavil and Prozac can cause dry mouth and systemwide dryness in addition to constipation. Muscle relaxants such as Flexeril, Soma, or Valium and Ativan will also slow down and relax the muscles you need to move your bowels. The good news is that according to some studies, very low doses of tricylcic antidepressants (such as Elavil) actually may help IBS because of its relationship with serotonin levels. (The newer class of antidepressants known as SSRIs have not yet been tested but anecdotal evidence seems to support the fact that they also are helpful.)

Dealing with the emotional side effects of IBS

It's not unusual for fibromyalgics with irritable bowel syndrome to suffer deeply both in their personal relationships and because they will often curtail activities for fear of not being able to control their symptoms. It becomes easier to stay home, where whatever symptoms you have can be dealt with privately. Staying in becomes a habit. It can also be embarrassing to go out to eat in groups of people because you have to have special food.

The basic problem with irritable bowel is the personal nature of the affected area. You may tend to keep to yourself to avoid discussing your problems, even at home, and certainly in the workplace. You may prefer to suffer in silence, not knowing how to explain your symptoms to others, except to say "I am having stomach trouble."

You will help yourself by having the courage to mention your illness to friends and the rest of your family. Explain that you have a medical problem. Make it clear to them that your symptoms can be controlled if you are careful with your diet. If they understand how important staying with your diet is to your health they can become your allies. Let your friends and family members know about your struggles and what you've learned about staying in control of your illness. You can't expect them to understand and support you if you don't tell them about it. Be patient with them, though, and explain things carefully and simply. Think about how long it took you to understand your diet and what you had to do to stay healthy, and then remember that they don't even have the condition. People will be much more willing to help you if you simply remind them gently of your needs. Be sure to be appreciative of all their efforts, even if some of them are misdirected on occasion. It's hard for people who haven't been sick to understand a chronic illness. There is a huge difference between having a bad stomach for a few days after the flu or food poisoning and having a chronic condition that affects your whole life.

Lots of people have IBS

There are millions of people in this country who have irritable bowel. You run across them all the time and probably never know it. You may be surprised, when you are open about your illness, how many others you know share it.

Several self-help groups, support groups, and information services exist to offer you support and guidance, some of them listed in the For Further Information section in the back of this book. Some people find it easiest to begin to socialize again in a group of people who already understand them. There is nothing wrong with this approach, especially if anxiety is one of your fibromyalgia symptoms.

Getting your irritable bowel under control on a daily basis is simply a matter of learning what to do, and doing it. The restrictions you need to observe will soon become second nature and will be assimilated into your everyday routine. Some things like vacations and holidays may require some advance planning and extra care, but you'll soon find out that a few simple precautions can make all the difference in the world.

IN A SENTENCE:

IBS is a disturbing and uncomfortable condition that can be kept under control by eating properly, managing stress, and implementing lifestyle changes.

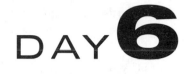

living

The Pain and Shame of Genitourinary Syndrome

OF ALL the cruelly debilitating symptoms of fibromyalgia, those classified under the blanket category that we call **genitourinary syndrome** are often the most painful, demoralizing, debilitating, and life-destroying. These are symptoms that occur in the bladder, urethra, and vaginal tract, and are the most difficult symptoms to resolve. Most physicians, despite their good intentions, aren't much help.

These were my first symptoms of fibromyalgia, and like many others, I spent years being referred back and forth between urologists and gynecologists, never really getting a satisfactory explanation for my pain. Numerous tests offered no clues that could help any of my doctors because fibromyalgia lay outside their realm of expertise. In the end, sicker from the medications they had given me than I had been before I started, I simply stopped taking the pills and gave up.

When I was finally diagnosed with fibromyalgia years later, the mystery was solved. In the beginning, not all my symptoms were associated with FM, but with each passing year more and more evidence accumulates to show the relationship between **Vulvar Vestibulitis,** Irritable Bladder, **Interstitial Cystitis,** and fibromyalgia. Thanks to open-minded physicians like my friend Dr. John Willems, who is head of OB-GYN at Scripps Medical Center, Paul St. Amand M.D., and others, women with

vulvodynia are now being steered in the right directions, which, I might say, is simply any direction away from surgery except as an absolute last resort.

What are the bladder symptoms of fibromyalgia?

The urinary symptoms of fibromyalgia include a constant urge to urinate, pain above the pubic bone, burning urine and pain while urinating, and despite an overwhelming urge to urinate, producing only a small amount of urine. Frequent bacterial bladder infections called **cystitis** are very common in fibromyalgic women.

About 25 percent of female fibromyalgics have had three or more bladder infections in their lifetime. I am certainly not the only woman who can report fifty or more attacks of cystitis and many more episodes of painful urination without any infection. I had my first bladder infection before I started kindergarten and had them without respite over the course of my entire life. My urinary symptoms traced a path from pediatrician to urologist, to student health centers in college to gynecologists, and back to urologists. If you're prone to bladder infections and urinary tract pain, you already know that intercourse can trigger your problems. Doctors popularly call this "honeymoon cystitis," because even healthy women can have this problem when they are more sexually active than usual.

You may not really have a bladder infection

It's also very common to experience all the symptoms of cystitis when your urine culture has shown no infection. You might have had same powerful urge to urinate that produces only a drop of urine and severe pain that may have caused you to run a slight fever. It's absolutely true that without a urine culture no one can tell whether or not they have an actual infection, no matter how many infections they have had. The symptoms really are identical. I'll tell you the truth. I am the Queen of Bladder Infections and I can't tell. The reason I mention this is because if you are a woman who is prone to yeast infections, then you should always get a urinalysis done before you start taking antibiotics that can trigger yeast problems. Request a urinalysis without a culture (you don't need a full culture to tell you whether or not infection is present) because that will be less expensive. Remember that even if your urine is cloudy you may not have an infection. You can't tell if you have an infection by how you feel or by looking at your urine.

• • •

Expect some testing to rule out other possible causes

If your bladder pain is severe or persistent, you'll be referred to a **urologist,** who will perform tests to make sure there's no serious cause for your misery. These tests include a **cystoscopy**, where a scope is inserted into the bladder in an attempt to check for abnormalities. You may even have a biopsy done of the bladder wall. You can expect to be screened for bladder cancer (especially if you are male or a cigarette smoker), kidney problems, endometriosis, and sexually transmitted diseases. Your doctor may also want to do a **hydrodistention of the bladder** under general anesthesia to confirm the state of the wall of the bladder. This is less painful than a cystoscopy and may be preferable.

Interstitial cystitis

If your symptoms are from fibromyalgia only, these tests will turn up normal or inconsequential findings of inflammation and you will be given the diagnosis of "interstitial cystitis."

IC is condition of the bladder wall marked by frequent urination (fifty times in twenty-four hours is not unheard of), urgency that can be accompanied by pain and/or pressure, pain in the lower abdomen, pelvic area, vaginal/urethral area in women, and scrotal or penile area in men. In both sexes, pain in this area can also come from muscular sources. Steady pressure and aching in the suprapubic area is often present and a muscular source should be considered when pain is present without urgency or painful urination. As you know from the previous chapter, fibromyalgia also regularly affects the inguinal ligaments, the cordlike structures that connect the hip to the pubic bone. When these ligaments are swollen they steadily tug at nerves and are the source of an aching sensed as deep pelvic pain. When the ligaments are swollen the lymph glands above them can be prominent and even painful. Occasionally, spasms in the area between the rectum and vagina known as the **perineum** can be the source of a heavy, dull, aching pain. Vaginal and rectal pains are also common.

Interstitial cystitis is *not* an infection like cystitis, so antibiotics will not cure it. It is a chronic condition in the bladder wall that occurs in people of both sexes and all ages. Interstitial cystitis is diagnosed much more rarely in male patients; only about 10 percent of patients are men. Because some physicians think of it as a woman's disease, in men it can be misdiagnosed as nonbacterial **prostatitis**, or prostatodynia.

Fibromyalgia and Yeast Infections

YEAST INFECTIONS are fairly normal occurrences in the general population, and fibromyalgics with their depressed immune systems may be more prone to them than others. Even knowing this, bear in mind that not everything that feels like a yeast infection is really an infection. If you have any doubts, your physician can do a culture for you. Symptoms of yeast infections include itching, burning, redness, and irritation of the vaginal area. Severe yeast infections may cause swelling of the vulva and you may experience painful, frequent urination caused by inflammation of the urinary opening. Vaginal discharge that is thicker than normal is the hallmark, and it will be whiter and cottage cheese-like. Self-treatment of vaginal yeast should not be attempted by any woman who has not first been diagnosed with at least one yeast infection by her physician.

DR. JOHN WILLEMS'S THREE RULES OF VULVODYNIA

Rule 1: Everything feels like a yeast infection

Rule 2: Not everything that feels like a yeast infection is a yeast infection

Rule 3: Refer to Rule 1

Treatment options include pills and a variety of creams used from one to seven days. Creams available include brand names such as Monistat and Gyne-Lotrimin. Homeopathic creams such as Vagisil may be helpful in reducing the itch. Diflucan is a one-dose oral medication obtained by prescription.

One of the best treatments, boric acid capsules, is very inexpensive and you can obtain them over the counter. In a study of one hundred women with chronic yeast infections that had failed to respond to treatment with over-the-counter or prescription antifungal medicines, 98 percent of the women successfully treated their infections with boric acid capsules inserted into the vagina twice per day for two to four weeks.

To use boric acid vaginally, simply purchase empty gelatin capsules in any health food store, size 0. Then buy a bottle of boric acid powder, available in most any pharmacy. Fill the capsules and close them up. Insert vaginally twice a day for two weeks, then, if needed, once a day for another two weeks. Boric acid is not messy like creams and other suppositories and you can use it every time you feel a flareup. In some women, this may be every month premenstrually.

Genital symptoms

The symptoms of vulvodynia or vulvar pain syndrome are severe pain, burning and/or itching in the area of the female's external genitalia, or vulva, which is extremely sensitive to touch. The area may or may not be visibly irritated. **Vulvar Vestibulitis Syndrome** is when pain occurs only in the vestibule, the area around the opening to the vagina. Patients may also experience shooting pains through the buttock and thigh areas. Dyspareunia, or painful intercourse, is very common. Pain may be continuous or intermittent.

So many women have both interstitial cystitis and vulvar pain that the overlap has caught the attention of researchers. They find that women with these conditions share fair, sensitive skin, are allergy and asthma prone, have **migraine** headaches, and are a hundred times more likely than the general population to have Irritable Bowel Syndrome. A connection with both fibromyalgia and chronic fatigue has also been made, and it is now thought that a common biological defect probably exists.[1]

The most common complaint of women with the vulvar pain syndrome is irritation of the inner vaginal lips near the opening. In the early stages or in milder cases this pain may only be present following intercourse.

Some common pain triggers include wearing clothes that fit tightly in the area such as blue jeans or pantyhose, and sitting in close quarters for prolonged periods. Long car trips and cross-country plane trips commonly cause flares.

VULVODYNIA, BY the way, is not a new syndrome, it has been mentioned in medical articles since the 1880s. In 1889, an English doctor, A. J. C. Skene, wrote about a syndrome of "excessive sensitivity." He recorded that when he examined the area with his fingers patients complained of pain "which is sometimes so great as to cause her to cry out." The treatment of his day was to remove the area surgically, which at least he honestly admitted resulted in only passing relief. More modern research has found the same **mast cells** present in vulvodynia as in interstitial cystitis, further suggesting that the syndromes are related.

You can expect to have more tests done

The diagnosis of vulvodynia is again made by exclusion. Testing excludes more serious conditions such as infections, sexually transmitted diseases, cancer, endometriosis, and nerve or dermatological damage. Luckily, this syndrome is not linked to a higher risk of any cancers.

Your doctor will first do a visual examination, and take some slides and/or cultures. It is important to rule out such things as vaginal infections, genital herpes or warts, some types of cancer, local irritations, or allergies. Superficial pain from the entrance of the vagina is known as vulvar vestibulitis. Diagnosis is made by touching the area with a Q-Tip. To dramatize how this feels when you have the condition I'll relate a little story. I was once at a lecture given by Dr. Willems where he explained how this Q-Tip test is done, that is, with the less painful end. One of the women in the audience spoke up and said "Which end is that?" I've never forgotten the question because it emphasizes how agonizing this is for women with vestibulitis. Remember, too, that often this area is sensitive with no external manifestations. While the area may be reddened or swollen, it just as commonly is not. When no other conditions are found, the diagnosis will be officially made.

Emotional aspects of the genital symptoms

Obviously, these genitourinary symptoms have a drastic effect on your quality of life, maybe more than any others. Vulvodynia especially can cause a terrible strain on marriages and other intimate relationships because it can result in **dyspareunia**, or painful sexual intercourse. For some women intercourse may be impossible. Men may have problems with pain and impotence. The hardest thing for sufferers is the fact that our culture is so sexually oriented. It is impossible to get through a day without being assaulted with jokes, stories, or articles about the subject. Billboards, magazines, commercials, TV shows, and movies bombard us with the joys of sex and make it look so easy. When you're suffering, these can be a slap in the face. We live in an era of easy sexuality, like it or not, which makes it doubly hard for those who cannot participate. It's hard for us not to feel like outsiders gazing into a wonderful, forbidden world.

Support is available

Support groups are located all over the world, and can be extremely helpful for both you and for your partner. These support groups can also help you to find caring, supportive physicians to help you manage your symptoms. Because these symptoms are so personal and intimate, it is important to find a special and compassionate physician who will help you learn about your condition and explain the alternatives that are available to help you.

I've already mentioned a most wonderful man and exquisitely kind physician, Dr. John Willems, M.D., Chief of Obstetrics and Gynecology at Scripps' Clinic in La Jolla, California. He has contributed to the education of both women and the medical profession about the treatment of vulvodyina as well as its connection with fibromyalgia. He believes that fibromyalgia is the cause of resistant vulvar pain, and has written articles on the subject that might help you talk to your gynecologist about your problems. You will find these articles listed in the For Further Information section.

Painful Intercourse

THERE ARE two types of painful intercourse: one is from pain at the entrance of the vagina, called superficial dyspareunia, or from pain deep in the pelvis called—you got it—deep dyspareunia. Superficial dyspareunia is the same condition as vulvar vestibulitis and intercourse is impossible because of the painful and irritated skin around the opening of the vagina. This type can also make oral sex and masturbation impossible to tolerate. Deep dyspareunia is caused by spasm of the muscles inside the vagina and pelvis, and so external stimulation is usually not painful with this condition. It is possible to have both types together.

Of course, although some forms of sexual contact may have become impossible and others difficult, there are other forms of sexual expression besides vaginal penetration. Physicians will cheerfully tell you this, but when you are exhausted and hurt all over, it's hard to feel enthusiastic about participating in any of them. Open communication with your partner and counseling may both be necessary and crucial, especially in the early stages of these conditions. Several online support groups offer pamphlets and material to help women and the men who love them with this problem. I don't mean to sound blithe here; it is disturbing and painful and not easy to live with vulvodynia and IC. And guilt about your partner's needs can be equally devastating.

Interstitial cystitis or irritable bladder can also take a toll on sexual relations. Sufferers often need to use the bathroom too often to relax and enjoy sex, and sex can also be painful. Bladder infections following intercourse are very common because of the sandpaper effect of urinary crystals.

Women with vulvodynia and bladder issues have yet another problem. Like Pavlov's dogs we have been conditioned to expect excruciating and long-lasting pain during and following intercourse. Men who are worried about performance and pain have the same expectation. It is very easy to condition yourself to forgo the pleasures of simple cuddling and of physical contact for fear that you will lead your partner on, or start something that you cannot finish. I have had people confess to me on more than one occasion that they have avoided forming meaningful relationships with the opposite sex because they feel that they would eventually be expected to perform sexually. Obviously high numbers of failed relationships are common to this group.

FIBROMYALGIA

IN A SENTENCE:

> The genitourinary symptoms of fibromyalgia are painful, embarrassing, and some of the most difficult to endure.

learning

Coping Strategies for Your Genitourinary Symptoms

WHILE WE are beginning to better understand the relationship between fibromyalgia and genitourinary symptoms, there still are no solid remedies for reversing these debilitating affects. The best course of action is to be extremely vigilant when the symptoms present themselves and patient in experimenting with the treatments that work for you, until you find the best remedies for your body.

Easing bladder symptoms and interstitial cystitis

Often, milder bladder symptoms can be controlled by local pain medications such as **pyridium** or its over-the-counter version, **phenazopyridine hydrochloride**. When urine is extremely concentrated, drinking large amounts of fluids may relieve some of the pain, and more relief can be obtained from drinking a six-ounce glass of water mixed with half a teaspoon of baking soda three times a day. Though your friends may tell you to drink cranberry juice, don't do this, and don't take vitamin C. Cranberry juice or tablets have been studied and it is true that they may inhibit infections in elderly patients. However, both cranberry juice and vitamin C raise urinary acidity and will make burning and irritation worse. Please, do not listen to friends and pharmacists' advice on this one.

There are other pain medications available as well. Urised and Prosed are both phenyl salicylate and shouldn't be taken if you can't use salicylates. Uristat is a nonsalicylate alternative, and all three require a prescription. Over-the-counter therapies include 1,000 mg of **chondroitin** daily, 1,500 mg of glucosmine, or an amino acid l-arginine. All three can be found in pharmacies or health food stores. This last supplement is taken three times a day (500 mg) for six months. Studies are divided about how well any of these therapies works.

An ounce of prevention

If you seem always to get bladder infections following intercourse, the first thing that you can do is to try to keep the bladder empty by always urinating before and after sex. While this may initially be embarrassing, it's much better than the alternative. This keeps pressure off your bladder and the urine will actually wash away any bacteria that may exist.

If this step doesn't work, another thing you can try is antibiotics. Some physicians will put you on a low-dose antibiotic for a whole year to completely kill off all the bacteria. Although these low doses don't usually result in yeast overgrowth, if your immune system is compromised enough by fibromyalgia this alternative may make you prone to yeast infections and cause you increased stress. If this is the case, you can ask your doctor for a stronger medication and take it prophylactically (for protection) each time you have sex.

Newer treatments for IC you can try

Interstitial cystitis is normally treated with **Elmiron (pentosan poly-sulfate sodium)**, which is the only oral medication that exists specifically for this condition and works by coating the bladder lining. This must be prescribed by a physician. Some patients benefit from bladder distention, which is performed under general anesthetic. Sometimes DMSO (dimethylsolfoxide), a chemical that works on pain and inflammation, is placed inside the bladder by a doctor, where it reduces pain. It can be used alone or mixed with other things (called a "bladder cocktail"), including steroids, heparin, and local anesthetics. There are several new medications in clinical trials for interstitial cystitis. **Detrol** is a prescription medication used for irritable bladder, to reduce the number of times you urinate in a twenty-four-hour period. It can be taken daily, or only as needed.

Diet affects your bladder pain

Sometimes IC can be managed with dietary strategies. This is generally accomplished by restricting caffeine, alcohol, and foods high in acid or spices. After you've stabilized your symptoms by avoiding all these foods, you can start to experiment. New foods should be introduced one at a time every seven days. Be sure to keep accurate notes about which foods you cannot tolerate, and mark down all the ingredients in each item. Keep track of your pain level, and also how many times you urinate in every twenty-four-hour period. Remember that an offending food can cause a flare within a day, and sometimes within an hour. The average person urinates about six times a day, and at most once at night. Your physician may suggest that you consciously try to extend the periods between urination to retrain your bladder. The Interstitial Cystitis Association offers a cookbook to help you with the diet, which is listed in the Resources.

Foods That May Trigger
Interstitial Cystitis Symptoms

DAIRY: aged cheese, sour cream, yogurt

VEGETABLES: legumes such as lentils, peanuts, lima and fava beans; tomatoes, soy beans, and onions

FRUITS: apples, avocados, bananas, cantaloupe, all citrus fruits, cranberries, guava, grapes, nectarines, peaches, pineapple, plums, strawberries. Also avoid: apple, cranberry, pineapple, citrus especially grapefruit juice, and grape juice

GRAINS: Rye and sourdough bread

MEATS AND FISH: aged, canned, cured, processed or smoked meats, anchovies, caviar, chicken liver, corned beef, and meats that contain nitrates or nitrites.

NUTS: avoid nuts (although almonds or cashews might be tolerated)

SEASONINGS: mayonnaise, ketchup, mustard, spicy foods such as chili and cayenne peppers, black pepper, soy sauce, miso, all vinegars

PRESERVATIVES: benzol alcohol, citric acid, MSG, Nutrasweet, saccharine

MISCELLANEOUS: tobacco, caffeine, all alcoholic beverages, chocolate, and medications containing ephedrine or pseudoephedrine, vitamin C (though you might be able to tolerate Ester C), B complex vitamins, calcium citrate[2]

Prelief might offer some relief

Recently, an interesting study by Kristene Whitmore, M.D., chief of urology at Graduate Hospital in Philadelphia, demonstrated that the over-the-counter dietary supplement **Prelief** (calcium glycerolphosphate) can help patients eat a wider variety of foods. Prelief is a powder that comes in packets so you can easily add it to acidy foods such as tomato sauce or coffee to make them more tolerable. Although it was designed for people with sensitive stomachs and not IC, the concept is intriguing. Information about this product can be found in the For Further Information section.

Finding support

There are online and in-person support groups for IC and for irritable bladder. By pooling resources such as observation of possible triggers, recipes, and experiences, you can save yourself considerable time in finding solutions. Support groups can give you shortcuts when you're frustrated and comfort you when you are feeling isolated.

Vulvodynia treatment strategies

Unfortunately, surgery is usually offered as a solution too quickly and too often. Dr. John Willems has had considerable success easing the symptoms of vulvar pain using topical **estradiol** cream to thicken and rebuild tissue. He discovered this when prescribing the cream to help women heal enough to tolerate surgery. So many of his patients felt so much better that he was asked why they needed to submit to surgery. As a result, Dr. Willems is outspoken in maintaining that surgery should be your very last resort. Consider asking your physician to put you on a trial run of estradiol.

Estrace, a prescription cream, is generally the topical treatment of choice, and does not contain plant extracts. Some women need more liquid formulas such as a vitamin E base and these can easily be made up by any compounding pharmacy. The healing process is slow because the tissue must be rebuilt. Dr. Willems says that it may take six full weeks before you can expect to see progress, and the pain can get worse before it gets better. Itching is a sign of healing, so whatever you do, don't take yeast medications or steroid creams. Just hang in there and keep going. If you're a numbers gal, he says he has about a 70 percent success rate. You should see definite progress in six months. When you have made good progress your doctor will probably start to decrease the dose to only one application

Things That Can Help with Vulvodynia

- Wear cotton underwear, white is best.
- Do not wear panty hose even with a cotton crotch area.
- Wear loose-fitting pants, although dresses are best.
- Don't use hot tubs or public swimming pools where you can smell chlorine.
- Don't put pressure on the area with activities such as bike riding.
- Don't sit for long periods without a substantial break.
- Don't sit in bucket seats for a long car ride. Use a piece of wood to level the seat out or sit on one of the foam donuts available at pharmacies.
- Use gentle laundry detergents in small amounts such as Ivory Snow and always double rinse all your clothes and sheets. Don't use bleach of any kind. Don't use fabric softener sheets in the dryer.
- Always use white unscented toilet paper but don't rub the area with it. Keep a spritz bottle in the bathroom and gently spray the area with cool water and then just pat gently until dry.
- Don't use bubble bath, body washes, or soaps with dyes or fragrances. Showers are really preferable to baths because all the chemicals from your body end up in the bathwater. If you want to soak in a warm tub take a shower first. Do not soak in hot water, keep it lukewarm.
- Keep body lotions away from the crotch area.
- Use pure cotton menstrual pads. Don't use tampons ever.
- Ask your doctor about lidocaine gel and Estrace cream for pain.
- Use a water-soluble lubricant for intercourse such as Astroglide.
- If you use a cold pack after intercourse make sure it is wrapped in at least two layers of towel so it doesn't burn the skin.
- Urinate and wash the vulva with a cool spritz of water after intercourse. If you have a bidet or a sitz bath you can use this instead. Do not rub. Very gently pat this area dry with a very clean towel. (Don't use toilet paper as it may stick.)
- Don't use wipes with a fragrance, and do not douche.

a day. If that goes well you will most likely use your cream every other day after that. Go slowly and you'll find your maintenance level. Bear in mind that Dr. Willems also says there is no single effective therapy for all women. Emu Oil and topical lidocaine cream for the pain (which requires a prescription) are two other topical modalities that you might find helpful.

Dietary measures may help vulvodynia

The Vulvar Pain Foundation of North Carolina advocates a first line strategy of dietary restrictions. This approach is based on the work of Clive Solomons, Ph.D., a biochemist from Denver who has focused on the effects of urinary oxalates as direct irritants to the labia. Oxalates enter the body from foods, especially vegetables, but are also produced in the body during normal metabolism, perhaps to excess. The director of the Vulvar Pain Foundation, Joanne Yount, has published *The Low Oxalate Cookbook* to help you make better food choices.

High Oxalate Foods

Beverages: coffee, chocolate (cocoa), beer, juice made from berries, tea, Ovaltine

Vegetables: legumes such as peanuts (peanut butter), beans of all kinds, tomatoes (tomato sauce and paste), soybeans (and tofu, miso), beets, celery, greens such as chard, kale, mustard greens, spinach, green peppers, summer squash, beets, leeks, sweet potatoes

Fruit: all berries, grapes, citrus fruit

Miscellaneous: wheat germ, pecans, black pepper, vitamin C

If you do experience vulvar pain and burning when you urinate, here's what works for me. I use a barrier of A&D Ointment or Vaseline on the external area just before I urinate (although some people use Desitin or Emu Oil). This will protect the tissue from being irritated by your urine. After urination be sure to pat the area gently instead of wiping. Some women pour a cup of water over the vulva while urinating because this both dilutes the urine and washes the area so that there is no trace of the acidic urine left on the skin. With small children you could always try what I recall my mother doing with me: Place them in a sink or basin of warm water and have them urinate into the water.

Topical cool compresses also help relieve pain and itching in the external vulvar area. Always make sure that these compresses are cool, not cold. Remember that your skin in that area is very, very sensitive. Cold can cause a burn or even frostbite. Because the cold will deaden the area you will not be able to perceive the damage being done, so be careful.

Coping with dyspareunia or painful intercourse

You can use support groups or Web sites as resources for help finding lubricants such as Astroglide that can be used even with condoms. There are also topical lidocaine solutions that some women have found helpful, and you can print out the information and take it to your physician. Do avail yourself of these support groups and their resources because as you will see in the For Further Information section there are very helpful booklets dealing with just this problem. I know from experience that the most important thing you will get from these organizations is the knowledge that you are not alone. Partners will benefit as well, because they also need understanding and to know that they are not the only ones living with this illness. The bottom line is that you should certainly only attempt what you are comfortable with, and use all the available resources you can find.

You may benefit from an antidepressant or other medication

Antidepressants are sometimes prescribed for **bowel** and bladder syndromes for the same reason they are used in fibromyalgia itself. Antidepressants have no direct action on the bladder or vulva, but generally increase pain tolerance and may help you sleep better at night. This is nothing to sneeze at because lack of sleep is stressful and certainly will make all your symptoms worse. You can't get enough rest when you have to make hourly trips to the bathroom. Although I can vouch from personal experience that it's possible to sleep sitting on the toilet if you're wrapped in blankets and have strategically placed pillows, I don't recommend it. Elavil is suggested because it can reduce spasms with its **anti-cholinergeric** properties and has **antihistamine** properties also. A last resort would be **opioid** pain medications and some of the muscle relaxants. If you use them, be sure to use them only when you absolutely need them or you will build up a tolerance. Remember too that constipation is one of the side effects of these medications and straining may cause severe pain and spasms.

Some physicians are now trying antihistamines for both irritable bladder and vulvar pain. This is because newer studies have shown that histamines are released both from the bladder lining and the vulvar skin. These histamines lead to the production of **cytokines**, which are what cause the skin to burn, itch, and be overly sensitive. Some of the medications used are Atarax (at bedtime because it can make you drowsy), Allegra, or Zyrtec. Patients usually begin with low doses and increase gradually to the maximum allowed if needed. Again, it will take six to eight weeks for you to see progress. According to Dr. Willems, continuous use of an antihistamine can make flareups shorter and less painful.

Nonmedicinal therapies can help, too

Warm baths, heating pads, and hot water bottles can help with pelvic pain and make it easier to relax so you can fall asleep. Anything you can do to help your muscles relax, like physical therapy, medication, or self-hypnosis, offers other possibilities for relief.

Biofeedback can help with chronic muscle spasms in the pelvic area, some of which are there because the pain causes women to tense up. Pelvic floor muscle rehabilitation can really help with the dull heavy pains. This technique can, of course, be used in conjunction with other therapies such as Estrace and diet.

Be cautious in trying new modalities

Be very careful when you and your partner are seeking help. It is tempting for us, in our desperation, to try some rather drastic "cures." There are some nasty treatments out there, so be sure that you research everything and seek a second opinion. Support groups will also warn you against some of these. I have heard stories from women who had alcohol or local anesthetic injections into the painful areas, or of skin being thinned permanently by steroid concoctions. Topical testosterone has also caused problems. There are even worse stories about the unsuccessful and sometimes mutilating surgeries women have undergone where parts of the **labia** or vagina have been removed. I call this the "right eye school of medicine" after the biblical phrase "If thy right eye offends thee, pluck it out." Don't be in a rush to try surgery or other intrusive therapies because these will certainly have an effect on your fibromyalgia. And never be afraid to seek a second opinion if you're confused. Some of your final options will be nerve blocks or surgery performed only by a physician who is a specialist and whom you can trust to be perfectly honest with you about the possible outcomes.

IN A SENTENCE:

> The discomfort and embarrassment of genitourinary symptoms can be combated with a combination of education, medication, topical remedies, and feedback from support groups and online Web groups.

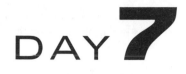

DAY 7

living

Dealing with All the Unanswered Questions and Symptoms of Fibromyalgia

IT'S NOT a news flash to those of us who have fibromyalgia that it affects every cell in the body. We know that nothing in our body seems to work quite the way it should. We've all experienced symptoms that don't fall into any of the neat categories we've just studied, and don't actually seem to fit into any category any researcher has ever devised! So before we move on, let's spend just one more day looking at some of the other symptoms that plague us. Just like the rest, these come and go, vary in intensity, and not every person has every one of them.

Skin conditions

Let's start with the skin because it's the largest organ of the whole body, and the most visible. The most common skin problem fibromyalgics experience is patchy rashes that vary in texture, location, and severity. Nearly all of us experience hives, as well as tiny dry bumps and tiny blistery patches of skin, usually on the fingers. If you visit a dermatologist it's likely you'll hear the diagnosis of eczema, a rash that's made up of scaly, dry, lined patches, usually in some shade of red. You'll be given cute little samples of various creams to try.

Skin symptoms may be different in different places

Your skin may be fragile, dry, and peeling in some spots, while in other places it's oily. Little patches of acne on the face, upper back, or chest called seborrhea can appear. In patients with oily skin, these breakouts can be quite severe at times and embarrassing because they're nearly always on the face. Others may break out in the places where they perspire, in a clear pattern that follows the location of sweat glands.

Itchy skin without visible rashes is both frustrating and common, and so are tingling and crawling sensations known in medical lingo as **paresthesia.** You may feel like there's an ant crawling on you, or as if there are threads hanging on your clothes. Around your face you may feel as if there's a hair bothering you that you can't quite locate. Burning on the back of the neck (usually where the tag to your clothes is sewn) is very common, and many of us can't bear to have labels touching our skin. Clothes and jewelry may bother you, and the bedcovers at night can drive you crazy. Sheets can feel like sandpaper, and itchy-crawly symptoms can be much worse when you're lying quietly and trying to sleep.

Changes in skin color and flushing are also common

Flushing and redness is often the first sign that a bad flare or cycle of fibromyalgia is beginning, especially in fair-skinned patients like me. Usually this is confined to the face, but often the neck, chest, and upper arms can be involved as well. Some patients even have a condition called **dermatographia** where scratching the skin results in raised white areas that stand out. In others, even minor scratching especially in the sensitive areas around the breasts can cause capillaries to break, tiny red dots to appear, or very faint spotty bruising under the skin.

Easy bruising all over the body occurs in women, and sometimes these bruises can be quite extensive and shocking. Other times they are faint, like a dusky ink stain, and you might try to scrub them off, thinking they're a smudge of some kind. You're not alone if you have bruises all over your legs and hips and have no idea how you got them.

Your hair will suffer too

In fibromyalgics, poor hair quality is a usual lament. Split ends, frizzy patches, and hair that seems to fall out in clumps are complaints I hear over and over. Your hair may break off all at once and seem to grow back slowly.

The hair can seem to change from dry to oily from month to month, and is often thin and limp, or coarse and frizzy.

Gunky eyes and stinging, burning eyes

Also included in skin complaints are problems with the really sensitive skin that lines the inside of our mouths, our eyes, and other orifices, and the mucosa that lines our moist tissues. The inner eyelids and eyes itch, water, and release mucus. During the day this is of no consequence because it's easily wiped away, but at night it dries and forms an unattractive, pale greenish-white crust. A little grit in the corner of the eye is normal, what my mother used to call "sleepy sand" (referring to the story about the sandman who puts kids to sleep). But in fibromyalgics this substance is gooey and thick and can actually glue the eyes shut by binding the upper and lower lashes together. In addition, since the eyelids are very sensitive skin they can be easily irritated and can swell with the indignity of burning tears. At other times the eyes will be the opposite, dry and itchy.

Your eyes can also burn and be very acidy. Many fibromyalgics can't wear contact lenses because they are too irritating, or because they are always cloudy or even covered with a very fine, soft grit. Bright lights are hard to tolerate, so it's normal for you to hate fluorescent lights. Sunlight can be irritating too, and it can be hard to see even with sunglasses because of peripheral glare. This glare can irritate the eyes and almost "burn" them, as well as cause headaches and eyestrain. Blurred vision is another problem, and you may also experience problems focusing at times.

You may experience a burned or metallic taste in your mouth

Your mouth may feel burned or scalded, and the saliva can be very acidic. I used to wake up sometimes with a rash around my mouth. Canker sores and cold sores, though a virus, break out when you're in a flare. Sometimes the tongue and the inside of the mouth can be one giant raw area. Your tongue can form a thick white coating, and dental calculus (tartar) forms very easily. Your teeth can hurt and may be X-rayed often to look for an abscess or infection, only to find out that none are present. A nasty metallic taste that is reminiscent of licking a battery is common, but others complain of an annoying salty taste that they can't wash away.

Solutions for the metallic taste in your mouth that drives you crazy is a tough one, and about the only thing you can do during the day is sip on something or use lozenges. Sipping might be a better solution if you're watching your sugar intake because although there are sugar-free candies, most contain **sorbitol**. Sorbitol or any sweetener that ends in "-ol" is a sugar alcohol and can cause gas, bloating, and diarrhea. There's also some evidence that excess sugar can make your mouth dry. If you can find hard candies with Splenda, that would solve your problem. Otherwise use a sugar-free drink mix like Crystal Lite. Tart flavors such as lemonade work best, or you can use a squeeze of lemon in regular water. You can keep it on your desk and take little sips as needed. You should also rinse your mouth often, and warm, salted water is best, although some people think baking soda works better. (Use ½ teaspoon in a cup of warm water). If this causes you to lick your lips and this makes them dry, use a water-based lubricant such as cocoa butter. At home, especially at night in your bedroom, use a **humidifier**. Remember that some medications (including antidepressants) can cause dry mouth so be alert to this and check with your doctor to make sure you aren't making the problem worse.

Acidy body secretions cause bodywide irritation

All bodily secretions are acidic and can burn. It's common especially in the area where you perspire to see red irritated spots. These usually occur on the forehead, under the arms or breasts, and behind the knees, especially if you wear nylon stockings. I used to be convinced that I was allergic to my own perspiration, but I knew this was too crazy to mention to any doctor so I kept it to myself. Acidic body secretions can also turn your fingers black under your gold jewelry. Sweat and urine can be dark and pungent with an acidic odor. The lining of the nose, bronchial tubes, vagina, and rectum all produce mucus that may be acidic and irritating. Women may notice red, chemically burned areas on their inner thighs especially following intercourse from their vaginal secretions, and in both sexes irritation around the anus can be red, itchy, or have a burned feeling.

Fingernail problems

Fingernails chip, break, and peel, and grow slowly. It's common for them to grow and then all break at once. Cuticles are dry, white, flaky, and peel and bleed. Hangnails are common, too, and if you aren't careful ingrown nails will follow. Even women who wear acrylic nails may have problems because the nails underneath are so flimsy.

What's going on?

Scientific studies have confirmed that there are measurable abnormalities in the skin of fibromyalgics, so this problem is not in your imagination. Biopsies show higher IgG (immunoglobin G) in the skin and more mast cells than in normal people. These cells release histamines in an allergic reaction, and this histamine release causes red, watery, itchy, puffy eyes, itchy nose, runny nose, and other symptoms common to allergic reactions. Allergies appear to be present more often in fibromyalgics than in the general population. Postnasal drip is an annoyance, as is a chronic nasal congestion. In some people, sudden nasal congestion (sometimes one-sided) is a harbinger of a flare or bad attack of fibromyalgia

Things you can try to heal your skin

Your skin symptoms can be treated as if they were unrelated to fibromyalgia, though if you get as far as a dermatologist it's a good idea to mention the connection. An over-the-counter cortisone spray or cream can help with the itching, and so can an antihistamine spray. You can also try an over-the-counter antihistamine pill for hives, especially if they are itchy or if they cover a big area and a topical remedy isn't practical. You may also be offered a prescription pill for itching. Some of these can make you extremely drowsy, so use these only at night and with caution.

If the itching is very bad, try a warm (not hot) oatmeal bath. When the itching is severe in one area, a cold compress will really help by deadening the area. If you have breakouts, keep your skin clean, and use a gentle acne medication, not salicylic acid, which is very harsh on older skin.

Be gentle with your skin

You should always treat your skin gently—less is always more. Stay away from harsh toners, cleansers, and alcohol. Use lukewarm water—never hot, which will make itching worse. Don't scrub, but gently clean. There are excellent gentle moisturizers for all skin types. You don't need to spend a lot of money, and if your skin is sensitive try fragrance-free baby products. You won't regret it if you baby your skin, and you might even find that there's more than one reason babies have baby soft skin. If you have skin allergies, one secret is to choose products with only a few ingredients. This way there's less chance something will irritate your skin. If your skin is dry and flaky, use a good quality alpha hydroxy lotion. I use one that used to be prescription but now is over the counter, a lactic acid formula called Amlactin. Lactic acid is the natural alpha hydroxyl in our own skin.

Don't succumb to the peel hype because that will leave sensitive skin even more sensitive. No matter how tempting it is to pick, squeeze, scratch, or rub, leave your skin alone! If you must seek help, ask a dermatologist and not an aesthetician or beauty consultant. Do not trust the advice you get at cosmetic counters, no matter how scientifically it is presented to you. The cosmetic industry is big business and it is not built on candid information. You can bank on the fact that you will be told whatever you want to hear, and be led to believe you have to buy lots of things to make your skin look good.

Trial and error, unfortunately, is the only way to find out what works best for your skin. If something irritates your skin, read the label and see if you can identify the culprit. It's worth the time to keep a little file of labels so you can learn which ingredients to avoid.

Commonsense things you can do to protect your skin

If your perspiration burns or irritates your skin, there are several things you can do. You can carry with you a baggie with soft cloths in it to wipe your forehead. Be sure not to use commercial wipes because they are loaded with chemicals and fragrance, and often harsher ingredients like alcohol or menthol. If you look, you can find cloths with baby wash on them that you dampen under a faucet. Using cool water with these really does a good job, and will even take off eye makeup without stinging or irritation. Avoid tight clothing in warm weather, as well as in winter if you'll be inside where it's warm. Nylon stockings and tight brassieres are major causes of rashes, so loose-fitting cotton pants and a cotton undershirt are better choices. Stay away from synthetic fabrics and stick with cotton and linen. You can find some very comfortable gauze clothing that will simplify things in hot weather. Baby powder or other body powder will help.

Protect your eyes, too

Sensitive eyes should be treated kindly as well. Consider wearing tinted glasses, which will ease some of the strain. You can get these in various tints and even wear them at work if fluorescent lights bother you. Always wear polarized sunglasses when you're outside and always keep an extra pair in your car. Another trick (and personal favorite) is to remove one of the bulbs from the fixture in your office so the light is not so bright. If you have your own work area or office you might be able to plug in your own lamp and leave the overhead lights off. At home, open curtains and let daylight in. **Beta carotene** supplements sometimes help with night vision but don't take more than the suggested amount because this could be dangerous. Artificial tears and saline nose sprays may also help with irritated eyes and nasal passages. Some studies suggest that lower melatonin levels might be associated with light sensitivity. You can certainly try a few milligrams of melatonin before bed for a week or two to see if you notice any difference. This natural hormone is available in health food stores and pharmacies.

Fingernails can be managed with a little care

If your nails split and break and your cuticles are ragged, you might consider getting a regular manicure once a month or so. A regular appointment isn't stressful, and you don't have to do anything fancy like acrylic nails. Your manicurist might want to put a strengthening coat on the nails you have; sometimes this helps a lot. If you have a support group you might consider helping each other with your nails every so often.

Gold jewelry turns my fingers black, but I don't have a problem with silver. (I've never tried platinum but it's supposed to be safe, too) Well-meaning people will tell you to paint your jewelry with clear nail polish, but that is a common allergen so this is not a good idea. I've had people tell me it isn't the gold in the jewelry; it's the alloy, like nickel, so purer gold should be better. This sounds like a good theory, but it never worked for me.

Hair today, gone tomorrow . . .

Hair loss is a very sensitive subject. If you notice that you're losing a lot of hair over a period of time be sure to tell your doctor. You'll need to have a thyroid test, and possibly some sort of workup to rule out some other possible causes, like lupus. Once those have been done and if they're normal, you can turn to the subject at hand, or rather, at head.

There isn't much you can do to make hair grow—though vitamin and supplement companies and dermatologists who advertise on the radio would have you believe otherwise. Hair loss is natural in both women and men as we age. It has to do with falling hormone levels. In women hair loss usually begins at about thirty, and becomes noticeable about ten years later. It is usually an overall hair loss, just fewer hairs grow. If women develop an actual bald spot, it's on the crown of the head, not like the receding hair line seen in men. If you don't believe me look at the hair of older women when you walk behind them. Very few have thick, luxurious hair. Some women have good results from **Rogaine**, a treatment developed from a blood pressure medication (minoxidil) that causes hair growth as a side effect. There is also a prescription medication, **Propecia,** used commonly by men that some women are experimenting with, though not women of childbearing age. It is also not an option for men whose partner may get pregnant. By all means discuss this option carefully with your doctor—it is a hormone and you need to make sure you want to accept the possible risks. You absolutely can't use it if there is any possibility whatsoever that you could get pregnant, that's for sure. It's not innocuous stuff; women aren't even allowed to touch the pill if it is broken and they are of childbearing age. Think about that.

Various forms of vertigo can occur

Vertigo isn't exactly dizziness, but we often think of ourselves as being dizzy when what we're really experiencing is vertigo. Vertigo is actually the sensation of movement: either of things around you, or you yourself. The sensation of balance, which arises from the inner ear, is just off. This is another symptom that can flare up when you're in a bad cycle. This problem seems to arise from the neurotransmitters in the brain. Over-the-counter sea-sickness medications such as **Marezine** will help with this. Just take them as directed for a few days.

Restless legs and leg cramps

The symptoms of **restless legs** are infamous for appearing at night, just when you lie down and are trying to fall asleep. It's more common in women than in men, seems to run in the family, and gets worse as you age, usually starting with menopause.

Restless legs are like little demons that wait until you start to relax to torment you. Symptoms actually can occur any time you are sitting still: on an airplane, in a theater, or riding in a car. They start with a general aching, and then the feeling that your legs are expanding. This sensation is described as a combination of tingling, prickling, crawling, throbbing, and twitching. It can feel like spiders are crawling on you, or inside you, just under the skin, or like an electric current is running through your veins. Although these symptoms occur most commonly in the legs, 30 percent or so of fibromyalgics experience the same sensations in their arms. An uncontrollable urge to move the affected area is part of the sensation and adds to your discomfort. After falling asleep, jerky movements often occur repetitively. Sometimes your whole body jerks when you're about to fall asleep and you feel as if you are falling. This jerk wakes you up instantly with a release of adrenaline.

Leg cramps at night are also often part of fibromyalgia. Feet may also be affected, causing the toes to curl apart painfully. This pain is intense and grabbing—it feels exactly like a charley horse.

Theories and modalities for restless legs

There are several theories for what causes restless legs. Often you'll hear it referred to as "restless leg syndrome," again, a collection of symptoms grouped together that includes various abnormal sensations such as prickling, pulsating, and crawling on the legs, as well as insomnia and daytime sleepiness. The simplest explanation of the cause is that during the course of the day, fluids settle into your lower leg because of gravity. Since fibromyalgics have marginally functioning systems, this fluid sits there and expands the tissue. This is a logical explanation for why it occurs so commonly at night, because then we're lying flat and the fluid is gradually pulled back out. Other abnormalities that could be involved include low dopamine levels, low magnesium levels, and slight anemia.

Restless leg syndrome is particularly awful because it tortures you when you are already exhausted and having a terrible time sleeping. There are support groups for this syndrome, and other resources for new research are included in the For Further Information section. You can keep track of new treatments by periodically checking them.

Certain medications can make restless legs worse. You should check with your doctor if you're taking any of these to decide if there's a reasonable substitute: **Calcium-channel blocker** blood pressure medications; most anti-nausea medications, especially **Reglan**; some cold and allergy medications (containing stimulants like pseudoepherine); and antidepressants are the most common culprits. (Some other symptoms experienced by fibromyalgics are actually helped by antidepressants, however.) Some rarely used medications that make the condition worse are major tranquilizers (including haloperidol and phenothiazines) and the antiseizure medication phenytoin.

Dietary Triggers of Restless Legs

Caffeine (coffee and tea)
Chocolate
Caffeinated soft drinks such as Mountain Dew
Alcohol

You may want to have a blood test for iron

Researchers have recently discovered that the symptoms of restless legs are often caused by a lack of iron. To find out if this applies to you, ask your doctor for a blood test to check your **ferritin level**. If this is less than 50 mcg/L, taking an iron supplement should help. Your doctor may also want you to take vitamin B or **folate**. You may also read that magnesium, calcium, or potassium will help. Be careful with these supplements because they can hinder your body's ability to use other minerals. Make sure your doctor approves of what you are taking, and that you do have a deficiency before taking a supplement. An amino acid, **L-theronine,** may be worth a try as well before turning to prescription medications. If sleep is the major problem, Tylenol PM is a good choice.

You can try prescription medications

Klonopin and other **benzodiazepines** are sometimes used, but during the day these can cause drowsiness (not a good thing for fibromyaligcs) and unfortunately these are habit-forming. If used at bedtime, some of the newer sleeping medications like Ambien or Sonata may be better choices if they are strong enough to help you sleep. **Neurontin,** an antiseizure drug, is also proving helpful. Pain medications should be used sparingly and only for particularly terrible episodes. Doctors often prefer to prescribe **Ultram**, a mild narcotic, than stronger opioids such as **codeine**. It's best to use the smallest possible amount of whatever you're taking to make you comfortable enough to sleep. You might want to vary your approach, using a sleep medication one night and doing without the next night, if possible. Some people do find that stretching or a massage helps if done before bedtime.

Some options for leg cramps

There are several good prospects for the relief of leg cramps. You can try flexing your foot upward if they only occur occasionally and are mild. Vitamin E has been shown to be effective at 400 milliequivalents at bedtime. It's safe to raise this to 800 milliequivalents if you only get partial relief. Benadryl (or diphenhydramine) at fifty milligrams before going to sleep is also a good suggestion. In a small percentage of people it can work as a stimulant, so try a small dose before going the whole hog. **Quinine sulfate** is an old standby, but now requires a prescription. Soma, also a prescription medication, has proven safe and effective even with long-term use.

Dealing with increased sensitivities

More and more research points to the conclusion that fibromyalgia results in some sort of sensory amplification. Pain is one of those sensations, but it is certainly true that we're overly sensitive to external stimuli as well. Like all the other symptoms of fibromyalgia, these sensitivities vary in intensity and are worse when other symptoms flare. Women generally have more acute senses and these symptoms occur predominately in us, although plenty of men complain of headaches from various sensitivities.

During a cycle it's common to be acutely sensitive to everything, including light. Florescent lights usually are the worst, due to a combination of the noise they make and the slight flickering and color of the light itself. Sometimes working in an area with no windows and only this type of light will result in a claustrophobic sensation.

Sounds also cause extreme discomfort, especially those of a certain pitch, generally those in a high register, or that are overly repetitious. Television noise is a common irritant (especially laugh tracks and sitcoms), as is the sound of children playing and screaming. Pounding or thumping when children play or workmen are working near you may drive you crazy. Women can get extremely sensitive to the pitch of certain voices, to the point where they have to turn the channel quickly on the radio or television when certain people start talking.

Strong odors can create strong symptoms

It's common for fibromyalgics to be very sensitive to smells, and stronger odors can cause nausea and headaches. These headaches may be so intense that you feel as if you are not able to see clearly, or it can be a dull omnipresent sensation that nothing can ease. Many fibromyalgics cannot tolerate perfume, first or even secondhand, and must use fragrance-free personal hygiene products. Cigarette smoke is extremely difficult to tolerate even when it is only on someone's clothing. Sometimes, for example, I take the stairs to avoid an elevator that doesn't smell right to me.

Chemical sensitivities

These sensitivities can be severe in some patients, leading to a diagnosis of "chemical sensitivities." While chemical smells can certainly trigger migraines and nausea, this seems to me to be only part of the problem. I can get the same symptoms from natural fragrances when I don't feel well, like gardenias or some jasmine plants. It isn't just synthetic chemicals that bother fibromyalgics. The smell of certain flowers in a vase can be overpowering, even when they're on the other side of the room, when you're not feeling well. Fish, especially tunafish, anchovies, or sardines can make you extremely nauseous.

Sensitivities are fairly easy to deal with on your own turf and tough everywhere else. At home keep your house uncluttered and carefully select the cleaning products you use. Buy unscented products for the whole family and use a very mild laundry detergent like Ivory Snow that won't leave an odor on sheets and towels, and if your skin is extra sensitive always use the extra-rinse setting on your washing machine. Don't use fabric softener sheets. Sometimes burning a plain candle in the kitchen can help with smells. I don't know why this is true, but try it, especially when you are chopping onions.

Communicate often about your sensitivities

Explain the situation carefully to your family members. Be patient and remember that they may not always smell what you smell. Remind guests that you're sensitive to odors and consider asking them not to wear perfumes or colognes when they visit. When you don't feel well stay away from stores and malls where there are lots of odors, noises, and crowds. It's also a good idea to cancel visits to people with pets, or who have smokers in the family. If you attend a support group or any other meeting, consider asking other members to refrain from using scented products. You'll actually find that this rule is commonplace for fibromyalgia support groups.

Intolerance to weather conditions

It's also no secret that fibromyalgics are temperature intolerant: sweating and boiling hot, or freezing when everyone around us is comfortable. You may feel as if you only have about a 10 degree radius of temperature in which you're comfortable, or that you're forever putting on and taking off clothes. During cycles it's common to run a low-grade fever as well. You may notice that hot flashes, sweating, and even cold sweats can happen a lot when you're not feeling well and trying to push yourself.

Try layering

There's no easy solution to your body thermostat problems except to layer your clothes. You can also keep extra clothing in the trunk of your car so if you get really uncomfortable you can change. You should always carry a blanket in case you get cold when you're sitting outside if you have children who practice and play sports. There are portable misters that will keep you cool in the summer, if heat bothers you. These are inexpensive and most drugstores or department stores carry them. You can also buy small heat patches to put in your pockets or socks when it's cold.

Don't underestimate the power of exercise

Exercise will reset your body thermostat, especially when you're cold. Sometimes in winter when I can't get warm I force myself to get up and walk around the block a couple of times. When I come back into the house, I'm always warm for the rest of the evening. When you're cold it may seem like a bad idea to go out into the cold, but it will really do the trick. Getting out to take a walk will also clear your head if odors are present in your house or a place you are visiting.

You may need to gently remind people of your sensitivities

Unless you live alone, your various sensitivities and intolerances will be an issue from time to time. It's part of human nature for the people who live with you to forget what they don't experience themselves. A family member who is in tune with your illness may notice a change of expression when you are in pain, or glazed eyes when you're tired. But they will probably not be able to sense the noise or odor that is giving you a headache. Be prepared to gently remind and work with those around you to make your home a comfortable place for all who live there. Being short-tempered when you're ill is natural, but if you are patient and willing to gently jog the memories of those around you, you will see better results over time.

SOME OTHER common complaints of fibromyaglics:

- O   Hypersensitivity to touch
- O   Problems with night vision
- O   Susceptibility to infection
- O   Catching every virus that goes around
- O   Easy bruising
- O   Swelling in fingers (rings may not always fit)
- O   Swelling of feet (shoes you suddenly can't wear)
- O   Sleep apnea
- O   Nighttime teeth grinding

IN A SENTENCE:

There are many uncategorized symptoms of fibromyalgia that you will encounter, but there are modalities for dealing with all of them.

learning

Frequently Asked Questions about Fibromyalgia

MANY PEOPLE have similar questions as they begin to learn more about fibromyalgia. Here are the ones that are asked the most frequently.

Is there a cure for fibromyalgia?

There is no known cure for fibromyalgia. Because the exact cause of fibromyalgia has not yet been identified, it is unlikely that any kind of cure will be found in the next few years. As it stands, it looks as if fibromyalgia is an inherited condition. Like diabetes, high blood pressure, and other conditions, it is most likely that effective treatments may be devised before a cure is discovered. As new research uncovers more information about the underlying causes of this condition, we'll all have more answers.

Does anyone know what causes fibromyalgia?

No. Fibromyalgia was once thought to be an inflammatory condition but no inflammation or arthritis has been found. It has been also called a psychiatric illness, but when depression and anxiety occur they are the result of the many symptoms of fibromyalgia rather than the cause. We know that patients with fibromyalgia are no more likely to be depressed than those with other chronic painful illnesses such as rheumatoid arthritis or lupus. Spinal fluid levels four times the norm of the main pain neurotransmitter, substance P, confirm that our pain is not in our minds. The body's immediate energy fuel, ATP, has been shown to be low in muscle cells. Neurotransmitter and endocrine changes have been seen in fibromyalgia, particularly involving serotonin and the pituitary-adrenal axis and may account for some fibromyalgia symptoms. Depression, irritable bowel syndrome, and migraine headaches are all associated with low serotonin levels.

Will my fibromyalgia get worse?

Although the pain and fatigue of fibromyalgia can be quite severe and can be exacerbated by certain health conditions, they do not result in the development of any deformities or lead to death. There is no actual destruction of muscle or any other tissue, and no deterioration of bones or joints. Patients with fibromyalgia do not become crippled, though their mobility may be affected by ongoing pain and stiffness. Fibromyalgia is not life threatening and does not involve the internal organs of the body. This is the reason you'll hear fibromyalgia referred to in medical texts as "non-progressive," despite the fact that you may notice that your symptoms get more severe over time. There is no evidence linking it to any form of cancer, or any life-threatening condition, and it has no known effect on life expectancy.

When I don't feel well, how do I know if it's fibromyalgia or something else?

Fibromyalgia, of course, does not preclude the possibility of other medical problems. You should never assume that everything that you are feeling or experiencing is from fibromyalgia alone. Because fibromyalgia is associated with widespread pain in all parts of the body, including the chest and abdomen, as well as severe fatigue, it is often difficult to know whether symptoms are related to fibromyalgia or caused by another medical condition. **Acute** pains, shortness of breath, and high fevers are among your body's warning signs and you should not ignore them. Follow up with your physician regarding any new symptoms you experience. He or she can then assess your history, conduct a physical examination, and perform any necessary laboratory testing to determine the exact cause of your symptoms.

Is fibromyalgia an autoimmune condition?

It's true that fibromyalgia is associated with certain immune system changes. However, these are not of the autoimmune kind seen in rheumatoid arthritis or Hashimoto's thyroiditis, but rather the immune system appears stimulated, as if your body were fighting a virus. Levels of certain **cytokines**, a class of immune system hormones, are elevated in fibromyalgia, but antinuclear antibodies and other connective tissue disease features are the same in fibromyalgics and normal people. Autoimmunity, from the Greek word *self (auto)* necessitates the presence of antibodies manufactured to destroy some part of one's own body that has been mistakenly perceived to be foreign tissue. These have not been found in any of the studies done on fibromyalgics.

Can my family catch fibromyalgia from me?

There is no evidence that fibromyalgia is caused by a virus or bacteria, or that it can be spread from one person to another by physical contact. For example, it is no more common in spouses of patients than in the general population. Extensive searches for a viral cause have turned up nothing. Many studies of the demographics of fibromyalgia confirm that it is not contagious, although it may be inherited. Genetic studies are currently being undertaken, and more on this topic will be known soon. But for the present, it's safe to say that no one can catch fibromyalgia from you.

Could my fibromyalgia be caused by my mercury fillings?

Mercury amalgam dental fillings have been mentioned by some sources in conjunction with multiple sclerosis, Alzheimer's disease, autism, and fibromyalgia because it's well known that mercury is toxic. However, the fact is "when mercury is mixed with metals such as silver it forms a stable alloy, similar to the way that sodium and chlorine—both hazardous in their pure state—combine to form an ordinary table salt," according to Frederick Eichmiller, of Paffenbarager Research Center in Maryland. The American Dental Association Code of Ethics has prohibited dentists from telling patients that having their fillings removed would treat any disease, and the AMA followed suit in 2002.

The NIH is two years through a seven-year multicenter study of the effect of mercury amalgam fillings. To date there is no indication that they are planning to stop the study, which is what would happen immediately if they had seen any data implying that fillings were causing problems. The American Dental Association, whose members stand to make a lot of money if it were suddenly suggested that we all have our fillings replaced, is launching a media campaign to discourage people from doing so.[1]

If this is of concern to you, then do your own cost/benefit analysis. The cost of porcelain composite fillings has gone down in the last couple of years and is only slightly higher than mercury amalgam, so you may consider replacing older fillings with the composite material (amalgam fillings have a life of about six years), or deciding to refuse amalgam material in any new dental work.

Is there a surgery to help fibromyalgia?

This is a common question because recently both the *Wall Street Journal* and the television show *20/20* did stories linking fibromyalgia with a deformity that can be helped by surgery. **Chiari malformation** is a congenital deformity where two parts of the brain (brainstem and cerebellum) bulge into the spinal canal, which can be seen on an **MRI test**. This $30,000 procedure, which is rarely covered by insurance, involves drilling bone away to decompress the area. The surgeons who popularized this surgery will allow you to mail your MRIs to them to see if you might be a candidate for their procedure. A new study by Georgetown University rheumatologist Daniel Clauw, M.D. et al. found more Chiari malformation in the control group than in the fibromyalgia group.

Why have some people benefited from this surgery? Dr. Clauw believes that there are probably people who have been misdiagnosed as fibromyalgics, who actually suffer from this malformation, **cervical stenosis**, or narrowing of the cervical spine. Since there is considerable overlap in the symptoms of these conditions, this is the most likely explanation. Meanwhile, the American Association of Neurological Surgeons has issued a statement saying, "There is no scientific evidence that chronic fatigue syndrome (or fibromyalgia) is a neurological disorder or that it requires surgical intervention. Therefore the American Association of Neurological Surgeons (AANS) does not recognize the use of cervical decompression as a treatment alternative."

I've been reading about tender points and trigger points. What is the difference between them?

Back in the 1980s when fibromyalgia was being defined, researchers found in excess of fifty locations in muscles and other soft tissue that caused pain when palpated. To simplify matters, and to make diagnosis easier, the most common eighteen were selected as representative of the situation all over the body. These eighteen are located symmetrically in all four quadrants of the body, and are known as tender points because they hurt more than surrounding tissue when pressure is applied to them.

Trigger points, a term sometimes used interchangeably, are actually something a little different. These occur all over the body, and produce pain that travels in reproducible patterns elsewhere in the body when pressure is applied. They are generally located in a taut band of tissue with a ropey texture that you can feel. Fibromyalgic patients have both tender points and trigger points. An easy way to remember the difference is that a trigger point, like a gun, shoots pain to another area.

What is the difference between myofascial pain and fibromyalgia?

Some sources refer to **myofascial pain syndrome** and fibromyalgia as separate entities and some say they are the same condition. Generally speaking, however, myofascial pain syndrome is considered to be a more regional form of fibromyalgia, because only certain areas in the body are affected. Most physicians feel that the difference between them is inconsequential and that they are either the same illness or have a large overlap in symptoms. Devin Starlanyl, the leading advocate today of myofascial pain syndrome as a separate entity, feels that it is an illness defined by trigger points, which appears to involve serious disturbances of nerve endings.

IN A SENTENCE:

> There's a lot to learn about fibromyalgia and its symptoms, so don't be afraid to ask questions.

FIRST-WEEK MILESTONE

By the end of your first week, you've come a long way in understanding and accepting your fibromyalgia:

○ YOU HAVE FOUND A DOCTOR WHO BELIEVES FIBROMYALGIA IS A VALID CONDITION AND WHOM YOU LIKE AND TRUST.

○ YOU KNOW WHAT FIBROMYALGIA IS AND ISN'T AND HAVE RULED OUT ANY UNRELATED HEALTH CONDITIONS OR ILLNESSES,

○ YOU HAVE MADE AN ASSESSMENT OF YOUR SYMPTOMS AND ARE INCREASINGLY AWARE OF HOW THEY RELATE TO YOUR FIBROMYALGIA.

○ YOU HAVE BEGUN TO EVALUATE YOUR ILLNESS IN ITS OWN CONTEXT AND ENVISION THE POSSIBILITIES OF REGAINING YOUR HEALTH.

○ YOU UNDERSTAND THAT YOU, ALONE, ARE ULTIMATELY RESPONSIBLE FOR REGAINING YOUR HEALTH.

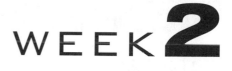

WEEK 2

living

Keeping Your Relationships Alive Even When You Don't Feel Well

YOU'VE SPENT the last week learning about what fibromyalgia is and now it's time to think about what having this illness will mean to you on a larger scale.

Now you know what you have, and that it's not because of something you did. Since it's not your fault, there's nothing you can do to make it go away, so what exactly *are* you going to do? How will you keep your life and your relationships from changing when you have such an unpredictable and debilitating illness? No matter how upset or angry you are that you have fibromyalgia, eventually you're going to have to give up on negative emotions. You might as well start now.

You're in the driver's seat

No matter how much help you get, you are ultimately in charge of yourself and your illness, and you are going to have to take care of yourself and make the important decisions. To a large extent, how you explain yourself and how you behave will determine how much support you will get. You can either use your illness to put a barrier between yourself and the world, or you can grow from your illness and embrace the world. There's no question that it's a great challenge to keep your relationships going when you have an illness like fibromyalgia.

Those who love you share you illness, too

It's time to think about your family and friends who have been worrying about you and wondering what they can do to help. If you have children, they may be confused because they see you changing: Sometimes you feel well enough to do things and sometimes you don't. These explanations are extra tough because you have an illness with a name that's hard to pronounce, that is invisible, and that most people have never heard of.

If you're still finding your own way, that's OK

Don't worry if you still feel confused about having fibromyalgia and what it really means. It takes a while to really accept that your life has changed in a way you can't control. Talking about your symptoms and giving your disease a name is an important step. When my husband was first diagnosed with diabetes he would get angry when I would mention it in public. In a restaurant if I told a waiter he was diabetic, he would sulk and ask me, "Why did you have to say that?" But as time went by and he accepted his illness, this changed. Now he is the first one to speak up when he is offered food he can't eat. I noticed that around the time he had the courage to say diabetes out loud he started taking his illness more seriously and taking better care of himself. When he was able to talk about it, I knew that he understood that his illness was real and was not going to disappear. The denial was gone and he was ready to take care of himself.

I think you'll experience the same thing as you work through this week. Issues will solidify in your mind and you will begin to think about how to ask for what you need, and how to be kind to yourself when you can't do something. In asking your friends and family to have compassion for you, you will learn to have some for yourself. And just as you will have to think about your responsibilities to them, you will begin to understand your responsibilities to yourself.

Put yourself in their shoes

You're going to have to prepare yourself for what your family and friends have to say about the impact your illness has had on them. You'll need to listen to their fears and concerns and try to comfort them. You have suffered a loss—your former healthy life—but they have lost something too.

You will have stages to go through with them—the same ones that you went through—anger, denial, grief, guilt, depression, and finally acceptance. You can't pretend you don't have fibromyalgia and neither can they. But fibromyalgia is not who you are. It has a place in your life, but it doesn't have to become your life or your identity.

"Some people never heal because they believe that if they healed they would be alone and abandoned. Being sick in this culture can be a very powerful way to get your needs met legitimately. Many of us don't know how to get our needs met without wounds," writes Christine Northrup, M.D., in *Women's Bodies, Women's Wisdom*. You can be a victim, but to have good relationships that are based on something real and solid, you have to do better and want more for yourself. If you think about it honestly you'll have to admit that it's not a good idea to cultivate relationships that are built on your illness and your powerlessness. There really needs to be more than that.

What your partner should know

How you approach the subject with your partner will depend on a couple of things. Some relationships will have changed a lot already by the time you're diagnosed because you used to be healthy. Other partnerships were formed when you were already ill, though perhaps less so than now. It will depend on where you started and where you are now in the scheme of things. Some people's fibromyalgia came on slowly, other people hit a bump in the road and never fully recovered. All of these things will have an impact on how you should deal with this.

Be honest with your partner about your fears, your sadness, and your anger. This will allow him or her to do the same. It's very important for this communication to go both ways. Neither of you should be a martyr, and both of you need to express your needs. Most of us feel as if we are betraying our family and friends because we've changed. However, you need to adjust your thinking. Remember that this is only one of the changes you will face in your relationship as time goes by. There is no way of knowing what health problems either of you will face, and other normal changes will occur as you both age. When I met my husband I had fibromyalgia, and many of our activities were colored by how I felt and what I could do. I plodded along bravely and it only slowly dawned on him how much of the time I didn't feel well. Now, ten years later, he is a diabetic, and his illness is a larger part of our lives than my fibromyalgia ever was. Now it is my husband who varies from day to day in what he feels able to do. Things have changed again.

Honesty can be hard

If you are honest and straightforward with your partner about your illness, though you both may feel sad from time to time, you will still have a strong relationship. Let your partner in to share your hopes and fears, disappointments and victories. And then you are better able to share his, or hers, as they are voiced.

Of course there are relationships that do not survive a partner's illness. I know this and I don't mean for this discussion to be all sunshine and roses. Seventy-five percent of marriages in which one person has a chronic illness fail. The only comfort I can give you is that relationships fail for many reasons, and you cannot help being sick. If you lose a mate as your illness unfolds, you will have to go on and rebuild your life. What happened to the relationship, what caused it to happen, and who should take most of the blame is, in the end, immaterial. Fibromyalgia is not a death sentence; you have a lot to live for, a lot to give to others, and suffering can make you even better at loving and sharing. You will have the capacity to build a stronger relationship with someone else. Letting go of things that don't matter can be easier because you don't have the strength to fight every battle. The stress of dealing with a bad relationship can make you sicker, and you don't have the energy for that.

It's normal to feel isolated

Chronic pain certainly changes your life. It brings a feeling of isolation, a belief that you are not like everyone else. You may not always feel like being around people. Other times you may resent being left alone. This also is in your control. You need those you have relationships with to believe you, and not second-guess you. Being honest and not acting like a martyr will make a huge difference. This is not the time to play games like saying no when you mean yes, or expecting someone to know how you feel. Remember that your pain is invisible, and when you suddenly start to feel awful you have to speak up and express yourself. Don't rely on your partner to read your mind.

Practice saying what you mean

I think this is the hardest part of having relationships when you have fibromyalgia. At least it is for me. On one hand I don't want to say "I'm in pain" every time my husband asks me what's wrong. I don't always want to be complaining about something. On the other hand, when I say "nothing," and I'm acting funny, then he doesn't know what to do. He thinks something else is wrong and starts to worry. I have to fight the feeling that he should know what's going on without asking. I know this is unfair, and I can't expect him to know if I don't tell him. But I don't want to complain all the time and have him worrying about me. This is the vicious cycle we find ourselves in. I've learned to use one simple phrase: "It's just my fibromyalgia again."

Making time for your partner

You do have to commit to spending special time with your partner. If you walk for exercise, maybe this could be something you could share. Or set aside a night on the weekend, so you can rest during the day if you need to, to spend together. On a good night it could mean going out to eat, or for a drive. On a bad night it could mean renting a movie and watching it together in bed. Don't let other obligations wear you down because you need to give something back to the person that loves you. Be sure to make it clear that you want to live life in spite of your illness. Fibromyalgia can take away the joy of living when each day seems like an obstacle and it might feel like it takes all your energy just to exist. So it's extra important that you stay in touch with the good things in life as well. Practice relaxing and focusing on a simple moment with someone you love. Don't waste that time worrying about what isn't getting done, or what you can't do anymore. You only have a finite amount of energy: Don't let worrying and being upset drain the small amount you do have. Practice consciously blocking negative thoughts. You have to learn to put things out of your mind.

When you set aside time to spend with your partner, take a break from talking about your symptoms. Make them off limits for the day. Remember that while you need to share important points, you both need to have other topics of conversation, and you'll have other concerns to discuss. You need to find a balance between sharing and burdening, so setting aside time when there is no mention of your illness is vital for both of you.

What to tell your children

You'll need to have a session with your children no matter what their ages. Tell them that you want to talk to them honestly about why you haven't been feeling well, why things have been different. Make sure you are clear that you are going to be all right, but that you'll have to make some changes and maybe sometimes you won't be able to do everything you'd like to do. Make sure they understand that your fibromyalgia is not your fault or theirs, and that people can't help it when they get sick. Be sure they can understand that they can't catch your illness. Explain to them that it isn't contagious. Let them know that your fibromyalgia isn't going to go away, so you have to talk about what's going on. Explain that you will find new ways to spend time with them, and that you'll still be available to listen, advise, and be a parent. It's important for you to show your children ways that they can help you, and to be grateful and thank them when they do. Make sure, though, that they don't feel that they have to "take care of you." Do not let them curtail their lives and their plans because you don't feel well and they feel they should stay with you. Let them know that you want to spend time with them when you feel better, not because you feel sick.

Be truthful but don't be too detailed

When you are crabby or irritable because you don't feel well, be honest. Children can understand that you feel cranky when you don't get enough sleep because you didn't feel well. Don't try to force yourself to do things when you shouldn't—find a way to do less and explain why are doing it. Don't forget your children need special time with you.

Explain about your sensitivities: Let your children know that one of your symptoms is sensitivity to noise, odors, and bright light. Show them things that they can do when you need them to be quiet. During the day, maybe you can sit outside in the shade a distance away and let them run and play. Evenings are hardest when you don't feel well, but with a little patience you can teach them how to help you.

Remind your children that your symptoms are changeable

Another thing that's important for them to understand is that you will feel differently from day to day. You don't want them to get their hopes up that you are well if you're going through a good period, and you certainly don't want them to think that you're worse, or that something else is wrong, when you're having a flare.

Last of all, it's important for them to understand that all people are different. Some kids like to play with dolls, some like computers or chess, some like sports. Not all moms and dads are the same, either. Some are old and some are young, some spend a lot of time with their families, some stay home, others have to work. Tell them that you and they will have a special relationship all your own. Explain some of the things that you can still do with them, and try to be part of their important activities. You can find ways to do this. I had two sons as a single mom so it was doubly important for me to be involved in their sports and scouting. I found that I could always find jobs that I could do. Don't approach the situation negatively. I knew I could never be a coach, or lead a hike, but I could pass out awards at the annual banquet or be a team mom and make the phone calls.

Communication is a two-way street, even with the smallest child

Always let your children ask questions and encourage them to talk about their feelings. Let them know that it's OK to be angry or disappointed when things can't be the way they want. Explain proper ways to let out their frustration. Be sure to let them know that you are angry sometimes and disappointed too. Encourage them to talk to you about their hopes and fears.

Occasionally spend some time sitting with each of them and let them talk to you about what they find confusing or about what worries them about your condition. Let them know that you're going to be truthful with them because you love them and having a good relationship with them is the most important thing in your life.

If for some reason one or more of your children is having trouble dealing with your illness, don't hesitate to get them help. Just a few sessions of talking to someone outside the family can make a difference, especially if you are a single parent. Understand that if you are raising your kids alone, they might be especially frightened of losing you, or of their life changing in intangible ways. It also may be much more difficult for them to experience the anger that is normal for them to feel about these changes because it's hard to be angry at the only safety net they have. Some schools have special support groups for children with various family problems, so you should explore this resource if you need it. Many hospitals have support groups for family members of those in chronic pain. Remember that the group you find need not be fibromyalgia-specific, especially for younger children who may be hazier on the details anyway.

Talking openly with your friends

We all have many kinds of friends. Some of yours may have already drifted out of your life because of your limitations. Maybe they were the kind of friends who were only in your life because you were in theirs. Now that you may not go where they are, you see them less and less. But we all have friends with whom we have a real connection, the thick-and-thin kind, and you will need to talk to these friends.

Take the initiative

We all understand a certain kind of fear—the fear of doing something wrong. Perhaps you know someone who has had cancer or a terrible loss like the death of child. Maybe you were unnerved at the idea of calling them up for fear of not knowing what to say or do. When my son Malcolm was born prematurely with a heart defect, the silence was deafening. No calls of congratulations, no girlfriends to commiserate about my labor. The phone didn't ring—until the afternoon my friend Patti called me. "How are you doing?" she asked. It was the most wonderful thing in the world—someone who wasn't afraid to pick up the phone and call me. I know that people were afraid of not knowing what to say, or of saying the wrong thing, but it hurt. If relationships are important to you, you'll have to make sure that your friends aren't afraid to call you—that they understand what is wrong and that you need to hear from them. Make it easy for them.

It's up to you to find a way to express your illness

Maybe you have friends who have heard about fibromyalgia. If not, they'll probably recognize the idea of chronic fatigue. You'll probably have to educate them a little about what your symptoms are. You don't have to tell them everything; start with the basics and go into more depth if they're interested. You might leave the explanation simple, letting them know that your symptoms will fluctuate but that you will not get worse. The important point is that although they'll need to understand if you're a little unreliable about making plans in advance, there's still a lot that you can do. Luckily, by the time you have enough complaints to be diagnosed, your friends probably aren't depending on you to play racquetball every Thursday!

If your friends help you out with things you can't manage, be sure to do something special in return. An old-fashioned thank-you letter can really make someone feel appreciated and doesn't take too much time or energy. It's important to remember that you have things you can give in return.

Don't expect all your relationships to emerge unscathed

You'll probably have to discard some friends and maybe even distance yourself from some of your family members. Very few of us are lucky enough to get through life without at least one person we can't really get away from who is convinced we're a hypochondriac and there's no such illness as fibromyalgia. Or maybe he or she just doesn't understand why you always seem to not be feeling well, why you can't just buck up and act like everybody else. If this situation persists after you have made a few gentle attempts to change the way this person feels, then move on. If it's a family member you obviously can't "lose" him or her, but you can keep your distance and firmly make the subject of your health off limits. You can practice some nice little phrases, or just bluntly change the subject. You may also have to endure busybodies who want to cure you. These folks always seem to have a cousin or a neighbor's daughter who has found a miracle cure that they want you to try. They clip articles and advertisements and just can't understand why you aren't leaping at their suggestions.

In the coming weeks and month, you'll learn about traveling and about support groups and getting out into the world. But before you are ready to do that, you have to take care of things at home. You'll have to figure out how to stay connected with the people that mean the most to you.

IN A SENTENCE:

> *Having fibromyalgia will change the relationships in your life, and communication is the key to working through these changes.*

learning

Introducing Fibromyalgia to Your World

IT'S TIME to think about what you need to say and how you want to say it. If you have a computer you can read some other people's suggestions on how to describe fibromyalgia to people who don't have it. The most well known is a letter by Bek Oberlin in Australia, which was written to describe chronic fatigue syndrome. Several authors have adapted it for fibromyalgia, including Devin Starlanyl in her book about fibromyalgia and myofascial pain. Reading these will give you some ideas of what you might like to say. You might also take a moment before you start writing to read Debbie's "A Letter to Fibromites" at www.fibrohugs.com. Think about what those who love you are going through as well. As Debbie writes, "So will we ever really understand what you're going through? No. Will you ever really understand what we are going through? No. But if each of us gives each other the time, love, and patience to find our own way in dealing with and accepting what fibro has taken from us, I think our relationship may be a lot better."

In the end you have to come up with your own explanation. A well-crafted letter about your symptoms can be adapted for a partner, a friend, or a family member.

*Feel free to adapt this, adopt it as your own,
or just use it for inspiration*

Fibromyalgia isn't all in my head, and it isn't contagious. It doesn't turn into anything serious and nobody ever died from fibromyalgia though they might have wished they could on really awful days. I can't control how often I feel good or how often I feel terrible. If you want to read articles about fibromyalgia I can show you some that I think are good. If you just want to learn as we go along, that's fine too. This is definitely going to be a process. The first step is for you to believe that there is an illness called fibromyalgia and that I have it. This may sound simple, but when you hear about some of the symptoms I don't want you to think I'm making this up.

Fibromyalgia is a high maintenance condition with lots and lots of different kinds of symptoms. There's no way to just take a pill to make it go away, even for a little while. Sometimes a certain medication can make some of my symptoms more bearable. That's about the best I can hope for. Sometimes I can take a lot of medication and still not feel any better. That's just the way it goes.

There's no cure for fibromyalgia, it won't go away. If I am functioning normally, I am having a good day. This doesn't mean I'm getting better, because I suffer from chronic pain and fatigue for which there is no cure. I can have good days, weeks, or even months. But a good morning can suddenly turn into a terrible afternoon. I get a feeling like someone has pulled out a plug and all my energy has just run out of my body. I may get more irritable before these flares, and suddenly get more sensitive to noise, or just collapse from deadening fatigue. Other times there may be no warning, I may just suddenly feel awful. I can't warn you when this is likely to happen, because there isn't any way for me to know. Sometimes this is a real spoiler, and I'm sorry.

Fibromyalgics have a different kind of pain that is hard to treat. It is not caused by inflammation like an injury. It is not a constant ache in one place like a broken bone. It moves around my body daily and hourly and changes in severity and type. Sometimes it is dull and sometimes it is cramping or prickly. Sometimes it's jabbing and excruciating. If Eskimos have a hundred words for snow, fibromyalgics should have them for pain. Sometimes I just hurt all over.

Besides pain we have muscle stiffness, which is worse in the mornings. Sometimes when I get up out of a chair I feel like I'm ninety *years old. I may ask you to pull me up. I'm creaky and I'm clutzy. I trip over things no one can see, and I bump into the person I'm walking with and I drop things and spill things because my fingers are stiff or my coordination is off. I just don't seem to connect the way I should. Hand-eye, foot-eye coordination; it's all off. I walk slowly up and down stairs because I'm stiff and I'm afraid I might fall.*

Because I feel badly most of the time I am always pushing myself, and sometimes I push myself too hard. When I do this, I pay the price. Sometimes I can summon the strength to do something special, but I will usually have to rest for a few days afterwards because my body can only make so much energy. I pay a big price for overdoing it, but sometimes I have to. I know it's hard for you to understand why I can do one thing and not another. It's important for you to believe me, and trust me about this. My limitations, like my pain and my other symptoms, are invisible but they are there.

Another symptom I have is problems with memory and concentration, which is called fibrofog. Short-term memory is the worst! I am constantly looking for things I have no idea where I put, I walk into rooms and have no idea why. Casualties are my keys, which are always lost, my list of errands, which I write up and leave on the counter when I go out. Even if I put notes around to remind myself of important things I'm still liable to forget them. Don't worry, this is normal for fibromyaglics—most of us are frightened that we are getting Alzheimer's.

I mentioned my sensitivities earlier and I need to talk about them again. It's more like an intolerance—to everything. To noise, especially certain sounds like the television, or shrill noises. To bright lights, to fluorescent lights. To smells like fish or some chemicals, or fragrance or perfume. I also have a problem with heat and with cold. It sounds like I'm never happy but that isn't it. These things make me physically ill. They stress me out and make my pain worse, and I get exhausted. Sometimes I just need to get away from something, I just don't know how to say it. I know that sometimes this means I will have to go outside, or out to the car, or home to sit alone, and that's really all right. Sometimes when I feel lousy I just want to be by myself. When I'm like this there's nothing you can do to make me feel better, so it's just best to let me be.

I have problems sleeping. Sometimes I get really restless and wake up and can't get back to sleep. Other times I fall into bed and sleep for fourteen hours. I'm sure that's confusing to be around, and I know there are times when my tossing and turning and getting up and down to go to the bathroom disturbs you. We can talk about solutions to this.

All these symptoms and the chemicals in my brain can make me depressed, as you'd imagine. I get angry and frustrated and I have mood swings. Sometimes I know I'm being unreasonable but I can't admit it. Sometimes I just want to pull the covers over my head and stay in bed. These emotions are all very strong and powerful. I know this is a very hard thing about being with me. Every time you put up with me when I'm in one of my moods, secretly I'm so grateful. I can't always admit it at the time, but I'm admitting it now.

I have other symptoms like irritable bowel and pelvic pain that will take their toll on our physical intimacies. Some of these symptoms are embarrassing and hard to talk about but I promise to try. I hope that you will have the patience to see me through these things. It is very hard for me too because I love you and I want to be with you, and it makes everything worse when you are upset and tired of dealing with all my problems. I have made a promise to myself and now I am making it to you. I will set aside time for us to be close. During that time we will not talk about my illness. We both need time to get away from its demands. Though I may not show it always I love you a million times more for standing by me. Having to slow down physically and having to get rid of unnecessary stresses will make our relationship stronger.

IN A SENTENCE:

> *Don't be shy about sharing your fibromyalgia and your daily struggles with family and friends—they can support you in myriad ways that will help you maintain a normal life.*

WEEK **3**

living

The Impact of Stress

DESPITE WHAT you hear and may have read in the media, stress does not cause fibromyalgia. Let's be clear about that. It's true that stress influences and can exacerbate a wide range of health conditions and illnesses. But there are plenty of stressed people without fibromyalgia, and your stress probably got a lot worse after you got sick. Everyone experiences a certain level of stress in life that can't be avoided. So in order to better cope with your fibromyalgia, you must teach yourself to respond appropriately to what you can't change.

Stress will trigger a flare up

There are many kinds of stress and all of them will make your symptoms worse. While this is true for all illnesses, keep in mind your finite energy stores with fibromyalgia. Stress can't give you any illness, but it does burn up energy, and the more stress you experience, the more energy you burn. (Don't forget that the brain uses more energy than any other part of the body.) You know from experience that you don't have enough energy even to get through the day sometimes, so clearly almost any level of stress can trigger a flare.

The effect of stress is so profound that about 50 percent of fibromyalgics can actually identify a huge physical stress, such as a car accident, or a period of profound mental stress, such as a divorce, as the event that pushed them into active fibromyalgia. They rightly feel that after a specific trauma, they never felt well again. The honest truth is that no accident can give you fibromyalgia unless you were predisposed to get it. However, stress can make you many, many times worse and push you from borderline symptoms into incapacitating pain and fatigue.

Just being sick is stressful

The sad reality is that living with fibromyalgia is, itself, stressful. The early period just after diagnosis is the toughest because you have so much to learn and deal with. But the stress doesn't end there. You have an illness that changes from day to day, and things need to get done in a world that doesn't slow down when you can't walk very fast. Learning to accept and manage as much stress as possible will help you in your recovery process.

Stress is often defined as a perceived inability to deal with a difficult situation. Yet stress is also the body's reaction to change, which means that it can be a catalyst for new thinking and new behaviors. The challenge can be physical or mental—the definition is purposely broad. And, because each of us has our own perception of what a difficult situation is, what triggers stress is different for all of us.

It's hard to separate fibromyalgia from stress. It's stressful to be in pain, worse to have unpredictable symptoms like irritable bowel. In fibromyalgics, chronic pain (not freeway traffic) is the number one source of stress. That doesn't even take into consideration the stressfulness of the fact that you have had a complete change in your life from your fibromyalgia. What you used to do and what you want to do are often impossible. It's even more stressful to have cognitive problems and to push yourself through fatigue. Add to this the normal fibromyalgia symptom of anxiety and nervousness and you can see the problem. Even without any added stress you're using up a lot of energy that you can't spare. Here's what you should know: Stress is in the body and in the mind. It makes us feel anxious, short-tempered, and overwhelmed. It's a vicious cycle that makes every single symptom we have worse.

Stress causes chemical changes in your body

Stress causes your body to release adrenaline (epinephrine), and other hormones like **cortisol** and **growth hormone**, which result in a surge of energy, raised blood pressure, higher blood sugar, and a faster heart rate. Hormones are powerful and they reach every cell in your body. They are useful when you need all your strength for "fight or flight," but if they're released over and over they'll eventually cause exhaustion. A heightened state of alert burns up a lot of energy.

Our physical responses evolved to ensure the survival of the human race, however, they were designed as protective measures against physical challenges that occurred when our ancestors came across an enemy and had to fight hard or run fast. Today, we face so many challenges on a regular basis that our bodies are often in a constant state of stress and are repeatedly assaulted by these same powerful hormones that were meant to be released only intermittently. In our modern world we run late, get stuck in traffic, watch our children play sports, get angry with co-workers, have deadlines on projects, and always seem to need to be somewhere in a hurry. And all of these things take a physical toll on our bodies. Even healthy people are exhausted after a stressful day. For fibromyalgics it's much worse because we have no reserves.

When stress is chronic, certain symptoms develop rather routinely. These include loss of appetite, exhaustion, heightened sensitivities to pain and other stimuli, disturbed sleep patterns, anxiety, and lowered libido. In extreme cases memory loss, depression, and obsessive thought patterns can develop. Muscle tension occurs because of the state of alert in the body, and chronic stress causes chronic irritability. Stress also depresses the immune system, at least in part because of the release of some of the adrenal hormones.

Changing your attitude about stress

Of course you can't get rid of your problems just by wishing they'd go away. Often things are out of your control. Everyone's tolerance to stress is different (and inherited) and with fibromyalgia all of our abilities vary greatly from day to day. You certainly can't control the world around you. You can't always manage your fibromyalgia symptoms. All that's left to do is to work on your *response* to the stresses in your life, to accept what you cannot change. We all know people with "hair triggers" who hop up and want to fight at the slightest provocation. We also know mellow, laid-back people who don't get riled up very easily. That's the kind of attitude you have to adopt so you can conserve as much energy as possible.

As you know, stress causes a powerful physical response in your body. You can usually feel the surge of adrenaline that makes your heart pound and can make you feel focused and pumped up. You can even feel the acute response in the pit of your stomach when you get upset. Your muscles tense up and you breathe more quickly—the "fight or flight" symptoms caused by the adrenaline release. In those moments it's easy to feel how hard your body is working; it's revved up into overdrive. You can feel the burst of energy that your body is forced to summon up, and after it passes, you can also feel how much your energy reservoir has been drained. It's normal to collapse after a stressful encounter, and because you have so little energy it's even worse for you when it's over. That's why it's important to keep your body from reacting physically to the negative things that life puts in your path.

Don't use stress to create energy

There are some fibromyaglics, myself included, who have used stress to keep functioning. The adrenaline gives off lots of energy when it's released, so some of us procrastinate and put off deadlines until we are frantic and have worked ourselves into a state because we can't possibly do what needs to be done. When we get crazed, we can ride the adrenaline surge to get our work done. The problem with this is that while it certainly works in the short-term, in the long-term you're draining off energy you need to use for coping, healing, and surviving. Some of us become "adrenaline junkies." Like any other addiction, it's very hard to break the cycle, but it can be done. And it needs to be done. A repeated alarm will finally exhaust the body to the point of a breakdown.

IN A SENTENCE:

> *Stress is a strong emotion that depletes your energy stores and must be controlled if you want to feel better.*

learning

Managing and Reducing Your Stress

WHAT ARE some of the things that you can do to successfully manage everyday stresses? The first thing you have to do is to teach yourself to take things one day at a time. Remember that there is no way to completely rid your life of stress. Preserve your strength to deal with what you can't avoid, and let everything else go. Dwelling on things you would do over, or wish you could change, is stressful and will not help you cope with today. Worrying about things that may never happen is also not productive and hence another waste of energy. Accept your fibromyalgia, your limitations, and what your abilities are right now.

Negative emotions are a waste of energy

Do not punish yourself for things you can't do. Concentrate on the positive things in your life and don't feel sorry for yourself. If you're having a bad day, give yourself a break. Read a book, watch a movie, or listen to music. Break your usual pattern and take a vacation away from the thoughts that are bothering you. Negative emotions are more than a waste of energy; they keep you from the positive thoughts that will release endorphins to help you feel better. You can consciously force your mind away from the thoughts that are dragging you down, and you must do it each and every time your mind starts down the wrong path.

HERE ARE SOME TRIED AND
TRUE STRESS-BUSTERS:

○ **Set up a routine.** Stress blows out the body clock, so give yourself a definite schedule. Remember how comforting routines are to small children. They can be that way to you, even if it's on a subliminal level. Your body will fall into a pattern and know what to expect. Go to bed at the same time every day. Set your alarm for the same time every morning. Even if you can relax in bed on a weekend morning, do it consciously. Wake up at your regular time and allow yourself to snooze or lounge in bed. Take breaks at the same time during the day. It will take some time for you to reap the rewards of this regularity, so be patient. Going to bed at the same time every night won't guarantee that you fall asleep every night, but it will certainly increase your odds.

○ **Exercise regularly.** Three times a week for twenty minutes or more will cause your body to release endorphins. Exercise gives the chance to clear your mind and enjoy the moment. If you're having a particularly tough time with stress, get out of the house and take a longer walk. Don't go to crowded or noisy places. Some people walk in the malls for exercise, but don't do this when your nerves are already overtaxed. If you live near the beach, this is a nice time to walk along the water. You can also wear headphones and listen to music. Select this music carefully, something peaceful or classical. Consider one of those nature tapes that you can buy in almost any music store. The water and ocean sounds are the most relaxing for me. If you like to sing, do it. I love show tunes, and when I'm all alone and listen to my music, singing really helps take my mind off my stress by occupying it with something else.

○ **Distance yourself from the problem.** Walk away, or go outside, and cool off. Put the problem out of your mind until the next day. Consciously steer your thoughts to some other subject. If a problem is wearing at you, it never hurts to sleep on it.

○ **Practice talking yourself out of your angry response**. Remember that mistakes will happen, and that sometimes everyone is unreliable. Teach yourself to be more easygoing. Remind yourself that whatever your problem is, it isn't a matter of life or death, and your health is much more important. Concentrate on the fact that nothing matters as much as feeling well.

continued on next page

○ **Slow down your thinking.** Most of us over-respond to injustices in a staccato burst of emotions. The fact is that every issue can be broken down into small parts. Step by step you can figure out a healthy way to handle whatever the problem is. Pace yourself by breaking down your tasks. Writing an outline of what I am thinking about works for me. It forces me to think only as fast as I can write.

○ **Rest before you are exhausted.** If you do this you won't crash and pass out for twenty hours. Take short breaks and catnaps if you need them. Learn that even just lying down and closing your eyes for a few minutes can really help. Putting a hot or cold water bottle behind your neck can be very soothing.

○ **Meditation can clear your mind**. It has proven to be extraordinarily useful for coping with many illnesses, including serious ones, but you have to practice. The power of the mind is incredible and this is your chance to learn a little about it firsthand. If you're having a stressful day with anxiety that is affecting your nerves, find a private place where you can relax alone and meditate. You may not need to do it for long—just a break and a few minutes of deep breathing may be enough. Relaxation tapes are available, as are good books about meditation at most bookstores and many online vendors.

○ **Learn to relax**. Meditation can help, but relaxation is an art. The good news is that it really isn't hard to learn and it can make your down time, your breaks, or your rest periods much more restful. Practice relaxing your muscles one by one starting with your toes and ending with the top of your head. Do your best to consciously think about every muscle group.

○ **Don't consume caffeine.** Caffeine, either in a drink or in foods like chocolate, can make you jittery even when you aren't stressed. Avoid sugar for the same reasons.

○ **Don't smoke cigarettes.** Nicotine is a stimulant.

○ **Check the side effects of medications.** Many can make you feel jittery or nervous. If you find something that you're taking could be contributing to the problem, confer with your physician.

○ **Don't forget that herbal supplements and vitamins can make you jittery too.** Some of them like ephedra (Ma Huang) have been implicated in raising blood pressure.

Meditation

Don't dismiss meditation as something "New Age," "out there," or something you just don't have the patience or time to do. For centuries, all peoples have found meditation to be healing and restorative. It doesn't matter what you call it—prayer, meditation, "taking a time out," visualization, or dedicated time focusing on your own rest and relaxation—it's some of the most valuable time you'll spend. I don't think you can get control over your fibromyalgia without learning to do this. You must recognize when you need to clear your mind, and then have a technique in place to help you do it.

Find a quiet place

The first thing is to find a quiet spot where you can be comfortable and where you won't be interrupted or distracted. If you have a telephone within earshot, unplug it. If you can close doors, close them. Pull down shades, or draw curtains to make the room where you're going to relax more peaceful. Hang a DO NOT DISTURB sign on the door if you need to.

Find a way to meditate that works for you

Most people find that sitting is the most comfortable position, although cross-legged on the floor like you may have seen on TV may not be possible for you. Since your pain areas will shift, each time you meditate, you will have to find a pose that feels right.

Take slow, deep breaths, in through your nose and out through your mouth. Clear your mind and concentrate on relaxing your body, starting with your toes. If you have trouble keeping your mind blank (I often do), you can repeat a phrase over and over in your mind. This is called a mantra—and it doesn't have to be Tibetan or anything like that. It can be a nonsense phrase, a poem, or just any thought. You could just think: "I am relaxing," "Stress is not important," "I can feel the quiet around me," or any simple phrase that comes into your mind. You can also do this while you're walking: Concentrate on your breathing and your stride and a simple thought, keeping stressful thoughts out of your mind.

There are many kinds of meditation and you can learn about these from other resources. Some people like a guided imagery technique where you visualize yourself taking a walk, detail by detail, in a beautiful, magical place. There are deep-breathing techniques and simple yoga exercises. Whichever one is comfortable and seems best for you is the one you should work with. With fibromyalgia, quieting your mind and taking your thoughts away from your pain and obstacles is important.

Simple activities can help to clear your mind

Some people (like me) have a hard time sitting still when they're upset. It just isn't natural for me—I even have a hard time sitting still when I'm relaxed and tired. I've discovered that the best way for me to relax is to take a walk. Just a few blocks and, often in spite of myself, I unwind and feel better.

A warm shower is actually another kind of enforced break. It is relaxing and will give you a quiet and insular place to calm yourself down. You can just take a long shower, or follow it with some deep breathing, or have a cup of tea.

Stress and insomnia go hand in hand

Stress is also the number one cause of **insomnia.** It's stressful when you can't fall asleep and it's even more stressful trying to function the next day after you haven't slept. When your mind starts going round and round in circles, and you know you have to get to sleep now or tomorrow will be a wasted day, the stress mounts. Then, inevitably, you starting tossing and turning and you can't lie still.

You can't ignore insomnia, so don't try

Be diligent in addressing insomnia if you suffer from it. Try the usual things like making sure that you're physically comfortable, have had a bath, a warm drink, and/or whatever relaxes you. Allow your physician to help you with medications or other therapies if you still have problems getting your rest, because it's so very crucial to your health.

Learn about the various medications that can help

When you can't relax by yourself, there are muscle relaxants that might help you and can be taken as needed. Soma is fairly mild and helps with anxiety and the sensitivities to sound and light that stress makes worse. **Flexeril** is a slightly stronger option and it's related to the tricylic **anti-depressant** family and so it helps with serotonin levels. The sleep hormone melatonin is enough for some people and is available over the counter in various doses.

Don't dismiss over the counter sleep aids like the antihistamine **Benadryl,** the active ingredient for which is marketed under many brand names. Buy Benadryl in tablet form so you can tailor your dose. Most nights a very small amount will do the trick and leave you free of morning drowsiness. On other nights, if you are anxious or feeling jumpy, you could take more.

Prescription sleep medications can be double-edged swords

There are many prescription sleeping pills available. Some, such as **Ambien,** are designed to give you a full night's sleep, while newer ones like **Sonata** are used to get you back to sleep after early awakening. You will need to discuss prescription approaches with your physician, who can take into account whatever else you may be using. Always remember that any sleep medication will cause you to be more tired the next day, and that the weaker and shorter-acting the medication, the weaker and shorter the hangover. Bear this in mind because if you are stressed due to your fatigue, dragging around the next day may add to your woes. Sleep is important, but many sleeping medications can sap your already faltering energy levels the next afternoon. This is why prescription medications should be used as the last resort instead of the first solution. In Month 4, we will take a closer look at all the medications used for fibromyalgia's many symptoms including insomnia.

How to beat stress

Keep track of what's stressing you out. It might be going to the doctor, or being on time for work. It might be going to a social function, or dealing with certain family members. Things to look at as possible contributors to your stress are people (certain family members, co-workers), activities (going to the mall, driving in rush hour traffic), and health lows (such as a period of decreased energy).

Make yourself a list and on a day when you don't feel stressed, examine it. Look at each thing you've listed and think of ways to defuse the event. You might need to get up earlier, take a long shower, or rest in the afternoon, or have someone drive you places when you're tired. If you look at issues when you're not in the middle of them, you'll be able to find some solutions that may not be obvious when you're upset.

De-stress your home

Examine what is stressful at home. For example, I get stressed out when my house isn't clean. It starts slowly and then escalates out of control. I open the refrigerator and see some drips at the bottom, and then I see fingerprints on the door. Then I start noticing that the floor is dirty too, and there's dust on the windowsill. Then I look and see that the kitchen trash can needs to be scrubbed. Suddenly I feel overwhelmed with everything I need to do.

An obvious solution for me was to hire someone to do some of the work, because I couldn't teach myself to relax about what I couldn't get done. I had to be firm with myself and remind myself that there are cleaning services I could call to come in. The problem I had to overcome is that my mind doesn't work logically when I'm upset. When I get that way, even simple things seem like too much to do. I make mountains out of molehills. How can someone help me clean if they don't know where things belong? The house is too much of a mess to let anyone come in to clean. While I'm feeling overwhelmed by the negatives you can be sure that someone in my family walks in with something I need to take care of now, and pow! Instant stress overload. So by committing to have someone come in once a month to do the heavy cleaning I have taken away a bigger problem—my overload, as well as getting the heavy cleaning done. Remember the parable about the straw that breaks the camel's back, and don't let your stresses stack up.

Triggers lurk in everyday places

Look closely at your everyday routines. See what triggers you can identify—what daily occurrences are likely to make you feel overwhelmed. For example, the day can get off on the wrong foot if you have problems getting your children to school. When you've identified a stressful part of your day, dissect the tasks involved so you can find ways to make them less difficult. Breaking things down into individual components when you aren't upset can be a big help.

You know the rush of adrenaline when something goes wrong in the morning, like when you oversleep or when your child can't find a shoe and you're late. Rushing to deal with this situation can leave you exhausted for hours, causing you to collapse when you get back home, and throwing off the rest of the day. There are things about this routine that you can change. Get your children into the habit of laying out their school clothes the night before. Supervise them in packing up homework before bed. If you have them put their backpacks in the kitchen or front hall before they go to bed you will see them there in the morning and know the job is done

Find ways to divide the tasks *between night and morning*. On your weekly check sheet of things to do, make a note to check their assignment sheets every Monday to make sure that no school project is going to get sprung on you at the last moment. Things like this can make for a lot less stress on a daily basis.

Take control of your responsibilities

Draw fair but nonnegotiable lines. It is absolutely in the best interests of all the people around you to understand what is and is not possible. For example, you might make a rule that if your child doesn't tell you about needed school supplies before five P.M., he'll have to do without them until you can take care of the problem. If a person dropping by your house unexpectedly is stressful, make sure you've told your friends to call first because of your health. If there's a specific time of day when you take a nap, tell everyone who calls you routinely not to call at that time. If you have family members that want to visit and you don't feel up to it, be firm. Compromise and meet them at a restaurant for a meal so you don't have to clean your house or shop for refreshments. Practice not being embarrassed because you can't do things other people can.

Get away from it all

Don't forget about distraction. Getting out and getting away are great stressbusters. You may not even realize how stressful it is to sit at home because it's usually part of an underlying layer of stress. All around you are things you should do, haven't done, need to do. And then the phone rings. Getting away for even a day can be incredibly restful. Sometimes local hotel chains have very reasonable weekend rates. Pick one with a Jacuzzi and check in overnight. If it's summertime and it's hot at your house, consider spending the weekend in an air-conditioned hotel. When there's nothing to do but relax, you'll have to relax. I know this is easier said than done. It's hard to force yourself to walk away from everything that you have to do. But you can, you really can. The things you have to do will wait for you. There is almost nothing that can't wait twenty-four or forty-eight hours—and that won't be easier if you tackle it in a more rested state. You don't have to drive far to get away, either. Look around your own area or in the travel section of your local paper for ideas. The Internet is a great place to find last-minute travel deals.

Don't forget laughter and friendships

This one is so important: Stay involved with family, friends, and support groups. Enjoy their company and interactions. Laughter will relax you, and cause you to release endorphins. True friendships will sustain you and comfort you in many ways. Resist the temptation to turn inward and believe that you have nothing to offer other people because of your illness.

At the same time it's necessary to step back from your relationships and look at them carefully every so often. It's important to identify things that drain your energy. Of course all relationships are give-and-take, but if the balance shifts and it's all give on your part, realize this. If the relationship is important, limit the time you spend with this person for now. Recognize that the best way to be a good friend is to stay centered and be in the best emotional shape that you can be.

Goals are important, too

Goals are like the horizon. You have to keep your eye on where you need to go and what you want to accomplish for yourself. Learn to set realistic goals for yourself. Take into consideration what suits your symptom level. Break each task down into parts and schedule a reasonable amount of work for each day. If you can do more than you've set aside, so much the better. Give yourself positive reinforcement.

Start projects early and teach your children the benefit of doing the same. If your health will not permit you to stay up all night desperately trying to finish building a dinosaur model from toothpicks—don't do it. There's a reason why a term paper is called a term paper. It wasn't meant to be written in one night. Your kids will thank you when they get to high school or college. Cramming is a not a healthy habit for anyone.

You must draw the lines and stand behind them

Be clear about your limitations when you have co-workers and others who expect things from you. Do not be talked into doing more than you can do. Explain the unpredictable nature of your symptoms and be firm. You are the one who must learn to say no and mean it. You are the one who has to take care of you. You won't be able to fulfill any obligations or help with any extra tasks if you don't do that first.

If you have a problem with someone, do the best you can do to resolve it, but recognize that you can't always do this. Don't let the situation brew in the back of your mind. If you make a mistake, apologize. Then let things go. Don't replay scenarios in your mind or try to convince people of your point of view. This will drain your energy quickly and serves no purpose.

Don't fall into a holiday trap

Holidays are stressful times. They can be difficult even for healthy people who feel overwhelmed without the added burden of unpredictable symptoms. This is where your practice of setting goals will really pay off.

Divide your tasks up into reasonable portions and stick to your list. If small, quiet holidays are the most you can manage, don't be pressured into changing your mind. Women, especially, are conditioned to believe that they must put together a great holiday. Don't fall into this trap. Share the burden of organization and preparation with your family members. You don't have to do everything yourself. Martyrdom is stressful; it takes a lot of energy to keep resentment going. Remember the saying about how many muscles it takes to smile and how many it takes to frown? Not only does it take less energy to go with the flow, but happy thoughts and good times will stimulate endorphin release and increase your sense of contentment and well-being.

Stresses at work

This isn't exactly a news flash, but *work can be very stressful.* Take all your scheduled breaks whether you feel like you can skip them or not. Get up and stretch. Walk outside and let the sunlight hit your face for fifteen minutes. Fresh air is good for you. Being away from the sound of telephones and office machinery will refresh you.

Examine your work area for causes of physical stress. Holding your body in an uncomfortable position will burn energy you don't want to waste on this. If you need a letter from your doctor to get a comfortable chair or computer screen, be sure to pursue this. Sometimes it's worth it to spend your own money if you have to. Footstools and armrests can often help. Telephone headsets can be very helpful if you tend to crook your neck around the phone. Look carefully at anything that feels uncomfortable to you and see how often you do it. If it's a routine task, look at a way to solve the problem. Physical tension and discomfort can make you much less able to cope with other things.

If your job includes tasks you can do at home you might be able to negotiate a slightly more flexible schedule in terms of when you need to be in the office. If your home is quieter or more comfortable it may be easier to get things done there when you are anxious or edgy during a flare. Distractions and noise around you can really get on your nerves and hinder your ability to concentrate. Talk to your supervisor or employer and ask for some trial tasks that you can try to complete at home.

It's important to your health to get outside

Some fibromyalgics suffer when they aren't exposed to enough daylight to help set their body clocks. If you're inside most of the day during the week, make a point of getting out and sitting in the daylight or taking a walk without sunglasses during your lunch hour or during a break. If you can determine that this makes you feel better and more cheerful but you live where winter is long and dark, consider daylight spectrum florescent light bulbs at home or at work. Some physicians will write prescriptions for light boxes that have been helpful for many fibromyalgics.

Learn to filter out noise

Noise makes stress worse. If you're out of sorts or having a tough time, close doors or wear earplugs. I have some rubbery ones I can wear even at the office to muffle the noise. I can still hear people around me, but it takes the edge off of the sound. It's abundantly clear to me that when I'm stressed out, noise can make me frantic and tip me over the edge. Some people also use headphones to listen to gentle or relaxing music.

Eat well

Good nutrition will help with all your symptoms including stress. Eating sugary or starchy junk food can provide instant energy, but it's false energy and you may be jittery and more nervous as a result. Many, if not most overstressed people abuse sugar to make themselves feel better. **Carbohydrates**, sugars, and starches pump you up by raising your blood sugar, a process that starts almost the second you put them in your mouth. The problem is that when your blood sugar rises it must also fall. The sleepiness or exhaustion that hits you in the middle of the afternoon can be often be traced to a heavy lunch. If your energy drops around the same time each afternoon, try eating more protein and skipping the heavy starches at lunch.

Some foods may make you feel better because they can increase your serotonin levels, which is itself a stress-buster. Both meat and vegetables contain this compound, but it's actually better absorbed from vegetables because meat contains many other amino acids. This is just another way that eating right helps you with your fibromyalgia. Warm milk is an old folk remedy that may really help you relax.

You must take control
to be successful in fighting stress

The most important and most fundamental key to fighting off stress is to take responsibility for yourself and your illness. Counting on other people is stressful. Use your family and friends to help you when you need it (learn to ask for favors in advance and express your gratitude), but in the end you must learn to count on yourself. I know many people whose major underlying stress is the fear that their partner will leave, or simply not be there to take control when things get difficult. There's nothing to do for this except to fortify yourself and learn to speak up and express your feelings. You have to take responsibility for as much as you can. You must count on yourself to say no when you need to, and to understand how to protect yourself. A preemptive strike against the things that cause you to feel stressed is the way to begin. It's like the old saying: "The best offense is a good defense."

Stress can't be vanquished in a day. It will take an ongoing, conscious effort to simplify and control what you can, and to let the rest go. Don't beat up on yourself when you fail, just resolve to handle the situation better the next time you are faced with it. Every day will always be a new challenge with fibromyalgia, but you can do it. Just take it one step at a time, one hour at a time, one day at a time.

IN A SENTENCE:

> *Stress will make everything about fibromyalgia worse, so it is imperative that you find healthy ways to reduce the stress in your life.*

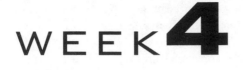

WEEK 4

living

Exercise Can Heal You

YES, YOU'RE tired. And yes, you ache. Undoubtedly, you won't be able to tackle your gym's new power spinning class or sign up for the local 10K run. But that doesn't change the fact that exercise is essential to your well-being. More than any other thing that you can do for your fibromyalgia, exercise will help you to lead a more normal life. If you've ever wished for something you could do to change the face of your illness and its effects on your life—the answer lies here.

The strong case for exercise

Exercise releases endorphins (the body's natural painkillers), relieves stress, helps you to maintain your weight, strengthens your muscles, protects your bones, and makes a healthier heart and lungs. Not only that, exercise will give you more energy and will also help you sleep better. Back in 1904, Sir William Gowers prescribed "perspiration" (or exercise) for his patients because in his experience it worked better than painkillers, a fact that has been corroborated over the years by many studies. The evidence is overwhelming that exercise will help you feel better. Yet most of us fight it tooth and nail. I know this because I did: tooth, nail, and with both hands and feet. I was dragged kicking and screaming to exercise, and I still don't love it. But like many other fibromyalgics, I do it. I'm a believer—I know it does what it's supposed to do.

Exercise is probably the last thing you feel like doing

When you don't feel well, exercise feels impossible. You feel like you are using every bit of your strength just to drag yourself through the day. Get up and exercise? You've got to be kidding. Just getting out of bed and taking a shower is tiring. Yet impossible as it seems, it is not impossible. Exercise is an essential part of any strategy to improve your health, no matter what your problem is or how many problems you have. It will work to your benefit to begin at any age, and any activity is better than none at all.

I used to firmly believe that doctors told people with fibromyalgia to exercise because they knew that they couldn't. Then, when these same folks came back complaining they still felt terrible the doctor had a trump card.

"Did you exercise this month?"

"No."

"Well then, how can you ever expect to feel better?"

I used to pump myself up telling myself that this exercise scheme on the part of doctors was unfeeling, guaranteed to make us feel worse and to give them a way out when they couldn't help us.

Observing the benefits

As I read more and more about the what exercise could do, and as I got to the age when the hot flashes started and I had to think about saving my bones, and when I began to gain weight (despite my best intentions), I took another look. I observed the people who came into our office—the ones who exercised and the ones that "just couldn't." I looked at people my parents' age—those that had stayed active and those who were couch potatoes. That's where the real dramatic difference lies. While there may be no evidence that exercise lengthens life spans, it certainly improves the quality of whatever time you have. Grudgingly, I came to the conclusion that I had to get up and get with the program. The one and only person I had to do it for was myself. I could no longer con myself into the notion that walking around the supermarket once a week or across the field at my son's football games would do the trick. Now I walk regularly and I know that the benefits are perhaps just as much mental as physical. It's no small matter that I really feel good about what I'm doing for my health. In this chapter I hope to persuade you to be as active as you can.

• • •

Even a little bit of exercise will do a lot for your health

The good news is that you don't have to do a lot of exercise to reap significant benefits. Many large studies have confirmed that regular moderate activity is nearly as beneficial for your health as the high-level stuff. So if you're not at least doing vigorous walking, that would be a great place to start, and you only need to build up to thirty minutes a day, or an equivalent amount done less frequently. This means that most people should have no difficulty working up to this level, and that the health benefits of exercise are within your reach.

You'll find that strengthening your muscles and increasing your endurance pays off in many ways. It not only releases endorphins, it causes hormonal changes in women, which helps balance their monthly cycles, improves the delivery of oxygen to the muscles, and helps clear waste products from the cells. A study in 2002 showed that regular exercise may even have an effect on raising **growth hormone** levels in women with FM.[1]

KATE'S STORY

I have had insomnia since I was a child, and we all know that getting good sleep is essential to our recovery. I have tried many substances to help me sleep, including Ambien, Restoril, Xanax, Flexeril, Benadryl, Melatonin, Calms Forte, Valerian, calcium, and magnesium. The only thing that has helped me consistently and measurably is aerobic exercise. It doesn't take much—a minimum twenty minutes a day, three days a week, preferably in the afternoon and well before bedtime.

"Aerobic" doesn't mean you pant and sweat and jump around, it just means your heart rate has increased. I don't even need to reach my "target heart rate" or take my pulse. I just walk or swim (warm pool, please!) until I am breathing a little harder. Since I started exercising regularly, I sleep soundly and sometimes don't even roll over more than once in the night! A big change. If I don't get my aerobic exercise, my insomnia comes right back, and the pain and fibro-fog increase the next day.

A portion of my twenty to thirty minutes "exercising" is actually spent stretching, since I can't go for more than a few minutes without stopping to stretch out a painful spot, but the exercise is still enough. And of course I always stretch a bit before I start and after I stop.

I never feel like I WANT to exercise—I'm always tired and in pain and often depressed. But I know I'll feel worse if I don't, so I do. It helps if I can get someone to walk or swim with me, but I usually can't, so I go by myself anyway.

I hope some of my fellow FM'ers will consider this and give this "good medicine" a try.

Love,
Kate

Rome wasn't built in a day— Start at a reasonable pace

You can and should start slowly. Do not strive to do too much at first, despite your good intentions, because it's easy to set yourself up for failure if you're overly ambitious. Remember, no effort is too small at the start. Now may not be a good time to join a gym or sign up for an aerobics class at the local park. This kind of overoptimism could defeat you. If you're not able to keep up, that could give you an excuse to feel like a failure and quit.

If you've exercised in the past, if you used to run marathons in your pre-fibromyalgia days, be sure to read this chapter carefully. Don't think that you can skip it because you know how to train and you know about exercise. In fact, it may be harder for you to figure out what to do simply because the rules have changed now that you're sick. You need to learn to hold back and do less so you won't be exhausted. You won't bounce back the way you used to. The purpose of exercise is to feel better, and it must be done differently when you have fibromyalgia.

How far you take your exercise regimen is up to you

When you get to the point where you've built up some endurance and you are enjoying exercise, you can think about making it official by joining a gym or an exercise class. Not everyone gets that far. Some people will continue at a moderate pace and won't graduate to that next level. If you decide you want to progress to aerobics, be sure to select the low-impact variety because you need something less jarring than the traditional type. Classes are held in many places, such as gyms, colleges, and local park and recreation centers. You can probably get information through The Arthritis Foundation for especially gentle classes (sometimes for senior citizens). Water aerobics is a nice addition to other activities and is gentle on the joints. Check out the For Further Information section for a list of videotapes you can purchase. Some video rental places even have tapes you can look at and try before you buy.

Remember that you can tailor an exercise program to any condition, and start at any level you need to. Robert Atkins, M.D., the cardiologist and diet guru, says, "If you still have the use of your limbs, you can exercise."

Take small, positive steps to start

In the beginning it's not a good idea to set a certain amount of time as a goal. Thirty minutes can seem like thirty hours if you haven't slept in two nights and your feet hurt. Checking your watch will really be discouraging. So don't start with thirty minutes. Start with a reasonable distance. Down to the corner and back, around the block, over to the park—whatever distance seems within your reach in the beginning. Something is better than nothing, and doing something enough times will teach you that you can do anything. Remember to stretch your muscles before you start any sort of exercise, and be sure to respect your body when it signals a different kind of pain than you're accustomed to experiencing.

Walking

For fibromyalgics (and most everyone else, too) the best exercise to begin with is probably walking. It's a lot safer for your joints than running. Though a warm pool and water aerobics may seem more inviting, swimming should be done only in addition to a walking program unless you have something seriously wrong with your legs or back, that is, something other than fibromyalgia. The reason I'm saying this is that weight-bearing exercise is important for women, especially during perimenopause or menopause and after. Women start losing bone mass at around age thirty-five. Though there are now some medications available that can build back some of the bone lost, they are expensive and have side effects. They also have not been on the market long enough to determine their long-term effects. Weight-bearing exercise will help you keep your bone mass. The same is true in men, for although osteoporosis is less common in men, it does exist. You will notice that men can also have the bent over, stooped look of osteoporosis and lose height as they age.

Make your routine easy

It is, however, important that you select a form of exercise that appeals to you. For most people it's harder to get motivated if they have to get dressed and drive to a gym and avoid the times when it's crowded with enthusiastic young people trying to impress each other. It's too easy to postpone the trip and to make excuses. That's why walking around where you live is a good way to start. If you live in a climate where walking outdoors isn't feasible year-round you might consider investing in a low-intensity exercise videotape so you can work out inside your home. You might also want to try a treadmill or an exercise bike. Before you purchase any equipment, rent it for a while and see if you like it. And because most people don't take this advice, you can also find used equipment of every description in your local paper or online for very reasonable prices.

Consider how you feel

If you decide to start with walking, you won't need any special equipment, you won't have to pay a fee, and you can just get up and get started without any preparation or fanfare. Each day you can tailor your distance to your physical abilities. You can do it alone if you feel like being alone or you can do it with a friend as a scheduled event. The latter is an excellent idea for at least one or two days a week. My friend Gwen comes to my house every Saturday morning for our long walk—we motivate each other to keep this schedule and it really helps. I look forward to seeing her, and it forces me to get out of bed. Other days I may go alone or with someone in my family. If I walk to the store for groceries I take my son to carry them back. If you decide to carry a few things, use a backpack because it will be much easier on your body than carrying shopping bags.

Pace yourself

With fibromyalgia, pacing is always the key to every endeavor. Even though you can push yourself to do more, don't do it. Your goal should be, in the beginning, to walk at least every other day. This keeps your muscles from tightening up too much and will actually make exercise easier. Remember that if you overdo it, muscle soreness will not appear until twenty-four hours following the activity and peaks between two and three days later. Fatigue, of course, will occur sooner. A good workout will release enough endorphins to last twenty-four hours. This is why small walks more frequently is more beneficial for out-of-shape muscles. If you find you're too sore to walk when the next scheduled day arrives, you'll know that you did too much. But always start out anyway. Fifty percent of the time you'll feel better once you get started and can talk yourself into continuing. The other half of the time you'll know it's just too much and you can do a little less. Sometimes if you feel achy, a warm shower before you head out can loosen you up, especially in cold weather. Be realistic, though, and understand that you will have setbacks and that you won't progress in a straight line to feeling better. You will move forward, though, if you stick with it.

It's crucial to warm up slowly

Before you start your exercise, you'll want to do some gentle warm-up stretching. Fibromyalgic muscles are tight so they're vulnerable to strains and sprains. Warming up means starting at a slower than usual pace. This allows your body to switch from **anaerobic** to **aerobic** exercise comfortably and smoothly. You don't want to contend with muscle cramps. So for the first five minutes of your walk, go slowly. If you're swimming or riding a bicycle, the same applies.

Track your progress

Keep track on a little calendar or jot down on a sheet of paper how long you've walked each day. This way you'll be able to see when you've done too much and suffered for it the next day. You'll also see how your workouts lengthen until you reach your goal. Concentrate on building up the duration of your exercise before increasing the intensity. When you reach the point where you are exercising the optimum amount, it will be up to you to decide whether to do more or just keep it up. You could graduate to a low-impact aerobics class, for example. Thirty minutes of moderate exercise a day will give you the benefits you need for your general health, but bear in mind that is the minimum amount of time.

Once you have established your exercise program, it gets easier to continue. Your body will reward you by producing endorphins, your muscles (including your heart) will get stronger, and you will feel better and more competent. Succeeding at something as difficult as exercise, especially when you're tired and achy, will certainly improve your attitude.

Balancing your exercise routine

There are two basic types of exercise, and eventually you'll want to try to do both on a regular basis, although the regular basis for some things might be once a month. Aerobic exercise is the activity we started with because it makes your **cardiovascular** system stronger. Your body requires extra oxygen for this kind of work, requiring your heart to beat faster and pump more blood around your body. The more you exercise, the more efficiently your body will learn to deliver this extra oxygen, and will strengthen your heart muscle. This type of exercise is what builds **stamina**, which becomes very important when you need to function and you don't feel well. Walking, running, and swimming are examples of aerobic exercise.

Anaerobic exercise is the short, intense type of activity that doesn't require extra oxygen—there isn't time to get it from your lungs to your muscles. Instead it uses the small amount of fuels stored within the muscles. Weightlifting, push-ups, sit-ups, and short sprints are examples of anaerobic exercise. This is the kind of exercise you might want to do later on, when you feel better, to build or tone muscles for a better appearance. If you bear in mind the distinctions between the two types of exercise you'll understand why you need to warm up before you start a session. If you start too vigorously you'll be doing anaerobic exercise—and you'll get tired very quickly. This is because it makes time for the increased oxygen you're consuming to get to your muscles. It takes a few minutes for the body to switch into the aerobic mode where sustained exercise is easily fueled by oxygen, and after twenty minutes, fat.

Flexibility exercises

You may also want to work on improving your flexibility if your muscles get stiff. You should have a stretching routine for the times when your muscles tighten up. Some people do gentle stretching just before bed and in the morning after a hot shower. They find this makes them much more comfortable during the day. Another good time for gentle stretching is after aerobic exercise, because your muscles are already warmed up.

Stretch your muscles carefully

The more stretching you do, the more you'll lengthen your muscles. You should aim to stretch at least four times a week. All stretching movement should be done very slowly to the point where you feel gentle tension. When you feel this tension you should start to work up to holding this position for thirty seconds. Do not bounce when you stretch because this will trigger your muscle to contract. If you feel sharp pain, ease up a little, and stop the stretch that is hurting you if necessary.

You must take charge of your exercise program

The truth is you can do more to relieve your fibromyalgia than any doctor. Exercise is one modality that, if done correctly, will improve the quality of your life. Healthy exercise is not a high-maintenance endeavor; it is a process that you can tailor to suit your abilities, and meld into the time you have available. If you want to feel better, you have to do it. Working with others in your support group or in special classes is a good way to feel solidarity and companionship on your journey with a chronic illness. But the beauty is that you can do it any way you like. If you prefer to work alone, that too is an option.

IN A SENTENCE:

> *Exercise is one of the most important things you can do for your health when you have fibromyalgia.*

learning

Planning Your Exercise Regimen

NOW THAT you understand the basics of what you need to do, let's look at the practical application. By now you should have selected which exercise you'd like to do — walking, cycling, or swimming, for example, and know that you're going to start with an eye toward building up to thirty minutes or more at each session. To prevent burnout, or overwork, I suggest planning your workouts ahead for the week. This will ensure that you don't overdo it one day and then have to skip the rest of the week.

You can start by walking out the door

Personally, I believe that walking is the best place for fibromyalgics to start. It is probably well within your physical capacity to walk at least a short distance, and it provides most of the health benefits you're looking for. But if you've selected swimming or bike riding, all of this information applies as well.

Again (and I can't emphasize this enough), start slowly. You need time for your tendons and bones to respond to their new workload. Trying to go too far too fast is the number one reason people conclude that exercise is too hard and they can't do it. It's also the easiest way to get injured. Start with something small that you can reasonably accomplish. You're going to have fibromyalgia your whole life and you're always going to need to stay active, so you have plenty of time to work up to where you need to be!

Create a reasonable workout schedule

You'll have to decide if you want to start with a once-a-day session or you want to break your exercise into shorter twice-a-day sessions. There are benefits to both. Once a day might be more convenient time-wise for you. For example, since I drive my kids to school early in the morning, the morning isn't a good time for me to get out and do anything. If you work, your lunch hour might be a time that's all yours that you could set aside to take a walk. This might be the best time of day to take a break and stretch your muscles. In summer, if it's hot, you might want to walk right after you get home in the evening. Whatever you decide, it's best to make a schedule and stick to it. Fibromyalgic bodies do best on a schedule, and if you set a regular time you won't have to figure out a way to fit it in every day when it's so much easier to postpone it or make an excuse.

How to increase your activity level

Most people can work their time up in weekly increments. If this seems like too much when you look at your exercise sheet, try two-week increments. Your schedule might look like this (or you might start out with much less time, like five minutes a day).

WEEK ONE: Walk 15 minutes a day (or ten minutes twice a day)
WEEK TWO: Walk 20 minutes per day (or twelve minutes twice a day)
WEEK THREE: Walk 25 minutes per day (or fifteen minutes twice a day)
WEEK FOUR: Walk 30 minutes a day (or twenty minutes twice a day)

NOTE: *The divided times are slightly longer because they are shorter, and you want to make sure to get your heart rate up to the point where your body will reward you with endorphin release.*

If you can't walk every day, then, for example, you could do three sessions a week and modify the times by adding them together. To do this it will take you longer to build up, but speed isn't the object. The object is to get to the point where your body will respond and you'll get the benefits you need. So you could start at fifteen minutes a day every other day or every third day. In the beginning, though, my suggestion is to walk a little bit every day to keep from getting too stiff or overwhelmed. Once you've

Walking/Exercise Tips

○ Wear comfortable well-fitting sneakers with socks.

○ Stretch lightly before your walk or activity and during if your muscles stiffen up or feel tight.

○ Go slow for the first five minutes each session so your muscles can warm up.

○ Slow down again three to five minutes before you stop so your muscles can cool down.

○ Carry water or a sports drink with you when you walk. Time your walks so you can take any medication more than an hour before you begin.

○ If you're walking alone or with someone else who isn't in excellent shape be sure to carry a cell phone so you can call for help if you need to. Some people like to carry pepper spray in case of emergency, such as encountering an angry dog.

○ Watch for warning signs that you're overdoing it (see warnings, below) and employ the "Conversation Test"—you should be able to breathe comfortably and carry on a conversation without gasping for air.

reached your target you can easily switch to an hour three times a week and leave it at that.

When to increase the intensity

Once you reach the optimum amount of exercise time, you should work on the intensity. You could try to walk a little farther in the same amount of time, for example. Most of us who walk regularly have a general route we take. I have a long walk, a regular walk, and a short walk for the days I just can't push myself the whole way. The long walk is what I aim for on weekends, and I try to do it in the same amount of time as my regular walk because it means I am going faster. Slow down if you get out of breath, or if your heart is pounding uncomfortably. Once again there's no benefit in pushing yourself too hard, only negative effects, because it will make you too exhausted for your next session. And every time you miss a session it's harder to force yourself out the door for the next one.

Try other disciplines for variety

Other weight-bearing options you may want to consider are yoga and Pilates, both of which focus on muscle strengthening, balance, and agility.

These require some study, but they offer many benefits. You may even find that your insurance company will pay for instruction. See Month 5 for more information.

Increasing intensity of exercise will benefit you

Once you are regularly exercising and meeting your goals in terms of duration, you can look at intensity if you want to get more physically fit. If you work up slowly, this is not a pipedream. Walking on a treadmill at a moderate pace can produce a good cardiovascular workout if you stick with it. To get the optimum benefit from your exercise, you'll want to aim for an increase of between 60 and 80 percent of your maximum heart rate. This number is calculated, and it's easy to figure out. You simply subtract your age from 220. If you are fifty years old, subtract 50 from 220 and your maximum heart rate would be 170. Your target would be between 80 percent of that number and 60 percent of that number or between 136 and 102 beats per minute. This means that you want to keep your pulse between 136 and 77 beats a minute. When you start out, keep your pulse at the lower end. Work up to a heart rate at the high end of the scale and concentrate on keeping it there. Take your pulse each time you finish exercising to see how well you've done.

Weight training

Working with weights is called resistance exercise, and it increases muscle strength and mass, which will help you lose weight and look better. There are internal benefits as well. Strong muscles hold the bones in place

---

Taking your pulse

PRACTICE FINDING the pulse in your wrist. The easiest place to feel your pulse is in your neck, so if you can't find it in your wrist you can always use the carotid artery on the front of your neck where your chin meets your neck on either side of your voice box. Use the pads of your fingers. Hold your right hand palm up. Place your left wrist on your right hand also palm up. The line where your wrist meets your hand should be parallel to your index finger. Now curl your index finger and your middle finger over the top of your wrist, just to the outside of the tendons there. Press in and you should feel your pulse. A little practice and you'll be able to do this easily, especially when your heart is beating more forcefully with exercise. What you want to do is count the number of beats in 15 seconds and then multiply by four to get your pulse rate, which is measured in beats per minute.

Warning signs that you should stop exercise:

○ Severe cramping or sudden stabbing pain in any muscle
○ Lightheadedness, feeling faint
○ Nausea with or without lightheadedness
○ Chest pain. If chest pain or discomfort in your chest, neck, throat, or left arm occurs, stop immediately. If this goes away within thirty seconds you may continue. If not, you should stop exercising and see your doctor right away. You may have coronary artery disease.

and this helps with posture and gait. The theory behind weight training is that when you work with weights you are putting more than the usual amount of strain on a muscle. This increased load stimulates the growth of certain proteins inside the muscle cell, which increases the muscle's force. Methods include use of free weights, weight machines, and **calisthenics**. The latter includes chin-ups, sit-ups, and push-ups—activities that use your own body weight as resistance. For women (and men) who are concerned with the loss of bone density, resistance training is very effective. Even people in their seventies or eighties can dramatically improve their strength and mobility with a proper program. This is why you'll see people walking with leg and arm weights. You can do this, or work with one of the many books or videos on the market for this sort of exercise. If you can do even one walking session a week with weights you'll notice a distinct difference within two months. Very light leg weights are the best to start with; you can get them in one- or two-pound increments. Arm weights may throw off your stride and will not do as much anyway. For arms you're better off doing some light exercises at home.

Begin very slowly

Fibromyalgics should start very slowly with weights. The best method is to use less weight and do more repetitions. This will increase your endurance and energy, which is the main purpose of the activity. Unless you're planning to become Mr. or Ms. Universe, there's no benefit to lifting huge amounts of weight, and doing so will increase your chance of a strain, sprain, or tear. You don't want to risk any serious injury that will cause a flare of your fibromyalgia and require time and energy to heal.

Sample Stretching Routine

NECK ROLL

Drop your chin to your chest. Stay in this position and feel the stretch in the back of your neck. Slowly roll your head to the right. Stay in this position and feel the stretch on the left side.

Roll your head to the front again. Now, roll your head to the left. Stay in this position and feel the stretch on the right side. **Do not roll your head backward! You could crush the vertebrae at the top of your spinal column.**

SHOULDER ROLL

With your arms relaxed at your sides, rotate your right shoulder backward in a circular motion. Be sure to complete the circle while keeping your arm straight at your side. Repeat the exercise with the left shoulder. Rotate both shoulders at the same time.

SHOULDER REACH

Hold your arms straight in front of you with palms facing each other. Interlace your fingers and rotate your palms so they face away from your body. Extend your arms forward until you feel a stretch in your shoulders and arms. Stay in this position for a few seconds, then relax.

VARIATION OF SHOULDER REACH

Raise your arms over your head with palms up. Push your arms upward and slightly behind your head. Hold on, then relax.

WRIST ROLL

Make a loose fist with your right hand. Holding your arm still, slowly rotate your hand in a circular motion at the wrist. Repeat the exercise with your left hand.

SHOULDER STRETCH

Stand with your feet slightly apart. Raise your right arm in front of you. Bending at the elbow, bring your right arm across your chest at shoulder level until you feel a slight pull in your shoulder. Gently apply pressure with your left hand at your right elbow. Stay in this position for a few seconds, then relax. Repeat the exercise with your left arm.

CHEST STRETCH

Stand just outside an open doorway (the doorway should be behind you) and face outward. Grab both sides of the door frame at chest level. Take a step forward and let your arms straighten behind you. Keep your head up and lean forward until you feel a stretch in your chest muscles. Stay in this position for a few seconds, then relax.

SHOULDER PULL

Stand just inside an open doorway (the doorway should be in front of you) and face outward. Grab both sides of the doorframe at the chest level. Lean back until you feel a stretch in your shoulder muscles. Stay in this position for a few seconds, then relax.

SIDE BEND

Stand with your feet apart, with knees slightly bent. Raise your right hand over your head and place your left hand on your left hip. Lean to the left, bending slightly at the waist. Stop as soon as you feel a slight stretch in your right side. Stay in this position for a few seconds and then slowly return to the standing position.

BACK ARCH

Stand with your feet slightly apart and knees slightly bent. Place your hands on the front of your thighs and bend forward slightly at the waist, without bending your back. Slowly inhale and arch your back. Stay in this position for a few seconds, then exhale. Straighten your back and return to the standing position.

BACK BEND

Stand with your feet slightly apart and knees slightly bent. Place your hands on your hips. Lean backward slightly. Be sure not to lean too far back! Stay in this position for a few seconds, then relax.

LOWER BACK

Lie on your back on the floor. Raise your right knee to your chest and hold. Raise your left knee to your chest and hold. Then put your arms around the back of both thighs and pull them into your chest.

CALF STRETCH

Stand facing a wall, with your feet about three feet away from the wall. Place your hands on the wall at about shoulder level. Keeping your feet flat on the floor, lean forward until you feel a slight stretch in your calves. Stay in this position for a few seconds, then relax.

FRONT THIGH STRETCH

Stand facing a wall, with your feet about three feet from the wall. Place your right hand on the wall at chest level. Bend your left leg backward. Use your left hand to grab the top of your left foot behind you. Gently pull your heel toward your buttocks. Stay in this position for a few seconds, then relax. Repeat the exercise with your right leg and hand.

LOWER BACK AND HIPS

Lie on your back with your knees bent and your feet flat on the floor. Rotate the knees to the right very slowly. Then rotate the knees to the left very slowly.

Water aerobics or aquatics

There are very few fibromyalgics who can't manage the amount of walking required for a basic exercise program. However, if you have post-polio syndrome, rheumatoid arthritis, or some sort of back injury or condition, walking may be too painful for you. Water exercise classes or swimming might be an answer. Though you won't get the same benefit for your bones, you will get the aerobic benefits to your heart and circulatory system, and endorphin release will occur. Water supports your weight—all but about 10 percent of it—and also offers some modest resistance. People who complain that they can barely even hold their arms up will find it much easier in water. In addition, water supports the spine and lower back if you have problems in this area.

The water you work out in should be chest high and warm (between 80° and 90° F). The Arthritis Foundation sponsors many water-based classes and they're usually inexpensive. You can also contact your local YMCA or any recreation center that has a heated pool to see what they offer.

Increase your range of motion

You should also do some gentle stretching to increase the length of your muscles and your range of motion. Most fibromyalgics are very stiff and a little stretching can help improve your posture and prevent injuries during more strenuous exercise. Just a few minutes a day can be very relaxing and helpful. You can do this on your own or you can purchase a stretching tape for fibromyalgics or attend a gentle class geared toward people with limited mobility. See the For Further Information section for information on where to find some good stretching tapes. A recent study in *The Journal of Rheumatology* showed that flexibility training alone results in overall improvement in fibromyalgics, although more benefit is seen when it's combined with other exercise.

You should plan to do a longer stretching session at least four times a week in a quiet place with shorter sessions at least once a day. Stretching should be done not only as the warm-up and cool-down parts of your workout, but also on days when you aren't doing any other exercise, or when you feel tight.

The basic rules of stretching

The basic rules of stretching are simple. Move slowly and gently, not vigorously or jerkily. When you've stretched to the point where you feel gentle pressure you must hold that position for three seconds breathing deeply and regularly. What you'll do as you progress is hold your stretch longer: first five, then ten, then fifteen seconds, until you work up to thirty seconds each. Start by doing just a few of each stretch, and gradually add to the number that you do.

○ Longer skeletal muscles need stretching the most.
○ Start with three repetitions per stretch and work up to more.
○ When your muscles are sore be very gentle and never work through intense pain. If something hurts in a way that you're not used to, ease back immediately.
○ Yoga exercises, which combine deep breathing with gentle stretching, are often very helpful to fibromyalgics.

IN A SENTENCE:

> It's important to remember that exercise is not a quick fix that will make you feel better right away, but something that you need to work at to increase the quality of your life.

FIRST-MONTH MILESTONE

It's been a month since your diagnosis, and you're beginning to get a handle on managing your fibromyalgia:

○ YOU HAVE LEARNED THE IMPORTANCE OF CARING FOR AND MAINTAINING YOUR EXISTING RELATIONSHIPS.

○ YOU KNOW THAT STRESS IMPACTS YOUR SYMPTOMS AND HOW TO MANAGE OR REDUCE IT ON A DAY-TO-DAY BASIS.

○ YOU UNDERSTAND THAT EXERCISE IS VITAL TO YOUR GOOD HEALTH AND YOU'VE BEGUN TO INCORPORATE IT INTO YOUR ROUTINE.

○ YOU BELIEVE THAT YOU ARE ON THE ROAD BACK TO GOOD HEALTH, AND IT'S A CHALLENGING JOURNEY BUT WELL WORTH THE EFFORT.

Working with Your Doctor

WHEN YOU have as many complaints as a typical fibromyalgic does, you definitely need a sympathetic, compassionate physician to work with you. You'll need someone to monitor your medications, answer questions about side effects, and rule out other problems when your symptoms flare up. It's very important not to assume that all your complaints are just another weird symptom of this mysterious illness. There are times when you'll need to make sure that nothing else is wrong. If you have a chronic illness, you are by necessity primarily in charge of your own condition, but you should not feel safe without a physician to support you. There are certain things that you will always know about yourself better than any doctor could, but there are important things that a doctor will know better than you do. You should not rely on support groups, Internet medical advice, or any book to take the place of a physician who can examine you when you need it. The problem is, it's not always easy to find a doctor you like.

Be your own advocate

Too often insurance policies tell us which doctors we can see and which ones we can't. Be sure that you know what your rights are according to your particular policy, and take the time to make the necessary appeals if you have to. If you have an exceptional physician in your area, you might consider paying out of pocket to go to him or her for periodic examinations. A reasonable compromise is to use your insurance-mandated physician for routine physicals, annual blood tests, medications, and any screening examinations you should have such as mammograms or prostate exams, and see a specialist if questions come up about your fibromyalgia. Make it clear when you see a doctor whom your insurance doesn't cover that you are paying out of your own pocket, and explain you'd like to come only when necessary. If you are honest and explain what it is that you need, you probably won't have a problem. Do not expect to get a discount for paying cash. This became illegal under the Kennedy-Kassembaum bill.

The best isn't always the most expensive

You don't need to see a physician of any particular specialty. A general practitioner should be able to handle prescribing medications and examining you to make sure you have no other medical problems. If you feel more comfortable with a specialist, that's okay, too. Specialists are often better informed on advances in particular areas, but you may find that they're more opinionated if you want to try something experimental. (Remember that I'm speaking in generalities and there are many excellent physicians in all fields.) The bottom line is that the important thing is to have a good relationship with the physician you select.

> **IT'S A** good idea to know which blood tests you need and how often you should have them done. You may find this information in the package insert that comes with your prescriptions. Especially if you are a member of a health maintenance organization (HMO), it isn't safe to assume that you're automatically getting the tests that you need. These organizations are cost conscious and it's important for you to be your own advocate.

Sometimes you need to be a patient *patient*

I work in the medical profession, and I can tell you that how you act is also important. When you find a good doctor, you'll want to make sure that you get off on the right foot. It's very easy to accuse a doctor of being too busy, or uncaring, but make sure that you don't contribute to the problem. Most doctors have many patients and are very busy. Good doctors have even more patients and are even busier. When you're eye-to-eye with the doctor, you don't want your time to be interrupted by phone calls or by people knocking on the exam room door. You don't want your time to be cut short because your doctor has to turn his or her attention elsewhere. Keep this in mind when you telephone the doctor's office, and make sure you are courteous and don't ask for instant attention for every symptom or concern that you have. Try not to be the patient who cries "Wolf," the one whose every symptom is an emergency. Be reasonable and be patient. When your concern isn't an emergency, allow the nursing staff to help you with general information and don't be mysterious. If you are going to leave a message for the doctor to call you, make sure your doctor knows what it's about. Calls need to be prioritized and doctors need to know how much time to set aside. If you're calling for general support, use the doctor's nursing staff. If you have a medical question, let the physician know what it is so he or she can have the resources ready to answer you.

Most doctors have the best intentions

I always tell people that doctors became doctors to help people, and by the way, I happen to believe this. Believe me, the money isn't all that good (unless you're a plastic surgeon to movie stars) and doctors work long hours and do a lot of unpleasant things you wouldn't want to do. (Trust me on this one, too.) Fibromyalgics tend to frustrate doctors simply because they have so many complaints and concerns, and nothing ever seems to help. You can help this situation if you take the time to thank the doctor for his or her effort and express gratitude for the things that do help you.

How often you go to the doctor may depend on your attitude

In Day 1, we talked a little bit about how to find a physician to treat fibromyalgia. But once you've found a doctor to help you, what should you expect from follow-ups, and how often do you need to make appointments? Part of the course will be steered by your physician, but since you're a partner in your health, you should have some input on this as well. Remember that individual doctors are different, as are individual fibromyalgics. Some people have lots of complaints and like to go to the doctor often, while others prefer to handle most things on their own, using a doctor only as a last resort.

How often your doctor will want to see you will depend on how many complaints you have, as well as the number of medications you are taking. Doctors are supposed to perform "good faith examinations" periodically, especially if they are prescribing new medications or making dosage adjustments. Expect that you will have to be examined at least once a year as a bare minimum and more often if you are taking medications that require blood tests or other evaluations.

When Your Symptoms
Aren't Caused by Fibromyalgia

HOW DO you know when to see a doctor? You have so many symptoms it's easy to assume a new one is just one more thing. But the truth is everything *isn't* fibromyalgia and assuming that it is can be dangerous. Here are some of the warning signs that you should have checked out:

○ Chest pain that gets worse with exertion, or crushing pressure that radiates down your left arm could signal heart problems.

○ Shortness of breath, wheezing, or a feeling that your airway is closing could be asthma.

○ Shortness of breath and a pulse rate that rapidly increases with exertion could be a coronary artery blockage.

○ A fever of over 101° F could mean a serious infection.

○ Red, hot, swollen joints may indicate gout or rheumatoid arthritis.

○ Blood in your stool, or dark tarry stool when you haven't been taking iron or Pepto-Bismol could be a sign of gastrointestinal bleeding.

○ Numbness, weakness, burning, or tingling of an extremity that does not change in intensity or location could be a nerve disorder.

○ Swollen glands that stay swollen could be a sign of infection or lymphoma.

○ Intense headaches in one area that affect vision, or any other sense, that does not let up could be a tumor.

○ Severe lower abdominal pain especially if accompanied by nausea, vomiting, and diarrhea, and rebound tenderness, which means that when you press anywhere in the abdomen it hurts. This could be appendicitis or diverticulitis.

○ Menstrual irregularities, excessive bleeding, or cramping could be a sign of hormonal problems, cancer, or **endometriosis**.

○ Any loss of bladder control or bowel control without cramps or urgency.

○ Skipping heartbeats that don't stop when you move around could indicate a heart problem.

○ Swelling of both ankles that when pressed on with your finger leaves an indentation could indicate heart failure or kidney problems.

○ Excessive thirst, urination, or frequent awakenings at night to urinate could indicate diabetes.

○ Unexplained weight loss could indicate various metabolic disorders.

○ Any loss of consciousness or strange sensation that is accompanied by slurring of speech or memory loss could be a transient ischemic attack.

○ A skin rash or discoloration that doesn't change could be lupus.

○ Any other symptom you are concerned about.

IF YOU haven't told your insurance company that you have fibromyalgia, should you? Many patients pay cash for all services related to fibromyalgia simply so that insurance companies will never carry that information in their files. More and more frequently insurance companies refuse to accept fibromyalgics, even for things like long-term nursing care coverage, and premiums for health insurance can go sky-high on individual policies. There is no simple answer to this question, but if you are insured on an individual policy and pay premiums out of your own pocket you might want to consider keeping your diagnosis a secret. You can do this if you see one physician only for fibromyalgia, and have another doctor to do your routine care. At the time of service for fibromyalgia-related issues you can pay cash so that insurance companies have no record that you have ever seen the physician in question. If you see one physician for all your other health care, when insurance companies request a copy of your records, this is what they will get. There will be no record in your files of fibromyalgia unless you have told your physician and he or she has written it down. So it's important to ask your doctor not to do that.

To make matters even worse, long-term disability insurance companies have begun a campaign to make it difficult for fibromyalgics. Even if you have a policy that you have paid into for years in good faith, they will try not to help you if you need it. It is to their advantage to insist that the disease and all of its variations stem from psychiatric disorders. If you've ever mentioned you were depressed or anxious it can be used against you. Insurance companies often have no difficulty in finding a psychiatrist who will agree that your problems are psychological. Since the vast majority of insurance policies do not cover mental disability beyond a specified time, there is a great deal of money at stake. Fibromyalgia cases have reached near epidemic proportions in the form of U.S. Social Security disability claims, workers' compensation, and accident litigation. This is being held against all of us. Do some shopping around and make sure the company you've selected is reputable. Support groups, including online message boards, are a good place to take a poll about which companies are best.

Monitoring your medications

It's an excellent idea to have one physician prescribe all your medications, and for that physician to also be aware of all the over-the-counter medications or supplements that you are taking. You should prepare an updated list to bring to each appointment. Include the milligrams of the medication and the number of times a day that you take it. Print or type this list up on a separate page so you can leave it for your file. New drug interactions and side effects of medications and supplements are being documented almost daily, so it's really a good idea to do this. Having all your prescriptions filled at the same pharmacy is also helpful, since pharmacists can often spot prospective problems. If you can't find one physician to do all your prescribing, then it's especially important for you to have a pharmacist you can trust. It's also a good idea to keep in your files a list of all the medications you've tried and how you responded to them. This will be very useful if you need your medications adjusted or modified. Remember that some medications are chemical cousins, so if you had a bad reaction to one member of the family you can save yourself some woe by not taking another related medication.

Keep track of when you have laboratory work done, and be sure to have it done at least once a year if you are taking medication of any kind. Even over-the-counter pain medications can cause abnormalities, so be sure that your physician refers to your list of them when blood tests are being ordered. Also make sure that you have received the results of all your tests—if you don't get a call within five days, it's a good idea to follow up. This is especially true if you use a laboratory that's separate from your doctor's office. You'll want to make sure that your results were actually received and reviewed. Doctor's offices can be busy, hectic places, so it's best to double check.

IN A SENTENCE:

> When it comes to your health you're in charge, so be your own best advocate.

learning

Follow-up Appointments with Your Doctor

WHEN YOU make a follow-up appointment with your doctor's office, be sure to ask how much time is being set aside for you. If it seems insufficient, you can request more. Don't suddenly arrive with a long list of concerns that can't be covered in the time you've been given. You should expect that your doctor will charge for this extra time, so if this is a concern, you should be sure to address it before you arrive for your appointment. If you want your doctor to read or review something beforehand, be sure to ask the staff if this is feasible and ask how long in advance the material should be submitted. If you'd like to discuss a new treatment or some research you've read about, you should check with the office staff to see if the doctor is aware of the study, and if not, you may want to supply a copy beforehand. It's never a good idea to arrive with a ream of paper and expect your doctor to read it while you are sitting there expectantly.

Your appointment was scheduled for a reason

When you go to see your doctor for a follow-up you should know why you are there. This should have been expressed to you at your previous appointment. For example, if you've just started on a new pain medication, your doctor may want to follow up with you in two months, possibly for blood tests. Thus, when you prepare for your follow-up, the first thing you should have ready for your doctor is a detailed description of what you've experienced and how you feel about the new therapy. If you have concerns, list them in the order of priority and mention them to your doctor one by one.

If you have something you want to discuss at your appointment, expect this to be the second thing you'll cover. Again, make notes and jot down the important parts of your doctor's advice. If you've just received a new medication, be sure you know how and when to take it, what to expect from it, and when your doctor wants to reevaluate you. Your notes might look something like this:

○ Reason for follow-up
○ Your input on this subject (what you have observed since your last appointment—be brief, an outline form is best)
○ Questions you need answered—any problems or concerns that have come up. Do you need to make a change?
○ Is there something your doctor can suggest?
○ What are the pros and cons of this suggestion (side effects, time it takes to see results, worst-case scenario, and best-case scenario)?
○ Is there anything your doctor wants you to watch out for?
○ When does the doctor want you to return?

The key to this format is to use an outline and keep each point concise. You will find that a little organization will pay off and make your appointments more fruitful. Don't be afraid to repeat instructions to make sure that you have them jotted down correctly. You don't want any misunderstandings. Some patients tape-record their office visits. If this is what works for you, ask your doctor to accommodate you.

Be organized

It may take some doing to find a physician you can work with, but if you are organized and centered and know what you need, it will be a lot easier. Be sure your doctor listens to you and takes your concerns seriously. If you use the above system to get organized, you'll be able to tell right away if your relationship is working the way it should. It won't be difficult to judge whether the doctor has answered your questions and listened to your concerns. You'll be able to see if your physician's instructions were clear and ideas were well thought out. Remember that listening is a two-way street, and that it's important you listen to each other's concerns. And always be honest. This will make it much easier for your doctor to help you and he or she will appreciate your honesty even if it isn't what he or she wants to hear. If you didn't do something you agreed to do, be sure to admit it, and ask for an alternative. Always remember that you are paying for the doctor's time and expertise.

Your medical records are your property

If you need to change from one doctor to another, you can get a copy of your records from your previous doctor to take with you. Your new physician may not need voluminous office notes scrawled in an unfamiliar handwriting, but copies of your blood tests or any other diagnostic tests need to be transferred. This may save you money down the line, as many tests do not need to be repeated. If you want to be even more thoroughly prepared, type up some brief one-page outlines of the development of symptoms and what you are doing for them and add them to your file as a quick reference for your new physician.

As a patient, under the law, you have the right to get copies of any records, but your signature will be required. Your doctor may charge you a small copying fee, but your records should be provided at no charge to any requesting physician's office, so have your new doctor request them. Be sure to allow adequate time for your records to be copied and forwarded, especially if your chart is large.

Under a new set of laws that just went into effect, patients have the right to examine their own medical records. You have the right to submit corrections to your file if you notice errors. This tip may become important if you have problems down the line with insurance companies.

Your doctor doesn't need to be a know-it-all

Above all, don't be afraid of a doctor who honestly admits what he or she doesn't know. Like a lot of seasoned fibromyalgics, when I encounter a doctor who doesn't know everything, I'm relieved. Most of us have marched from one doctor to another getting lots of strongly stated answers and lots of information that somehow didn't work for us or apply to us. Fibromyalgics often feel like their individual concerns get buried in what a doctor is convinced is true for every patient. So if your doctor takes the time to look something up during your visit to make sure the information you're getting is accurate, be pleased. This doctor is expressing concern for you, and is trying to help. You may have found the doctor you've been looking for!

FIBROMYALGIA

IN A SENTENCE:

> A little perseverance will help you find a doctor that's right for you and that you can work with.

Hypoglycemia and Fibromyalgia Can Go Hand-in-Hand

NOT EVERYONE with fibromyalgia has **hypoglycemia** or is intolerant to carbohydrates. However, for reasons that are still being debated, a great number of fibromyalgics are prone to blood sugar swings. Physicians who believe that the cause of fibromyalgia is a flawed **autonomic nervous system** believe that it may cause low blood sugar at times. Those who subscribe to the theory of a problem with the **hypothalamic-pituitary-adrenal axis** believe hypoglycemia is caused by the effect adrenal hormones have on blood sugar levels. Most physicians who treat fibromyalgia patients in any numbers have noticed that limiting sugars and starches in the diet can help them to feel better. Since eating right is a relatively easy way to boost your energy, let's look at fibromyalgia and diet in more detail.

Pay attention to your blood sugar

Endocrinologist Paul St. Amand, M.D., who believes that fibromyalgia is the result of faulty energy production (a slightly different twist to the theories mentioned above), has done considerable research about the interweaving symptoms of fibromyalgia and hypoglycemia. He believes that the overall drain of energy he sees in fibromyalgia leads to carbohydrate cravings that give way to a larger problem in many patients. His statistics, tabulated in over a thousand patients, show that over 40 percent of women and about 20 percent of men need to be concerned with this entanglement in a serious way. For them, controlling fibromyalgia alone will not restore well-being. A larger number of patients have what's called **carbohydrate intolerance,** which means that although they are not out and out hypoglycemics, they feel better following the diet for reasons we'll discuss later in this chapter. Both groups must address their blood sugar problems seriously in order to feel better, no matter what else they do to control their fibromyalgia symptoms. Other physicians have produced similar numbers, so while the mechanism is still being debated, the fact that hypoglycemia and fibromyalgia frequently coexist is not.

Hypoglycemia is also a syndrome

The word *hypoglycemia* simply means low blood sugar, but the condition it causes is a syndrome, which means that it is defined by a related set of complaints. Just like fibromyalgia, these can be used to diagnose the condition much more accurately than any tests your doctor can perform. Symptoms neatly divide into two types, but only one set is distinctive enough to confirm the diagnosis. These are known as the acute symptoms of hypoglycemia, and these are the ones that occur three hours to four hours after eating, when your blood sugar falls.

Acute symptoms are the easiest to identify

The acute symptoms of fibromyalgia are the easiest to spot, so let's look at these first. Dizziness and faintness usually occur first and can be quite severe, so that occasionally people even pass out. Then, as the blood sugar continues to fall, the next thing that's experienced are the symptoms of **adrenaline** release. Adrenaline, the "flight or fight hormone," gives us the sensations we recognize from when we feel frightened or threatened: the rapid pounding of the heart and head, shaking, trembling, hand tremors, sweating, and anxiety. When these symptoms are forceful enough, you've experienced a panic attack. You may also feel confused or weak and turn pale.

Chronic symptoms of hypoglycemia

The chronic symptoms of hypoglycemia are always present no matter what your blood sugar reads, although they vary in intensity. They are a result of the physical stress this syndrome puts on your body. You can't use

CHRONIC SYMPTOMS OF HYPOGLYCEMIA

Fatigue

Insomnia

Nervousness, irritability

Depression

Blurring of vision

Ringing ears

Gas, abdominal cramps, bloating, diarrhea

Numbness and tingling of hands, feet, and face

Flushing, sweating

Foot and leg cramps

Frontal headaches

Impaired memory and concentration

ACUTE SYMPTOMS OF HYPOGLYCEMIA

Pounding heart

Palpitations or heart irregularities

Panic attacks

Nightmares and severe sleep disturbances

Faintness and actual **syncope**

Acute anxiety

Hand or inner shaking or **tremor**

Sweating

Frontal headache or pressure

them to make the diagnosis because they're not very distinctive—as you can see on the chart above, the symptoms are almost identical to fibromyalgia and several other conditions. In addition to the symptoms listed, you may also experience vague feelings of nausea, anxiety, nasal congestion, and ringing in the ears. Midafternoon headaches and fatigue are very common—headaches usually occur right across the front of the forehead and feel like you have a rubber band around your head. Muscle stiffness and leg cramps can be severe, but no tender points exist when you look for them. You may have bad dreams, or wake up a few hours after going to bed, as well as problems getting started in the morning mentally and physically without caffeine. When you have a sudden surge of fatigue it, like your headaches, can be relieved by eating. You will feel faint, have palpitations, and get anxious and irritable when you are hungry. Hunger pains can be very intense, and a few hours after lunch you may be hit with a wave of sleepiness or a craving for sweets or caffeine. In fact, most hypo-glycemics have a strong craving for sweets or starches such as bread, and feel better after they eat.

There are no shortcuts

The first thing you'll have to do if you believe you're carbohydrate intol-erant or hypoglycemic is to get very familiar with the diet below. You must take responsibility for eating correctly, and now is the time to start. You will have to stick to the diet religiously—no cheating for two months. If you make a mistake or deviate from the dietary restrictions below, your two-month period will start over. It takes this amount of time on the diet for your body to heal and for your hormones to settle down. There are no short-cuts to controlling your hypoglycemia, and I promise that if there is a mir-acle solution to sugar craving and carbohydrate binging we will all hear about it. In fact, look for my picture in the advertisements because I'll be there, first in line.

Getting started

When you start the diet, be prepared. The good news is that you will start to lose your cravings after about a week and you should start to feel more energy in about two. But the honest truth is that these first two weeks can be very tough, especially if you've relied on sugar and caffeine for energy. There's no doubt that coming off carbohydrates (if you're intolerant to them) is hard, like a drug withdrawal. More and more studies are equating the effects of carbohydrates on the body to an addictive drug, and of course caf-feine is already considered one. It might not be as tough for you as I'm describing, but it's best to prepare yourself to battle at least some cravings, fatigue, and even headaches. Be extra gentle with yourself for the first few weeks and persevere. It's worth the effort because in the end, you'll feel much better. Bear in mind that the worse the effects of withdrawal from car-bohydrates are for you, the more you need the diet you are adopting.

Have plenty of food available

The most important thing is to have things around the house that you can grab and eat when you're hungry. Make several large containers of sugar-free Jell-O, a few baked apples, or some egg salad at the beginning of each week. Make quiches or fritatas, egg custard, or crème fraiche with fruit to snack on. It's important not to feel deprived, and with a little effort you won't be.

The Basic Hypoglycemia Diet

MEATS

You can have all meats, fish, fowl, and seafood, **except for cold cuts that contain sugar.** (Bacon and ham are acceptable even though their ingredient labels list sugar. Most of this is lost in the curing process, or cooks off.)

DAIRY PRODUCTS

You can have milk (nonfat, low fat, whole, or goat), cream (sweet and sour), all cheeses, including cottage, ricotta, and goat cheese. You can have butter, margarine, and eggs. Yogurt must be unsweetened, though you can add your portion of fresh fruit or a sugar-free syrup or sweetener.

FRUITS

You can have one piece of fruit every four hours from the following list: apples, apricots, cranberries, grapefruit, lemons, limes, nectarines, oranges, papaya, peaches, pears, plums, strawberries, tangerines. You can have ½ cup every four hours of any type of berry. You can have a large wedge of any type of melon every four hours. You can have an unlimited amount of fresh coconut. **No fruit juice** except tomato juice, V-8 juice, unsweetened coconut milk, and unsweetened orange juice. **You cannot have bananas, grapes, pineapples, fruit juice, or dried fruits.**

VEGETABLES

You can have the following vegetables in unlimited quantities: artichokes, asparagus, bean sprouts, beets, broccoli, Brussels sprouts, cabbage, carrots, cauliflower, celery, chard, chicory, Chinese cabbage, chives, cucumber, daikon, eggplant, endive, escarole, greens (all including salad, mustard, and beet greens), jicama, kale, leeks, lettuce, mushrooms, okra, olives, onions, parsley, peas, peppers (all colors), pickles, pimiento, pumpkin, radicchio, radish, rhubarb, sauerkraut, scallions, snow peas, spinach, string beans (yellow and green), squash (winter and summer), tomatoes, turnips, water chestnuts, watercress, zucchini.

    You cannot have potatoes (any color), yams, parsnips, lima beans, lentils, black-eyed peas, baked beans, refried beans, kidney beans, black beans, barley, garbanzo beans, or corn.

NUTS

You can have any kind of nut, including soy nuts.

BREADS

You can have a total of three slices a day of bread as long as it has no sugar, honey, or any other carbohydrate sweetener added. **You cannot have more than two slices at one time. You can substitute one serving of sugar-free flatbread, unsweetened puffed rice cakes, or a corn tortilla for a slice of bread.**

MISCELLANEOUS

You can have low-carbohydrate products such as snack bars (2–3 g. of carbohydrate), low-carbohydrate bake mixes, protein powders (with no carbohydrates) carob, gluten, soy or almond flour, 1 cup of popped popcorn, pork rinds, wheat germ, puffed rice, shredded wheat, or other sugar-free cereals. You can have tofu, soybeans, and nuts. Soymilk is OK unless it is sweetened with one of the forbidden sugars. You can have all oils, vinegars, spices, herbs, and any condiment that has no added sugar, including all imitation flavorings, ketchup, mayonnaise, mustard, and soy sauce. You can have only one ounce of unsweetened chocolate at a time because of the caffeine content. You can have low-carbohydrate chocolate bars and candies if they are made with chocolate liqueur and do not contain caffeine. There is also a caffeine-free cocoa called Wonder Cocoa that's very tasty. You can have no-sugar-added nut butters and 1 tablespoon sugarless jellies every four hours. **You should not have caramel coloring because it is made from burned sugar or corn.**

BEVERAGES

You can have sugar-free drink mixes such as Crystal Light, club soda, zero-carbohydrate flavored soda waters, decaffeinated coffee, weak or decaffeinated tea, and sodas with no sugar or caffeine like Diet 7-Up. **You cannot have hot chocolate unless it is sugar- and caffeine-free (such as Wonder Cocoa) or Ovaltine.**

NOTE ABOUT ALCOHOL: *After two months on the diet, try having a glass of dry wine or one drink: Bourbon, cognac, gin, rum, scotch, vodka,with a nonfruit juice or unsugared mixer. You should not mix alcohol and fruit juice because it is too high in carbohydrates.*

YOU **CANNOT** HAVE: CAFFEINE,* SUGAR (ANY COLOR), CORN SYRUP, SUCROSE, FRUCOSE, DEXTROSE, MALTOSE, HEXITOL, MANNITOL, MOLASSES, HONEY, MAPLE SYRUP, RICE SYRUP (ANY COLOR), WHITE RICE, CORNSTARCH OR OTHER STARCH, CORNMEAL, PASTA OF ANY KIND, FLOUR, SWEET WINES, OR CHAMPAGNE.

This includes medication that contains caffeine such as Anacin, Excedrin, Fiorinal, Caffergot, and Midol.

Eating properly is not as hard as you might think

The media is full of stories about how badly Americans eat, but there are still many of us who don't indulge in junk food, processed meats, or sugary baked goods. There are health food stores, farmers' markets, and co-ops with a wide selection of fresh produce, cheeses, and unsweetened dairy products. There are many excellent low-carbohydrate cookbooks and stores and Web sites that sell condiments and other supplies, like low-carbohydrate bread and muffin mixes. There are several excellent support groups online and Web sites that offer free cookbooks as well as a wide array of books for sale. As you feel better, your options will multiply and avoiding the foods that make you feel worse will become a way of life.

IN A SENTENCE:

> Hypoglycemia, or low blood sugar, is a common companion to fibromyalgia and can be diagnosed easily by symptoms such as panic attacks, night sweats, and hunger tremors.

learning

What You Need to Know about the Hypoglycemic Diet

HYPOGLYCEMIA DESCRIBES the situation in the blood, so it is not really a very accurate name for the entire syndrome. The blood is not responsible for symptoms; the culprit is your brain, which relies primarily on **glucose** for fuel.

Many hormones play a role

Your brain works night and day directing all your bodily functions and for this it needs abundant fuel. Because of its huge need for glucose, when the brain senses a drop in blood sugar it gets frightened. It orders the release of a barrage of hormones to stop the blood sugar from falling—growth, **cortisol**, and **glucagon** in turn, but they work slowly. Finally in desperation, with its proverbial back to the wall, and fearful for its own survival, the brain orders the final assault—**adrenaline** release. Adrenaline is amazingly effective, it stops the blood sugar's fall within a minute or two, but the victory is bittersweet because of the dramatic symptoms that accompany it.

What causes the blood sugar to fall?

The same thing that causes blood sugar to rise is eventually responsible for making it fall: consuming carbohydrates. The carbohydrates we eat are mostly chains of glucose molecules. Some are long, complicated strings, others are short and sweet—the shorter the string the sweeter the taste. Table sugar (sucrose) or sugars from fruit (fructose), honey (maltose), and milk (lactose) are known as simple carbohydrates, because of the simplicity of their structure. Starches such as bread, pasta, rice, potatoes, cereals, peas, and beans are known as complex carbohydrates because they are composed of longer chains, sometimes with branching arms. When eaten, all carbohydrates are quickly broken apart into glucose molecules and used for energy, but if there is an excess, it is distributed all over the body for storage.

Carbs cause blood sugar to rise rapidly

Carbohydrates raise blood sugar very quickly. Breakdown begins in the mouth with an enzyme in our saliva. Simple carbohydrates go directly into the bloodstream without being digested and **complex carbohydrates** are digested in the stomach. Simple carbohydrates—foods derived primarily from plant sources—have the same effect on blood glucose levels that table sugar does because they are all strings of glucose molecules. It doesn't matter whether you eat a potato, a slice of bread, or a candy bar or drink a soda, your blood sugar will start to rise almost immediately, which is why you need to stay away from these foods.

Insulin lowers your blood sugar

Another powerful hormone is responsible for clearing this glucose out of the bloodstream and ferrying it into the cells to be used as fuel or to be stored. This hormone is called insulin, and it is secreted from special cells in the pancreas and heads to the liver first. There, carbohydrates are eventually converted to glycogen and nourish the muscles and other organs.

Insulin, also called the storage hormone, is strong and efficient. It ushers glucose into fat cells to be changed and stored as fatty acids. It also takes glucose to muscle cells to be converted to glycogen, which is stored for a time when a quick burst of energy is needed.

• • •

Sometimes insulin works too well

Even after eating a carbohydrate-packed meal, unless you're a diabetic, the blood is rapidly cleared of excess glucose within a couple of hours. In diabetics, for a variety of reasons, insulin does not do its job very well. In hypoglycemia it's the opposite—the blood sugar falls as it should, only it continues to fall until the brain is alarmed. There are actually two ways in which blood sugar can fall too low. One is if too much insulin is released, and the other is if the hormones that are excreted to put the brakes on insulin don't do their job well enough. The end result is the same: The brain frantically orders adrenaline release to stop the blood sugar from going any lower.

Frequent episodes of low blood sugar cause even more problems

A single episode of hypoglycemia can leave the brain confused. But when this happens frequently, the brain starts to get wise to the false alarm, as do the other organs. Finally, the adrenals refuse to release adrenaline, because now they know that the brain is crying wolf. When this happens, the body must now rely on the slower-acting hormones we mentioned before: cortisol, glycogen, and growth. This is why over time, hypoglycemics feel rotten all the time, and lose the ability to experience panic attacks. While this sounds like an improvement, the fact is that the exhaustion that this process causes is much worse because you never feel 100 percent.

Unfortunately, there's no blood test for hypoglycemia

If you're wondering why there's no test to diagnose these blood sugar abnormalities, remember that adrenaline is so powerful that it works within two minutes to correct a low blood sugar. To catch hypoglycemia on a blood test, you'd have to have the blood drawn at the exact moment just before adrenaline is released, and clearly this is virtually impossible. Some physicians try to do this with what is called a **Glucose Tolerance Test**, which is actually better used to diagnose diabetes. For this test, the subject drinks a beverage laced with glucose and then blood samples are drawn periodically over the next five hours. Even when blood is frequently sampled, it's easy to miss the moment when blood sugar is at its lowest. In addition, research has shown that each person may have his or her own individual

Cheat Busters

WHEN YOU first begin the diet, you'll be tempted to cheat. It's probable that you'll feel pretty lousy and inside you'll know that if you could just eat some sugar you'd feel better. The fact is, the more you need this diet, the more you'll crave carbohydrates. In general a little high-fat splurge may help you cope. Some people swear that Macadamia nuts work wonders when they're tempted to cheat. I make a little mousse of whipped cream and flavored protein powder (or plain protein powder with sugar-free flavored syrup) and sprinkle it with nuts, which usually satisfies my cravings and my sweet tooth. You can also have your portion of fruit sliced with sour cream, a splash of sugar-free syrup, and chopped nuts. Here are a few other secrets that might help you, although in time you'll certainly come up with your own.

If you crave something crispy, try:
- Pork rinds. These are all protein, with no fat. You can buy some that you can microwave like popcorn. (www.microwaveporkrinds.com)
- Cheese crisps. There are various fancy ways to make this, but I just heat a nonstick frying pan on the stove over medium to high heat. Then I slice cheese and lay it in the pan. It will melt together and bubble. Cook it until it is firm, and brown around the edges. You can peel it up with a spatula and flip it. I turn the heat off when I flip it, let it sit a minute, and then slide it out of the pan and pat it with a paper towel. I slather this with guacamole and hot sauce.
- Try making fried chicken with a pork rind crust.

If you are craving potatoes:
- Steam cauliflower with a few cloves of garlic, and when it's soft, puree it in a blender with cream and butter and you have fauxtatoes. You can also throw in a spoonful of bleu cheese.
- Steam celery root and follow the same instructions as above.
- Make patties out of this mixture and coat in pork rinds and fry for croquettes.

If you crave a creamy texture:
- Try egg custard.
- Whip heavy cream with a sugar-free syrup such as English toffee flavor.
- Whip heavy cream with a flavored protein powder to make a mousse.
- Make sugar-free ice cream.
- Have a serving of carbo-lite yogurt or sugar-free ice cream.

If you crave sweets:
- ○ Make a sugar-free cheesecake.
- ○ Have strawberries and sour cream.
- ○ Have a baked apple.
- ○ Have some sugar-free Jell-O with whipped cream.
- ○ Make a float by pouring a diet soda into a glass with whipped cream in the bottom.

If you crave chocolate:
- ○ Have a sugar-free (Carbo-lite) chocolate bar. There are other types too, such as Atkins Endulge.

If you crave pasta:
- ○ Cut a spaghetti squash in half and steam until soft. With a fork, peel out the strings and top with sugar-free tomato sauce and meatballs or butter and parmesan cheese.
- ○ Make lasagna using cabbage leaves as pasta.
- ○ Make ribbons from zucchini with a vegetable peeler, salt, and let sit on a paper towel for a few minutes. Sauté with cheese and butter or tomato sauce.
- ○ Have eggplant parmigiana.

Noodles
- ○ In the Japanese section of your supermarket or in a specialty store, you can find yam noodles with no carbohydrates. These work in soups only.
- ○ Make egg noodles out of egg. Spray a nonstick frying pan with oil. Scramble a few eggs and pour into the pan, a very thin layer. When it's set, flip it. If, like me, you aren't adept at this, just slide the pan under the broiler until the top cooks too. Slide it out of the pan and roll it up. Then slice the roll horizontally. The thinner the slices, the thinner the noodles will be. Do not recook these noodles. Drop into soups when you're ready to serve them.

Rice
- ○ You can chop water chestnuts or cauliflower to the size of rice and microwave for a minute. This works in casseroles, fried dishes, and even as stuffing.

number that defines hypoglycemia. Many people release adrenaline well above 50 mg./dl, the number that was once considered the standard for hypoglycemia. They experience all the nasty symptoms of hypoglycemia without the magic reading that convinces doctors that they're hypogyclemic. Much as we'd like to make it so, hypoglycemia, it turns out, is not a disease you can diagnose by the numbers.

As you can see, once again you're faced with a syndrome that is best recognized by its symptoms. If the complaints I've listed sound familiar to you, then you should consider the possibility that you are hypoglycemic, or prone to swings in blood sugar levels. If you don't have *all* of the complaints but you still notice that foods affect how you feel, you may simply be less tolerant to carbohydrates than others. You can consider yourself carbohydrate intolerant and the same diet that controls hypoglycemia will make you feel better, too.

The hypoglycemia diet

The solution to hypoglycemia sounds pretty simple. All you have to do is eat properly so that your body never has to deal with a carbohydrate load that will start the metabolic cascade of errors. It's as simple as Newton's Law: "What goes up must come down." In carbohydrate-sensitive terms, this means that if we don't allow our blood sugar to go up too high, then it won't fall precipitously and cause nasty symptoms. The good news is that proteins and fats, the other two foodstuffs, do not cause blood sugar to spike upward.

The wisdom of a high-carb diet is now in question

By now you're undoubtedly aware of the philosophy that our modern diet is not what we were designed to eat. Evolution simply hasn't kept up with modern science. Airplane travel has given us year-round fresh fruit; factories churn out sweets and processed, refined foods, and stores are loaded with them. Desserts, cereals, and pasta are inexpensive and easy to prepare. Fast food is handy, we're all too busy, and no one feels like preparing and cooking meals when they don't feel well. Caffeine occurs only in small quantities in nature. Our much-maligned Western diet is high in starchy, overprocessed, sweetened foods. The American per capita consumption of sugar has risen dramatically and that doesn't even take into account the sugars we consume through so-called "healthy foods" like baked potatoes, pasta, whole wheat bread, and fruit juices. When our bodies are under stress, it's especially hard for them to cope with this avalanche of foods we were not designed to eat.

Certain symptoms will improve on this diet

Ending the repetitive hormonal surges caused by hypoglycemia will improve certain symptoms of fibromyalgia dramatically. You will probably notice fewer problems with fibrofog, or the afternoon drowsiness that wiped you out a few hours after lunch. If you experience the more intense symptoms of headaches and shakiness when you're hungry these will also improve. Morning fatigue may ease dramatically simply by avoiding the heavier carbohydrates before bed, which can improve your sleep. Irritable bowel syndrome almost always gets noticeably better within in a few days.

You'll have more energy

Most people start to feel more energy in about ten days, and then are 75 percent improved within one month. Within two months all the symptoms that you experience from hypoglycemia or low blood sugar will be gone. But remember, you'll still have fibromyalgia, so you'll still be saddled with whatever fatigue is part of that illness.

Experimenting with forbidden foods

After two months on the diet with no cheating, you will have repaired the damage that repeated bouts of fluctuating blood sugar levels have caused in your body. Congratulations! Now you can start experimenting or cheating, as I like to call it. You can start slowly adding some of the milder carbohydrates back. Cheating does not mean scarfing down three beers and three slices of pizza. It means a small amount of the forbidden carbohydrates to see if they will have an effect on the way you feel. Start with foods that are the least likely to cause problems. The safest are those with a low **glycemic index**, which simply means that your body produces a smaller amount of insulin when you eat them. Potatoes, pasta, and sucrose are high on the glycemic index charts and may always have to be limited, according to the degree of your problem. Brown rice is a pretty safe place to start. Next you might try a small amount of white rice or no-sugar-added ice cream. Always start with small servings at first. Chocolate syrup, potatoes, and candy bars remain off limits, unless you're prepared to pay the piper for a few days afterward.

Cheating is a learning process

Venture slowly, and if your symptoms return tighten up your diet for a few days until you recover. Before too long you'll have learned what foods you can tolerate and understand the price you'll pay if you cheat too exten-sively. If you've eaten too much, or a particular carbohydrate is too power-ful for you, you'll know it fairly quickly. You will feel more tired, perhaps more achy, and you may get a headache. Some people complain of feeling drugged and confused, or you may experience the adrenaline release symp-toms like a panic attack, especially at night. If you've cheated at dinner you may wake up in a cold sweat or have nightmares. When you experience these symptoms within three to three and half hours after eating, you will know that you've gone too far. It won't take long for you to figure out what you can and can't tolerate.

It's really important to remember not to overdo it when you start this process. Your symptoms *will* return if you don't practice self-discipline. Back off immediately at the first signs of trouble. It's tempting, believe me, to start grabbing things indiscriminately when you start to crash and feel lousy, but that will only make it harder for you to get control again. When you've gone too far, resume the diet as it's written for a few more weeks until you feel perfectly well. On your next attempt cheat less frequently and be more careful.

Remember that stress makes all symptoms worse

When you're under stress, either mentally or physically, you will be more sensitive to carbohydrates, just as you will be if your fibromyalgia is in a flare. Women will find they are more sensitive during the week before their menstrual period, when the craving for sweets may be much stronger. Ill ness and injury will also drain your energy and make your body more vul-nerable to hypoglycemia. During those periods you may have to tighten up on your diet to avoid compounding your problems.

Learning what you can tolerate

Part of the process in this first year is learning to pick your poisons. We all have foods we don't mind giving up, and these you should always avoid. Remember that each time you cheat makes you more vulnerable, whether or not you enjoyed it. Be smart and save your cheats for the foods you hate doing without. For instance caffeine, once you've gotten through the ini-tial withdrawal period, may never be worth the risk. When symptoms return, back off early and regain your equilibrium before there's a disaster and you crash and burn. A slice of pizza or brown rice are two examples of a cheat you might begin with.

• • •

The bottom line

I want to emphatically state that *you must adhere to the dietary restrictions of the hypoglycemic diet just outlined if you are sensitive to carbohydrates and you want to feel better.* Sorry, but there are no shortcuts. This one you have to do for yourself, by yourself, each and every day.

IN A SENTENCE:

> *If you are hypoglycemic or have an intolerance to carbohydrates, changing the way you eat is crucial if you wish to regain your health.*

Medications
and Fibromyalgia:
A Double-Edged Sword

ALL OF us are looking for relief from our symptoms. You wouldn't have picked up this book if you had found a way to control them on your own. And, as you've probably figured out by now, using medications to relieve your fibromyalgia symptoms is complicated. You just have too many symptoms to be easily handled. Even getting a respite from your two major symptoms may require an arsenal of medications with potent side effects. Here's what you need to know.

Picking the right medications
for your symptoms

Unless we just give up and medicate ourselves into oblivion, every day becomes a serious challenge when you have fibromyalgia. Control becomes a balancing act: what you need to accomplish versus how you feel, taking into consideration what you can cope with at this moment, and what is just too much to bear. The fact so many fibromyaglics take vast amounts of drugs and supplements, and in so many different combinations, is ample proof that none of them are very effective. To make it worse, what seems to help one person may be inef-fective for another. As I tell everyone who asks me: "If there was a simple answer, a medication that worked for all of us, we would know it, and we would all be using it."

There are no medications specifically for fibromyalgia

If you open the *Physicians' Desk Reference for Prescription Drugs* and look for the word *fibromyalgia*, you won't find a thing. There are plenty of effec-tive medications for other chronic illnesses so, in this respect, fibromyal-gia is in a category all by itself. This does not mean that no drugs have been tested on fibromyalgics. On the contrary, double-blind, placebo-controlled studies abound. However, the results of these studies have been so unim-pressive that they haven't made their way into any of the drug databases.

You will be prescribed medications based on your symptoms

There's only one approach left to take, and that is to treat your symp-toms. Doctor and patient confer: "Would you feel better if you could sleep?" (sleeping pills) "Are you depressed?" (antidepressants) "Are you in more pain than you can handle?" (pain pills) "Do you need more energy?" (stimulants). Before you know it, you'll have a medicine cabinet full of pills. **Polypharmacy** is a real and present danger to fibromyalgics, who may end up more miserable than they started as well as financially strapped by tak-ing a pill for each of their various complaints. Side effects and interactions become a concern, and because none of the medications work very well anyway, it's common to wonder if anything is really helping at all.

Medication side effects can make your other symptoms worse

One of the problems with treating symptoms with medications are side effects that can easily make your existing symptoms worse even while they make others more tolerable. For this reason treatment is often a double-edged sword. Medications that help you sleep make you more tired by day, and pain pills that dull your senses may make you constipated. Headache medications can make you jittery; antidepressants can further suppress your already pitifully low **libido.**

• • •

The final responsibility is yours

I've tried to be fair in listing the good and bad effects of the many kinds of medications in this chapter. Some of the side effects listed occur more frequently than others, and in the interest of time I haven't detailed all the potential problems. Some medications have important bold text warnings on their packaging. This is only one of the reasons why it's absolutely imperative that you get your own hands on the package insert of every medication you're considering. In many instances you can get this information off the Internet, if your doctor or pharmacist can't, or won't, oblige you.

I can't say this more urgently: Read for yourself about the medications you're considering. They are going into your body, not your doctor's. Weigh consequences with the possible benefits. Be aware that wonder drugs hit the market with a splash of publicity and some are consequently withdrawn because unforeseen effects are found when they're used in a larger population. While I know that medications can improve the quality of our lives, I am often appalled at the list of drugs people have been given and the toll they have taken on their lives. Pharmacists will say that they can't tell you what the interactions are between three drugs, let alone four or five. Remember that no combination of drugs is going to take away all of your symptoms. There are no short cuts when it comes to your health. Medications can help you, but only when they are used carefully.

In this chapter we'll look at some of the most common classes of medications used for fibromyalgics. For specific information on each medication, there's an appendix in the back of this book.

A respite from pain

Pain is often fibromyalgiacs' biggest complaint. There are a few high-pain-threshold people who don't notice anything more than stiffness or an occasional minor headache, but they are certainly in the minority. There's a good reason why pain is so awful and so impossible to ignore. The brain gives the pain signal priority over all other sensations and feelings because it is a warning sign. If it were possible to ignore pain, it would be a lot easier to hurt ourselves or do damage to ourselves without noticing. The purpose of pain, simply put, is to grab your attention, and keep it until you do something to make it stop. The longer it lasts, the more frantic it makes you. It's supposed to. There are biological reasons why it should.

• • •

Fibromyalgia pain isn't easy to relieve

As you can guess, this doesn't bode well for fibromyalgics because there's nothing we can stop doing to halt our pain. We can't pull the splinter out of our finger, or pull our foot out of a too-tight shoe. Our hand isn't resting on a hot stove and we're not slicing our finger with a knife. Since we're not doing anything to cause our pain, we can't stop it ourselves, either. That's why chronic pain is the most difficult pain to relieve. It wears down the body and exacerbates many other symptoms by making it difficult to be active, to sleep, and to lead a normal life.

Analgesics and anti-inflammatories

Acetaminophen, or Tylenol, is usually the first choice for pain. Nonsteroidal anti-inflammatory drugs **(NSAIDS)** are commonly used for their **analgesic** effect, in addition to their anti-inflammatory properties. Keep in mind though, that with FMS there is no inflammation. NSAIDs, including ibuprofen (Advil, Aleve, Motrin) and Naprosyn (naproxen) are not safer than acetaminophen, which can cause liver or kidney damage when used to excess. NSAIDS can also cause stomach bleeding and liver damage both in the short and long-term. Newer studies of both NSAIDs and acetaminophen suggest that they may interfere with basic energy production. NSAIDS also disrupt the deepest stage of sleep in some patients, a special concern for fibromyalgics. Some of the newer anti-inflammatories, a category called Cox-2 inhibitors (Vioxx and Celebrex), have proven to be easier on the stomach. These drugs are *not* stronger, so if prescription strength Motrin doesn't help you, these won't either. Their main advantage is that they cause fewer stomach problems and last longer—one pill can work for twenty-four hours.

Aspirin is another alternative for pain if you can take salicylates. This oldfashioned remedy for pain may help, but you should watch for gastrointestinal bleeding if you use it in any quantity or for over a month of continuous use. Aspirin is contraindicated with alcohol and anti-coagulant drugs. It may alter the way other medications work such as gout medications and oral hypoglycemics taken by diabetics. You should not take aspirin with NSAIDs because of the greatly increased risk of gastrointestinal bleeding.

Acetaminophen and NSAIDs
work together to help with pain

You may already know that you can take a combination of acetaminophen and nonsteroidals. The combination of the two works synergistically

---

Botox Party Anyone?

BOTOX (BOTULINUM TOXIN TYPE A) was originally developed by the U.S. military as a potential nerve agent, but was approved by the FDA for cosmetic use on facial muscles where it works by relaxing the furrows and lines that develop as we age. The next logical step was to try using it to treat conditions where painful contractions are a problem, such as cerebral palsy, multiple sclerosis, and stroke. Some recent studies have shown that it may also help some of the symptoms of fibromyalgia. Botox has been shown to have some value in intractable headaches, neck, back, and pelvic pain when it is injected into the taut muscles—it works by causing selective paralysis and weakness. Newer studies have been done demonstrating several months of relief after injection into tender points. It takes about eight days to see any results, and the effect peaks at about three weeks. It's possible to build up immunity to botox. Side effects include weakness, headaches, and bruising. It is also quite expensive at $400 per shot, and there's not enough evidence to convince insurance companies to pay for it. If you decide to try it, make sure the physician you select has lots of experience with it.

---

and is actually quite effective, especially for a dull headache or all-over aching. Combined with a hot or cold pack (and if you can take a break, a moment to lie down), you may find that these can manage most of your pain by day. Simple combinations like this will certainly help you function, at least on one of your better days.

Stronger medications for pain

Most doctors can be persuaded to give you something "a little stronger" for days when your pain can't be controlled with over-the-counter drugs. The idea behind this stronger medication is that you should only use it when you really need it, when other modalities have been exhausted, preferably only in the evenings, and not every single day. In theory this is a great idea, and, in fact, if you stick to it, you'll experience a reasonable amount of success. The point here is that the less pain medication that you use, the less you will need, and the more relief you will get. You won't build up a tolerance, so you won't eventually be stuck battling your doctor for more or for stronger compounds to provide relief.

Mild narcotics can help you cope with difficult pain

The first step up from over-the-counter pain medications are mild **narcotics**. These include various acetaminophen and codeine compounds such as Vicodin or Lortab, or darvon (propoxyphene) and darvocet (propoxyphene combined with acetaminophen). You'll need to have periodic blood tests to look for liver or kidney damage. Most fibromyalgics find that while no pain medication takes away all their discomfort, these mild narcotics make a big difference when they are in a cycle of pain. Side effects are usually mild: drowsiness and constipation, as well as some decrease in mental agility.

Tramadol

Tramadol (Ultram) is a mild analgesic that works in a different way than other older pain medications. It is the first medication of its kind and is thought to be less addictive than **narcotics**. It has a few side effects including nausea and at higher doses, some dopiness, but in double-blind studies tramodol had distinct benefits for fibromyalgia in both the long and short-term. Tramadol lowers the seizure threshold, but has caused seizures in only a small number of people. It is marketed in a combination with Tylenol, called Utracet, because the two drugs have been shown to work synergistically.

Nerve pain requires slightly different medications

Epilepsy and fibromyalgia are not related, but a group of medications marketed for seizures have been shown to help with nerve pain. Neurontin (gabapentin) is the most commonly prescribed; others are Tegretol (carbemezine), Topramax (topiramate), and Depakote (valproic acid). These work on nerve impulses in various ways and help control burning pain, pins and needles, and the feeling of electricity in the extremities, as well as other types of nerve pain or **neuropathy**. Baclofen (lioresal) relieves painful muscle spasms by decreasing spinal cord reflexes. Regular blood tests need to be performed if you're prescribed these medications. Side effects include dizziness, nausea, blurred vision, and tremors.

Headaches and migraines have specialized medications

Headaches are a common complaint of fibromyalgics, from vice-like tension headaches to **migraines** that cause nausea and visual disturbances. Studies have shown that over-the-counter Excedrin (a combination of aspirin, acetaminophen, and caffeine) is often as effective as prescription drugs. Butalbital combinations such as Esgic or Fioricet are used for tension headaches, but can have a rebound effect, causing a headache the next day. Midrin is a combination drug that has been shown to be as effective as the newer triptans in relieving migraine and tension headaches and

Topical Pain Relief Options

○ **Trigger or tender point injections:** a technique in which a local anesthetic in combination with synthetic cortisone is injected directly into the painful area by a physician. Most useful when only a few areas are painful.

○ **Botox injections:** purified chemical from botulism that causes a disruption of the nerve-muscle junction when injected. Improvement can last for months.

○ **Nerve blocks or epidurals:** anesthetics injected directly into nerve tissue used for severe localized pain.

○ **Topicals containing NSAIDs:** compounding pharmacists often sell creams that contain an anti-inflammatory that when applied is absorbed through the skin.

○ **Topical lidocaine (also available in patch form):** local anesthetic that when applied topically can block pain for several hours.

○ **Topical salicylates:** menthol, peppermint oil, and methyl salicylate are forms of aspirin that are absorbed through the skin. Because they bypass the stomach these can be used if aspirin causes gastrointestinal distress.

○ **Topical capsaicin:** (Zostrix, Dolorac) derived from chili peppers, reduces the level of substance P and dulls pain receptors in the area where it's used.

is much less expensive. Imitrex (sumatriptan), Maxalt (rizatriptan), and Zomig (zolmitriptan) are some of the triptans, a newer class of drugs designed to treat migraines. Side effects include nausea, fatigue, and chest pain. The triptans have generally replaced the older ergotamines like Cafergot because they have fewer and milder side effects. For those with frequent headaches, two classes of blood pressure medication, calcium channel and beta blockers, are used with minimal side effects as a prophylactic measure.

If you need them, there are stronger pain medications

Stronger narcotic pain medications such as Oxycontin, Duragesic morphine, Demerol, and methadone are making their way into fibromyalgia treatment, but they haven't arrived without controversy. A vocal group of fibromyalgics have demanded these drugs for stronger pain relief and sometimes can get doctors to prescribe them. More often, despite escalating use and greatly diminished cognitive function, even these drugs do not provide complete pain relief. Safety for long-term use of these medications is far from established and they certainly have an effect on cognitive function. Though they may take away more pain than their weaker counterparts, your life will certainly be more circumscribed when you take them. For many of us, simply because we have children and have responsibilities that require us to function at a certain level, these medications are not realistic options for us most of the time.

The Opioid Controversy and Fibromyalgia

Opioid is a term that was originally used to describe synthetic substances such as methadone, but now is increasingly used to describe the entire category of these drugs. **Opiate** is used to describe only natural compounds—medications derived from the opium poppy such as opium itself, morphine, and codeine, which is derived from morphine. Opioids and opiates are both narcotics—they occupy the same receptors and have the same action upon the body. We tend to be shocked when we hear the word *narcotic* because we tend to associate it with drug educations programs like "Just say no!" Narcotic is not a synonym for illegal, but it does mean something potent. The dictionary defines the term as "an addictive drug, such as opium, that reduces pain, alters mood and behavior, and usually induces sleep or stupor. Natural and synthetic narcotics are used in medicine to control pain."

Opioids are true double-edged swords. Habituation and dependence are real threats, and addiction is no joke. But just as not everyone who drinks becomes an alcoholic, not everyone who takes narcotics develops a problem. Daily use increases the chances your body will become dependent. Occasional use and careful self-monitoring decrease the chances you will have a problem. The less often you use these medications, the more potent their action will be. Physically, over time, we develop a tolerance to narcotics, which means that with regular use we may require more and more to do the same job. This is a medical fact, not a judgment. With continued use your body develops a desire for them, and will create pain in an effort to convince you to produce them. If you have drug addiction or alcohol problems in your immediate family or in your own past you should not use these drugs. It's no secret that Vicodin, Percodan, and Oxycontin are among the most abused drugs today.

Devin Starlanyl, who strongly advocates the right to receive adequate pain medications including opioids, writes: "Only when other therapies fail should you and your doctor consider them, and they should not be used alone. The healing regimens of diet, bodywork, mind work, lifestyle modifications, and so forth must be continued, and hidden perpetuating factors must be identified and treated. If the central nervous system has been sensitized to a great degree, and other medications and therapies either don't work or aren't tolerated, then narcotics should be considered as a legitimate option for pain control."[1]

Stronger pain medications have stronger side effects

Side effects of narcotics are another aspect of the double-edged sword because many of them are already complicating with fibromyalgia. These include nausea and stomach problems as well as constipation that can be very severe in some people because these drugs slow intestinal motility. Narcotics can also cause mental confusion, memory problems, and increased fatigue, depression, and listlessness. This all means that many of the symptoms you experience from fibromyalgia may get much worse.

Antidepressants are not just for depression

Even before you're offered pain pills, your doctor will probably suggest that you try an antidepressant. This may confuse you, especially if you don't think that you're particularly depressed. Despite their rather bleak performance in studies of fibromyalgiacs, these are the drugs of choice for the majority of physicians. Tricylic antidepressants have been shown to be between 25 and 37 percent effective in fibromyalgia, and the newer class, SSRIs, have been shown to be slightly less.

The theory is that antidepressants are advantageous because they help with other symptoms besides depression—they can suppress pain perception by up to 50 percent, help with deeper sleep, increase energy, and some can even help with weight loss.

The oldest antidepressants seem to help the most

The older antidepressants are known as **tricylics**, and include amitriptyline (Elavil) doxepin (Sinequan), and nortriptyline (Pamelor). These are the oldest class on the market, and have been studied the most. They are not considered addictive, and are usually started at a low dose. Tricylics can help achieve deep sleep, heighten the effects of endorphins, and make more serotonin available. Because they can cause drowsiness, they are usually taken in the evening, before bedtime. Other side effects of this group include: weight gain, fatigue, constipation, dizziness, and weakness. They can also cause sexual dysfunction, and more seriously, heart rhythm abnormalities.

Newer types of antidepressants

The second, newer class of antidepressants is called **selective serotonin reuptake inhibitors (SSRIs)**. They are more expensive, and there are five on the market right now, including Prozac, Paxil, Zoloft, Celexa, and Luvox. SSRIs cause less drowsiness than the older drugs, may help modestly with fibrofog, and help the body to release more endorphins. Side effects are nervousness, insomnia, loss of appetite, headaches, diarrhea, and reduced sexual desire. (Some doctors suggest discontinuing the medication for a few days periodically to enhance libido. Since they are long acting, they'll still help with symptoms over those days.)

The last group of antidepressants contains the drugs that don't belong in either of the other two categories. These are Wellbutrin, Serzone, Desyrel, Effexor, and Remeron. Of these, Serzone has no effect on pain but also does not have the sexual side effects, and Wellbutrin has recently been proven effective in weight loss. Desyrel (trazodone) is commonly used to help patients with sleep problems. They all can cause dry mouth, constipation, and listlessness.

Antidepressants can be used in combination, too

Since the various types of antidepressants work differently and help slightly different sets of symptoms, it's common for doctors to use them in combination. Generally low doses are used to keep the side effects in abeyance. The tricylics are usually presecribed at bedtime to help with sleep and SSRIs by day to help with energy and cognitive function.

Muscle relaxants and anti-anxiety drugs

Muscle relaxants and anti-anxiety drugs are another common group of prescription drugs used by fibromyalgics. Double-blind studies have been hard to conduct because their side effects are so obvious. Most patients can tolerate them in only very limited quantities because of the level of fatigue they induce, but they provide a certain amount of relief from muscle spasms and may help with sleep. Morning drowsiness and mental fogginess are the two main reasons why patients discontinue them.

Options for muscle spasms and tightness

Because physicians can easily palpate contracted muscles on the back and necks of fibromyalgics, muscle relaxants are often prescribed. Taken at night these can help with sleep and if taken in smaller doses generally do not cause too much daytime drowsiness. Carisoprodol (Soma), Skelaxin (metaxolone), or Flexeril (cyclobenzaprine) are the most commonly used because they have far less addictive potential than do the **benzodiazepines**, which are actually hypnotic sleep medications. Norgesic is a combination of orphenadrine, aspirin, and caffeine that may result in less

WHAT ARE GENERIC DRUGS? Generics are medications for which the patent has expired meaning that any company can market them. They must pass FDA testing but this doesn't always mean that the absorption and fillers are the same, and some variation is legally allowed. However, don't dismiss generics out of hand if you're paying for your own medications as they can potentially save you thousands of dollars. But if a generic doesn't seem to agree with you in the same way the brand name did, be sure that you explain this fact to your doctor who can order that no substitution should be permitted.

also may cause rebound symptoms. Any medication that relaxes muscles will cause some degree of daytime drowsiness, fatigue, and constipation. The latter occurs because muscle relaxants act indiscriminately, and relax the muscles of the bowel as well. Zanaflex (tizanidine HCL) is a newer drug on the market that reduces muscle spasticity and is being prescribed by some doctors for fibromyalgia. It has been tested less than the older medications and drug interactions should be carefully checked. It's much more expensive than the others for which generic brands are available.

Benzodiazepines are widely used for sleep and muscle pain

Benzodiazapines (sometimes called tranquillizers) such as Valium (diazepam), Xanax (alprazolam), and Ativan (lorazepam) are given to fibromyalgics primarily because they may eliminate abnormal brain waves that cause sleep problems. These drugs will also reduce anxiety and muscle spasm. Klonopin (clonazepam) and Ativan also may help decrease pain because of some analgesic action on the brain and help with restless legs. On the downside they have the potential to cause physical dependence, irritability, depression, lethargy, and fatigue, as well as mental fogginess. For instance, you can't discontinue taking Xanax abruptly—you must be weaned off it.

Barbituates are not generally used in fibromyalgia because of their side effects and the potential for abuse. Benzodiazepines, which have taken their place, act on specific receptors involving a neurochemical GABA (gamma aminobutyric acid). Several sleeping pills like Halcion (triazolam) and Dalmane (flurazepam) are benzodiazepines. Side effects of this group are lethargy, drowsiness, irritability, nausea, and disturbing dreams.

• • •

Sleeping well is essential for health

Sometimes a little sleep can go a long way to increase your tolerance to pain and the other nasty symptoms of fibromyalgia. Over-the-counter sleeping aids include the antihistamine Benadryl (diphenhydramine). It's the active ingredient in Tylenol PM, Just Sleep, Sominex, and Unisom. It's not habit forming, and can even be safely used by children. Effective doses range from 12 mg to 100 mg, but sometimes doctors suggest higher amounts. In some people this compound can cause agitation, and if it does this to you, obviously you should not try to use it for sleep. If you find it leaves you tired by day, try a lower dose. I generally find that 12 mg works well for me. New studies have shown that antihistamines may have some painkilling effect because they counter the release of histamines, which are a pain promoting substance.

Atarax (hyroxyzine) is a prescription strength antihistamine used for fibromyalgia as well, to relieve hives. It also has a slight pain relieving effect.

Benzodiazapines are also prescribed sleeping aids

If over-the-counter sleep aids don't help you, you should talk to your doctor. Benzodiazepines are the most commonly prescribed sleeping medications, particularly a subset known as **hypnotics**: ProSom (estazolam), Dalmane (flurazepam), Restoril (temazepam), and Halcion (triazolam). (The last of these drugs has been withdrawn from the market in several countries because of severe side effects including aggressiveness and anxiety.) There are also two newer compounds that are hypnotics but not benzodiazepines: Ambien (zolpiderm) and Sonata (zaleplon). This class of drugs acts by enhancing the action of a neurotransmitter, GABA, and Ambien has the most selective action. The duration of action also varies, and in fibromyalgia shorter duration is considered better to reduce morning fatigue and the rebound effect. Ambien has a six-hour effect; Sonata has only a four-hour action. For people who wake up in the middle of the night and can't get back to sleep, Sonata would be the best choice.

Side effects of benzodiazepines include nervousness, anxiety, lack of energy, and headaches. It's easy to become dependent on sleeping medications, so most physicians will encourage you not to take one every night. Usage for a period of over four weeks can cause certain kinds of memory loss. Withdrawal, manifested as insomnia and agitation at best, and seizures at the worst, can occur if you've been taking them regularly and suddenly stop.

Stimulants can be prescribed to create some energy

Stimulants are medications chemically related to the natural hormone adrenaline. A newer drug called Provigil (modafinil) seems to be the most popular. It can be taken as needed to increase energy. Other people have been given older compounds such as Adderal (destroamphetamine sulphate) or Ritalin (methylphenidale HCL), which are usually used in attention deficit disorder (ADD). The downside of these stimulants is that they result in a rebound fatigue. The body must recover from the huge expenditure of energy these stimulate. Other side effects are headaches, **tachycardia,** nausea, diarrhea, dry eyes, dry mouth, a bad taste in the mouth, insomnia, and nervousness.

USE A commonsense approach to your medications

○   Always ask your physician if there are older medications that might be generic and thus less expensive.

○   Ask for a small amount before you fill a full prescription. If something doesn't agree with you, you won't be stuck with half-full bottles you don't know what to do with.

○   Convince yourself that there is no combination of drugs that is going to take away all of your symptoms, and that many combinations of medications can add to them.

○   If you're going to try something new, ask your doctor how long you should stay with it to give it a chance to work. If it doesn't seem to help within that period, ask how to go about discontinuing it.

○   Try things one at a time and reevaluate your list periodically.

○   Don't stop medication on a whim. Talk to your physician because it's dangerous if you don't know exactly what you're doing. Some medications must be tapered off gradually. Be sure you know how long a drug stays in your system. Some antidepressants stay in your system for several weeks, so going off them for a day or two won't tell you anything.

IN A SENTENCE:

Many medications are used for the symptoms of fibromyalgia and it's up to you to educate yourself about their effects and side effects.

learning

The Guaifenesin Protocol: A Possible Treatment Option

WHILE RESEARCHING medications for fibromyalgia, you'll probably come across a treatment using a medication called **guaifenesin.** Since this has proven effective for many fibromyalgics, it is worth looking at. You should know that this treatment is experimental, although guaifenesin has been on the market for many years and used for other illnesses. To date there has been no successful double-blind study of its use for fibromyalgia, but you will read that it has helped many people. Guaifenesin was formerly a prescription medication, but now it is an over-the-counter preparation.

The guaifenesin protocol

The **guaifenesin protocol** is the work of Dr. R. Paul St. Amand, M.D., an endocrinologist in Marina del Rey, California, who has dedicated over forty years of his life to treating fibromyalgia. He himself, as well as several members of his family, have the illness.

Dr. St. Amand believes that fibromyalgia is an energy-deprivation disease. He postulates that it's the inability of each cell to make abundant energy that is the cause for all the

---

IN 1994 a bit of serendipity brought a medication called Guaifenesin to Dr. St. Amand's attention. In a short period of time it proved more effective than any of his previous fibromyalgia medications with a wonderful postscript—it had no side effects!

> **GUAIFENESIN**: (gwy-FEN-e-sin) is an expectorant that thins mucus and helps to loosen phlegm. Guaifenesin generally comes in a 600 mg tablet, but is also available in both lower and higher strengths. Since July 2002 it has been available over the counter; you just have to ask a pharmacist for it.

---

symptoms we experience, and this is why so many systems in our body malfunction simultaneously. Without enough energy, all our systems function marginally and we have many complaints. He believes that this underproduction of ATP is caused by a slight excess of phosphate inside the power stations cells, known as the **mitochondria**.

How guaifenesin works

According to Dr. St. Amand, taking guaifenesin starts a reversal process in fibromyalgia by causing the kidneys to pull the excess phosphates from cells. This causes all of your symptoms to come and go in turn: pain, fatigue, fibrofog, irritable bowel and bladder. Symptoms will exacerbate, diminish, and then clear in this cyclical fashion. Eventually, as time progresses, you become asymptomatic.

There is a specific way to find your dose of guaifenesin

When you start guaifenesin, the proper way to begin is with 300 mg twice daily. You should remain at 300 mg twice a day for one week. If you feel distinctly worse within a few days of starting your guaifenesin, you have started your reversal and there is no need to change your dose. Don't be discouraged if you don't feel any differently during this first week. The fact is that the vast majority of patients don't. *Six hundred milligrams a day will only reverse fibromyalgia in about 20 percent of people, according to Dr. St. Amand.*

At the end of the first week on guaifenesin, if you have felt no differently, you should raise your dose. The correct way to do this is by moving up to 600 mg twice a day, or doubling the dose you started at. Dr. St.

Amand has his patients stay at this higher dose for three more weeks. Again, a worsening of symptoms indicates that you have begun your reversal. If this is the case, you would stay at this dose, and not change it. Roughly 50 percent of patients start reversal at this level.

Let's say you're one of the 30 percent of people who hasn't felt any worse after a month on 1200 mg of guaifenesin. It's normal to be afraid that this is just another treatment that isn't going to work for you, but you should just raise your dose to three pills a day. At this point it's highly likely that your symptoms will exacerbate. Only 10 percent of patients will need more guaifenesin, and will have to raise their dosage still higher, to 2400 mg a day.

Once you find the dose that causes your symptoms to escalate, there's no need to change it. All you have to do is continue to take guaifenesin. Your symptoms should cycle—that is get better and then worse, better and then worse. Like a bouncing ball, they will get less dramatic, and good periods will become more pronounced. Eventually you should have all your symptoms under control.

You'll need to learn about salicylates

Guaifenesin's effect on the kidney is blocked by the chemical **salicylate**. Renal tubules, where the guaifenesin must act, have receptors just like other cells, and salicylates and guaifenesin compete for the same sites. Just as pain signals are blocked when pain medications dock in pain receptors, guaifenesin is blocked when salicylates park in the receptors it uses.

Avoiding salicylates means reading labels. It means you'll have to know what is in all the products you are using in and on your body. Both synthetic salicylates, like aspirin-containing medications and some topical exfoliants and natural salicylates, like plant oils, gels, and extracts, will block guaifenesin's action.

GUAIFENESIN BLOCKERS:

Salicylate, salicylic acid, octisalate in medications or topical products
Oils with plant names (except soy, wheat, corn, oats)
Gels with plant names (except soy, wheat, corn, oats)
Extracts with plant names (except soy, wheat, corn, oats)
Mint flavor, mint oil, menthol
Plant compounds such as camphor, bisabol, pycnogenol, or bioflavinoids
All herbal medications

Before you try guaifenesin, decide if it's right for you

There are several excellent sources for more information about using guaifenesin. I recommend you read the book I coauthored with Dr. St. Amand, *What Your Doctor May Not Tell You About Fibromyalgia*. On the Internet, you'll find Dr. St. Amand's papers and more information at www.fibromyalgiatreatment.com.

IN A SENTENCE:

> *Many medications are used to treat fibromyalgia, and with a little research and perseverance, you can find the right ones for you.*

Alternative Therapies

ALTERNATIVE TREATMENT for fibromyalgia is something of an oxymoron, since there is no standard treatment. Still, certain therapies fall in that category, and no doubt you hear a lot about them from various sources. This may sound strange, but because there is no accepted effective treatment, there are many alternatives. If this sounds like a catch-22, it is. It's something you should bear in mind as you read this chapter. When mainstream medicine has no concrete solution, people with other ideas step in to fill the void. People with chronic pain and fatigue are desperate, and when physicians can't help them, they often search for any promise of relief they can get. If you haven't tried alternative treatments yet, you probably will—it's estimated that over 90 percent of fibromyalgics try some kind of alternative to conventional medicine.

What exactly does alternative medicine mean?

Alternative, complementary, or natural remedies are terms used interchangeably when describing treatments that fall outside the scope of the usual medical practice. Of course, this definition changes with the times and is often dependent upon who is doing the defining. Some physicians will refer to acupuncture as an alternative; however, these days many insurance companies that won't cover anything considered experimental will pay for it. In some cases, insurance companies are also paying for some dietary supplements.

Analyze information about treatments

Whether or not you'll decide to try some of these alternatives, it won't hurt you to be informed about how to evaluate information that comes your way. As time goes by you'll certainly have lots of well-meaning friends and acquaintances talking to you about things they think you should try. Sometimes when you're not feeling well, or you're going through a flare, you may consider taking their advice. Hopefully you'll remember some of the things you've read here, or refer back to them if you need to.

Make no mistake about it; dietary supplements are big business in the United States, the single most popular form of alternative therapy. We buy about $5 billion worth of these products a year and that number continues to grow. One expert estimates that there are more than twenty thousand herbal products available in this country. These supplements have physiological effects on the body because they contain active chemical compounds. These compounds, or collections of chemicals, are not inherently more or less toxic or beneficial than the often synthetic chemicals that make up prescription drugs, simply because they are extracted from plants or animals. This is a basic and important point to understand. Heroin is a plant product. Oxycontin is synthetic. Endorphins are made in your own body, a natural compound for humans. Yet they all occupy the same receptors and thus have similar effects on our bodies.

We don't know everything about prescription drugs

We don't always know how prescription drugs work. They're supposed to be pure but as we know, mistakes can be made. Sometimes batches of drugs have to be recalled because of identifiable errors. Even carefully controlled FDA-approved drugs can turn out to be more dangerous than they appeared in trials; some have even been withdrawn from the market, as you may have heard. When you take a medication, you get a package insert telling you how the drug works, and a list of possible side effects and the frequency with which you should take it. You do not get anything similar with most supplements because they have not been tested or approved in the same way.

Laws that govern the marketing of supplements are different

Dietary supplements (herbals, vitamins, minerals, amino acids, and tissue extracts) are all regulated by the same law—the Dietary Supplement

Health and Education Act (DSHEA) of 1994, which is somewhat controversial for a few good reasons. This law does not require the manufacturers of products to submit proof of efficacy, or proof of safety, and it sets no standards for quality control. Prescription and over-the-counter drugs, on the other hand, must perform detailed studies proving that they are safe and effective for a particular use before they can be marketed.

What the standards for supplements do regulate is what labels can say. Supplements cannot claim to be therapeutic—they cannot state that they treat any disease. The only legal statement they can make of this sort is to indicate which of the body structures or bodily functions the product "supports" or "maintains." All supplements are required to carry a disclaimer from the FDA on their labels, and can be removed from the market if they are proven dangerous.

Getting the required amount of vitamins and minerals

Some people think extra vitamins are not necessary for anyone who eats normally, but others will insist that living in the modern world somehow robs you of necessary vitamins. Other studies insist that the soil our food grows in is depleted of nutrients so we need to take supplements to make up the difference if we want to be healthy. If you're sick, and concerned you're not eating correctly, or if you're on a special diet because of food sensitivities, you may be concerned.

Unlike with some other forms of supplements, a lot of research has been done to determine how much of each vitamin and mineral is needed by humans to avoid deficiencies. The general consensus is that taking vitamins in a quantity that's close to the RDI (reference daily intake, a new term that replaces the old USRDA, or recommended daily allowance) is not harmful. On the other hand, it is certainly not wise to take vitamins and minerals in much larger amounts, or more than 10 or 100 times the daily suggested amount. At that dose their effects, especially long term, are unknown. We do know that large doses of some vitamins may be harmful: An excess of vitamin A can cause liver disease or bone abnormalities, too much vitamin B_{12} can cause nerve injuries, and too much vitamin D can lead to kidney stones.

Strive for good nutrition

The best way to get vitamins and minerals is to eat properly, consuming protein and vegetables. For one thing, it's quite possible that our foods contain nutrients that haven't been added to vitamin pills. In food form they may be absorbed in different ways since we get them gradually over the course of a day. Plant foods, the ones most people are concerned they don't eat enough of, also provide fiber, which is necessary to healthy digestion, and you can't replace fiber with a multivitamin.

It makes sense that if you're worried about nutrition, you should make an effort to eat better. It doesn't take as much as you think to fulfill the daily requirements—and you might find that you actually eat a lot better than you think you do.

Long-term benefits

Results of studies on the long-term benefits of taking vitamins and minerals on your general health have been mixed. Certain illnesses do cause certain deficiencies that can be corrected with the proper supplementation, but fibromyalgia has not been shown to be one of these. There are no documented vitamin or mineral deficiencies in fibromyalgia—and hundreds and hundreds of studies have been done trying to find one.

One of the problems with studies about vitamins is that not one single person is getting no vitamins at all. We are all getting, at the very least, a large portion of what we need from what we're eating—there's really no way to design a true control group!

Your body needs balance

An important thing to remember when consuming vitamins, minerals, or any other supplement is that the body has many complicated mechanisms for maintaining the right chemical balance. Even very well informed researchers are learning more every day about some of the ways this is done, so you can't expect a pharmacist, or your personal doctor, and especially not an employee in a health food store, to provide you with these kinds of facts. For example, high levels of vitamin C can cause a depletion of copper and increased absorption of iron.[1]

You do need to check with your pharmacist or doctor about whether or not your vitamins or minerals might interfere with any prescription medications you're taking. For example, some antibiotics may be rendered ineffective when taken with a calcium supplement. Vitamin C can affect the

MANY COMPANIES make extravagant claims about the vitamins they market, including a case for natural vitamins being more beneficial than synthetic ones. The fact is that there is no evidence that natural vitamins are better in any way. However, they are certainly more expensive.

accuracy of several blood tests. People taking blood thinners should check with their physicians before taking higher doses of vitamin E. Bear in mind, however, that all the facts are not yet known.

What you should know if you want to take vitamins

There are two basic types of vitamins, and the distinction between them is important if you're going to take supplements. Water-soluble vitamins can be taken safely in larger amounts because they are eliminated easily by the body through urination. It's extremely difficult to take too much because your body can't store them. To put it simply, you may not be able to raise the value of your blood, but you can make some very expensive urine. Our bodies simply extract what we need from these pills, and excrete the rest. Water-soluble vitamins are measured in milligrams, and include the B vitamins and vitamin C.

Fat-soluble vitamins, or vitamins A, D, E, and K, can be toxic if they are taken in large amounts because the body stores them. These are measured in international units (IU). Some rather large studies have implicated vitamin A in some cancers, or the possibility that it may cause cancer to grow more quickly. It would seem prudent to avoid vitamin A in supplements, and also to treat all these fat-soluble compounds with respect. Beta-carotene, a slightly safer, water-soluble precursor of vitamin A, is the compound that can turn you orange if you eat too many carrots, so it's obvious that your body can't easily excrete the excess, or this wouldn't happen.

Always try one vitamin at a time

If you're taking vitamins for some sort of therapeutic effect, and not simply as insurance that you're getting proper nutrition, bear this in mind. Try things one at a time. If you take a vitamin pill with twenty-seven different vitamins in it, you will not know which of the compounds helped you. Down the line you will be paying for something that you don't need. This does not apply to multivitamins, but simply to large quantities of vitamins marketed to treat a certain condition.

Herbal supplements

Less is known about herbal supplements because even less research has been done on them than on vitamins. In some cases, with more exotic treatments like algae from the Arctic Ocean, or fungus from the slopes of Mt. Fuji, there's been almost none.

It's hard to do accurate research on herbal supplements. Because of the varying potency of many herbal products it's even more impractical to run studies on them than on vitamins. Still, you'll see references to "scientific studies" and "data" peppered throughout their publicity blurbs and official-looking handouts. It will be your task to read though these booklets and try to evaluate what's written there. Make sure that the published source that's used is not someone affiliated with the company that sells the product. In research from other countries this can be hard to find out, but look at the name of the company that's done the research or is marketing the product. Sometimes it's obvious that they're one and the same. Many manufacturers have a Ph.D. or a medical doctor on staff who conducts his or her own "research," sometimes with some rather novel techniques. You can also get a clue from the publication that is cited. Some are independent publications, or pamphlets put out by these corporations. Other times you'll see a reputable journal reference like *Science, Nature,* or *The Lancet,* which is the premier British medical journal. If you're interested, you can read more about the research by getting copies of the actual articles.

Know exactly what you are taking and how it works

First of all, learn what is in the supplement you'd like to take. Some contain only one ingredient, like evening primrose oil. Others contain what's called "proprietary blends," meaning that the company has mixed together some compounds and patented it as unique. This rather common practice occurs because, of course, no one can patent red clover or tea tree oil. All they can do to get you to buy their brand is to make it look unique and somehow better that the competition.

Once you get the ingredient list, you'll have to research them. The *Physicians' Desk Reference* series publishes a paperback volume on herbal medications. This is a good resource because it's impartial and only deals with documented material. There are also publications about herbs and supplements in bookstores—another good place to start. The Internet has dozens of drug and supplement information Web sites. Be careful, though—you can get a lot of information off the Internet, but much of that material is written by people who sell supplements and therefore tout their safety.

Keep in mind that studies done in vitro (in glass or in a test tube) may not translate to in vivo, or real life. Also studies on mice, pigs, and other animals may not apply to humans. Look for data on humans, and look for data that pertains to your age group and your sex. If you're a twenty-year-old woman, the effect of growth hormone on eighty-year-old men may not be particularly pertinent to you.

You should also try to find out how the supplement works—if you have an objection to taking a certain kind of medication because it has side effects like

Possible Relief for Migraine Sufferers

THIS YEAR a study was published suggesting Coenzyme Q-10 as a prophylactic measure for migraine headaches. According to this study, after three months of 150 mg a day, 61 percent of patients had a 50 percent or more reduction of days with headaches. No side effects were reported. Obviously this is not an overwhelmingly positive study, but it certainly merits a closer look, especially since it lacks the side effects we're accustomed to with current therapies, like fatigue and rebound headaches.

Source: *Cephalgia, vol. 22, pp.137-141, 2002.*

possible liver damage, make sure the herb you're about to take doesn't work in the same way and have the same risks. Many women who are adamantly opposed to taking hormone replacement therapy (HRT) are taking plant supplements that contain those same compounds, which logically could carry exactly the risks that scared them away from HRT in the first place.

The cost of treatment

Cost is another factor to consider. Herbal medications and supplements are generally not covered at all by insurance companies, which makes them much more lucrative for pharmacies than their prescription counterparts. These days, pharmacies generally only receive a "filling fee" from insurance companies, which is usually three dollars or less for prescription drugs. So when someone purchases a fifty-dollar supplement, the establishment makes a much higher profit. Make sure it's really true that the supplement can do something that a regular prescription drug can't, especially if you have to pay cash for it, and especially if your finances are a little shaky. It may not be worth the added stress of trying to figure out how you're going to pay for your supplements every month.

How to check up on products

Potency and purity of herbal supplements is important, and since these aren't regulated, be very careful. Some companies are certainly more reputable than others. There are also independent laboratories that test supplements and publish their findings to help you. One of the easiest of these to use and to access is Consumer's Lab, at www.consumerslab.com. You'll find information on recalls, reviews, and test results for vitamins, minerals, herbs, and other products.

Hormones and fibromyalgia treatment

There are various types of hormones on the market, both over the counter and by prescription. Since it's been written in medical journals that some hormone counts may be low in fibromyalgia, some doctors and chiropractors will suggest that you try supplementing them.

First you need to make sure that the level of the hormone you're looking into trying is actually low. There are extremely accurate blood tests for all hormone levels, so that you do not need to test your hair, saliva, or urine. All of these substances are composed at least in part of waste products and are not reflective of the current level of anything in your bloodstream. You also don't have to put a thermometer under your arm. Basal body temperature is normally different from person to person, and a lower basal body temperature is not a sign that you have a thyroid deficiency. You can do a little research on normal body temperatures if you want to confirm this.

Taking hormones may suppress your own gland

There's another simple fact that escapes the notice of many people. If you add hormones, your own glands quite normally stop producing them. That's the theory behind taking thyroid medication when you have an enlarged thyroid gland, or goiter. Taking a supplemental hormone simply puts your own gland to sleep, and it shrinks and stays asleep as long as your body is getting that hormone from an outside source. So you can see that taking adrenal hormones (or adrenal extract) or thyroid hormones won't raise your own levels unless you take an abnormal amount. Abnormal amounts show up on blood tests; an abnormal level of any thyroid hormone, high or low, has risks. Low levels can cause hardening of the arteries, high cholesterol, and fatigue. High levels are also dangerous: heart problems and osteoporosis, or thinning of the bones, can result.

Natural hormones may not be natural for you

These days many people refer to plant hormones as "natural," and some groups highly tout this concept. Plant hormones (any hormone with the prefix phyto) are certainly natural, they occur in nature, but they are not bio-identical to anything produced in the human body. In fact, some of them (especially steroids, or sex hormones) have to be chemically altered so that the human body can derive any benefit from them at all. In addition, not all hormones can be taken orally. There is no pill for human growth hormone on the market, no matter what any advertisement says. Growth hormone, like the hormone insulin, must be injected.

Our bodies release hormones differently than supplements

Whatever method you use to get supplemental hormones into the bloodstream is imperfect and unnatural. Our own glands release small amounts throughout the day, some, like adrenal hormones, occur in very specific patterns because they are part of the sleep-wake cycle. With an injection, a huge slug of the hormone pours into the bloodstream immediately, and with a pill, they enter the bloodstream in a surge about one hour after ingesting them. So, though they perform certain positive functions for us and work to keep some people alive, they do not act in exactly the same way when they are put into the body by any unnatural means.

Hormone supplements should be handled by an expert

What I hope you understand is that hormone replacement or supplementation isn't a simple, straightforward proposition. Even the oldest hormone on the market, Premarin (an estrogen), has surprised researchers in recent studies. Other hormones haven't been on the market nearly as long, some of their effects may be unknown, and where all their receptors lie is still being discovered. Hormones can only act on cells via receptors that are specially designed for them. They can't act on cells that don't have these, but they do act on all the cells that have them. That's why estrogens pose a risk for breast tissue. Some newer forms are inactive in the breast, however, because they are tailored carefully so that they only fit in very specific estrogen receptors. These new compounds, as far as is known, won't raise the risk of breast cancer because the receptors in the breasts won't accept them. Other hormones are meant to decline as we age, and no matter how natural the substance is that we use, having them after a certain age is unnatural. So, as you can see, it's wise to make sure you're in the hands of a physician who specializes in this field.

Animal extracts as treatments

The theory behind taking animal extracts as supplements is made pretty clear on their labels. Bovine (cow) spleen is supposed to support your own spleen, bovine adrenal glands are meant to boost your own adrenal gland, and so on. In some cases they will work (although in the case of bovine adrenal glands they only work to suppress the human gland) and in other cases they are simply digested like any other protein. It takes a knowledgeable physician to know which is which. Consumer's Lab (www.consumerslab.com) and Quackwatch (www.quackwatch.com) are sources that can help you to research this on your own.

To top it off, many scientists feel that people should look at these products very carefully because they are actual animal glands. If you've heard of mad cow disease you'll understand why you should be concerned about the possible risks. This is especially true of extracts associated with the liver, which is the organ that detoxifies the body, but also true of others such as pituitary extracts. Any toxins and certain illnesses in the desiccated organ you're consuming could very well be transferred to you via a mechanism called **prion transfer.** Prions are proteins that have been altered by disease and are impervious to heat, detergents, and your digestive tract, meaning they can carry disease between species.

Homeopathy

Homeopathy is a system that's been around for about two hundred years, based on something called "the law of similars." The premise here is that by using an infinitesimal amount of a substance that's known to cause a certain symptom, you can relieve that symptom and facilitate the body's ability to heal it. This system shares the philosophy that the smaller the dose, the more powerful the effect.

Due to a loophole in a 1938 law, products that are listed in a book called *Homeopathic Pharmacopoeia of the United States* can be marketed as drugs, yet they are only regulated by the very lax laws that govern supplements. These remedies are usually marketed in pharmacies, health food stores, and by certain practitioners.

Homeopathic medications are extremely diluted

Homeopathic products are usually minerals and plant substances, diluted with either water or alcohol if it's soluble, and crushed and mixed with lactose if it isn't. The original dilution is made with one part of the original substance to ninety-nine parts of what it's mixed with. Then one part of this solution is taken and diluted again, and this is done over and over. When you look at the label you'll see the strength listed as a number followed by the letter X, telling you how many times this process has been done. What you end up with is an incredibly low number, for example, a 30X dilution means that the original substance has been diluted 1,000,000,000,000,000,000,000,000,000,000 times. In homeopathy it is believed that even when a substance is diluted this completely it's still effective because the memory of the substance is still present in the homeopathic medication. Since most of these products don't contain detectable amounts of any active ingredient they are impossible to test for anything.

Because they're diluted to such a degree, homeopathic products are marketed as a kinder, gentler sort of supplement to people who are afraid of harsh medications with nasty side effects. Most health food stores do a bumper business in them, and you can find them in pharmacies as well. There's no proven risk in using these products for an illness like fibromyalgia, although attempting to treat cancer or high blood pressure with them might be a problem because it could cause people to deviate from more proven therapies.

Naturopathic medicine

Naturopathic doctors (ND for short) do pre-med training, and then complete further training in natural therapies. Not every state licenses them, though by 2008 it is expected that NDs will be available in every state. Insurance will sometimes cover their services, which include diagnostic lab and X ray. Naturopathic medicine is based on the prevention of illnesses (a little late for us!), and there are various specialities such as Chinese and Native American. Homeopathy, nutrition, physical medicine, psychological counseling, botanical supplements, and lifestyle changes are among the various methods that are used. Prescription drugs are not used at all. To find an ND in your area, or to learn more about naturopathic medicine, contact the Association of Naturopathic Physicians at 866-538-2267 or go to www.naturopathic.org.

IN A SENTENCE:

Many dietary supplements and treatments are marketed with extravagant claims that you should evaluate carefully before you buy.

learning

Physical Therapies That Might Help You

MODERN PHYSICAL therapy began as a discipline in the wake of World War I as a way to rehabilitate amputees and other injured servicemen. They were taught new ways of moving and adapting to the physical changes their lives required. As time went by it became obvious that these same modalities could help other people with physical limitations, especially during the polio epidemics. Today there are many forms of hands-on or movement training modalities as well as physical exercise disciplines that have proven helpful to many fibromyalgics. Some are considered entirely alternative or complimentary; others, like acupuncture, are making their way into Western medicine, and still others are handled by physicians and are now considered part of mainstream medicine.

Massage and other hands-on treatment

When you hurt, it's natural to be afraid of someone touching you, and the thought of someone pressing, pulling, or stretching you might be downright scary. Sometimes, however, hands-on therapy can really provide some relief: from heat and cold therapies to massage to techniques that utilize machines such as **biofeedback**.

Heat and cold therapies

Trying these modalities on your own is very easy to do, and usually people have natural preferences for one or the other. Warm baths and showers definitely relax muscles, and heating pads or hot water bottles are an extension of this therapy. A bag of frozen peas wrapped in a small towel can do wonders for headaches. Physical therapists can use whichever you prefer.

> **YOU DON'T** even have to be able to sew to make a hot/cold pack for use in the freezer or microwave. Simply take a long tube sock or a knee sock and fill it with dried beans, such as kidney, lima, or pinto. Knot in the open end and *voila!* It's ready to be heated or frozen. Always make sure that the pack is not too hot or cold for comfort, since either extreme can numb the skin and prevent you from feeling burn damage.

Massage therapy

Since recent studies have shown it to be valuable, physicians and insurance companies are both capitulating and are prescribing massage therapy for fibromyalgics. *Gentle* massage is the key, so be sure that the therapist you see has experience with fibromyalgia. Check with your doctor or support groups for referrals. If you can't afford a professional massage, you'll find many machines on the market from chairs to mechanical massagers that might be helpful. On most of these you'll want to use the medium setting, as the higher one may be too painful. Remember that you may not be able to tell until a day or so afterward if any technique was too vigorous for you. Also, be advised that not every fibromyalgic can tolerate massage therapy no matter how gentle. A gentle Swedish massage, which combines kneading, stroking, and friction, is the best for your body. Do not allow any therapist to attempt to press out lumps, press too firmly, or use elbows on your body. Massage therapists can be located through the American Massage Therapy Association at 888-843-2682 (www.amtamassage.com).

Other techniques

Two so-called release therapies are often performed by massage or **physical therapists**. The first is called Myofascial Release. This is a specialized stretching technique that concentrates on the **myofascia**, a thin tissue that covers all the organs of the body and holds them in place. Therapists are guided by feedback from the patient's own body. To learn more, www.myofas-cialrelief.com is a good resource.

Craniosacral release concentrates on the membranes and fluids that surround the brain and spinal cord. This therapy includes the bones of the skull, and face, and the spinal cord down to the tailbone. It is especially helpful for neck, face, and jaw pain. It sounds a bit frightening, but in fact a very light pressure is used, so gentle that patients sometimes can't even feel it and can fall asleep during sessions.

The Bowen Technique, which was developed by an Australian named Thomas Bowen after World War II, is a massage therapy that uses no force, simply extremely light touch through the clothing. Each session focuses on several areas of the body and targets areas that are tense. The therapist takes breaks that allow the body to "absorb" the changes. Sessions normally last a little over half an hour. For more information visit www.bowenther-apy.com or call 530-823-5759.

Occupational therapy

Many people mistakenly feel that this form of therapy is for assistance in the workplace, but it isn't. It is a type of therapy developed after World War I that uses productive or creative activity in the treatment or rehabilitation of disabled people. Basically, it promotes healing by occupying both your body and your mind. The idea is that performing tasks that focus both the brain and the body will speed rehabilitation. The goal is to restore muscle strength and mobility throught the use of special tools, materials, and equipment. Simple activities such as arts and crafts are examples of things that can be incorporated into the therapy. Information about this therapy and tips on finding therapists can be found through the American Occupational Therapy Association at 301-652-2682 (www.aota.org). Most insurance companies, including Medicare, usually cover this form of therapy.

QUESTIONS TO ASK YOUR PHYSICAL THERAPIST

○ How many treatments will I need to feel a difference?

○ How often must I have treatments?

○ Will my insurance cover the cost of my treatment/how much will my treatments cost? (Bear in mind that your insurance company may refuse to pay, in which case you will be responsible for the cost.)

○ How will I benefit from this therapy?

Chiropractors

A chiropractor is not a medical doctor but instead is a licensed professional who has received specialized training in the skeletal and nervous system. Chiropractic medicine is based on the theory that if the body is properly aligned, it can heal itself. These days many insurance companies do cover selected chiropractic services. Chiropractors on the whole are very knowledgeable about fibromyalgia, and in fact many fibromyalgics were originally diagnosed by a chiropractor. Despite this, since chiropractors do manipulations and alignments, you should be sure the one you have chosen understands the need for gentleness. Studies show that this modality may be most beneficial if you have severe neck and shoulder pain.

Chiropractors cannot prescribe medication because they are not physicians, but many recommend and sell a number of dietary supplements. You should be aware that your insurance will not cover these items. Visit www.chirodirectory.com for more information.

Doctors of Osteopathy

Doctors of Osteopathy have earned a degree similar to a medical doctor and can prescribe medication. However, their emphasis is on manual palpation, hands-on therapies, and natural medications. They believe strongly in the body's ability to heal itself, and focus on the musculoskeletal system. Like chiropractors, they perform manipulations to realign the body, but they use other therapies as well. For more information or to find a practitioner in your area call 301-652-2682 or go to www.aota.com.

Acupuncture

Acupuncture is an ancient Chinese healing art that involves the careful insertion of needles into specific points in the body. Studies on the benefits of acupuncture have produced mixed results, but many fibromyalgics do get some relief of symptoms from this process. It is not painful, but it does cause the body to release more endorphins. Insurance often covers acupuncture if you have it done by a medical doctor. The American Academy of Acupuncture can direct you to a licensed practitioner. You can contact them at 800-521-2262 or www.medicalacupuncture.com.

Acupressure

Acupressure is a therapy that involves firm, direct pressure using fingers, knuckles, and palms over certain areas of the body. If you're afraid of needles, this might be worth a try. Many fibromyalgics do a form of self-acupressure for back pain. This technique involves placing a tennis ball on the floor and lying on it. Moving around, pushing down, and putting pressure on the area will press out some of the fluids around tender points and provide some temporary relief. Visit www.wholisticonline.com for more information.

T'ai Chi

T'ai Chi is an extremely gentle, graceful, low-impact martial art form that originated in China. It is popular with fibromyalgics, who get relief from the gentle stretching and relaxation techniques that are part of this healing art. The exercises are called forms, and consist of poses based on animal forms. Classes are often given at adult schools and parks and recreation departments. Because it is so gentle, some senior citizen centers offer classes as well. It's also simple to learn on your own; several excellent instructional tapes are available at www.activevideos.com.

Yoga

Don't be intimidated by the word *yoga*. Pictures you've seen might have looked downright scary with poses that hurt just to look at. However, there are yoga classes for all levels of fitness. Of all the physical therapies fibromyalgics try, yoga is the one that gets the most rave reviews, because of its combination of stretching and mental relaxation.

Yoga exercises relax the major muscle groups and stimulate circulation. Deep, rhythmic breathing is part of the discipline, which is an important technique for relaxation and meditation. Yoga before bed can help with sleep, and during the day it can help make your lunch or coffee breaks more relaxing.

The National Yoga Alliance will refer you to registered teachers (www.yogaalliance.com) or you can look around for classes in your area. Be clear that you want gentle classes, and talk to your instructor before you start any class. Make sure that he or she knows about fibromyalgia or other chronic pain conditions such as arthritis, and is willing to guide you properly at your own pace. If you want to try it on your own, you can find great yoga self-help tapes and books at most bookstores and on the Internet.

Pilates

Today, Pilates is quite the celebrity rage in Hollywood, but it is based on the century-old teachings of Joseph Pilates. The goal is to improve posture and flexibility as well as increase stamina by using slow, controlled movement.

According to several fibromyalgics I know, "the body awareness takes your mind off your pain." You are taught through exercise the job of each muscle group and how to strengthen them through exercises that isolate your core muscles. There are many Pilates classes taught especially for fibromyalgics at health clubs and fitness centers.

Pilates exercise tapes can be purchased in bookstores and online at various sites, including www.gaiam.com.

The Alexander technique

Frederick Alexander, a professional orator born in 1869, developed chronic hoarseness that he discovered was caused by poor posture. The technique he developed, once used by George Bernard Shaw, teaches the release of muscle tension through "posture, breath, and movement." Much of the work is concentrated on the head and neck area, which makes this helpful especially for headaches and face and neck pain. Sessions last about forty-five minutes and you are personally coached in relaxation. For more information, visit www.alexandertechnique.com or call 800-473-0620.

Feldenkrais

Moshe **Feldenkrais** was a Russian physicist who suffered a severe knee injury that threatened his ability to walk. He combined his interests in judo—he was a black belt—psychology, biology, and physics into a discipline that got him walking again without pain. The technique that bears his name teaches awareness of the muscles and skeleton, and can be especially helpful because it increases your range of motion, helps you move more efficiently, reduces stress on your joints, and develops your flexibility. For more information, contact the Feldenkrais Guild of North America at 800-775-2118 (www.feldenkrais.com).

Trager work

Milton Trager grew up in Miami, Florida, where he studied dancing, gymnastics, and boxing. He discovered he had a natural gift for massage, and became a physical therapist and then a medical doctor while developing a technique called Trager Work.

Trager sessions begin with table work, where you are dressed in a flowing garment and are gently stretched and rocked into deep relaxation. Then you are taught simple exercises that can be done anywhere and will help you reach a relaxed, meditative state. This system is called Mentastics, for mental gymnastics. Training involves about six once-a-week sessions, but you are given homework. You are instructed to practice your technique each day for two or three fifteen-minute sessions.

Trager Work combines both hands-on and physical movement training, which are two methods that have been shown over and over to reduce pain and benefit the quality of life for those with chronic pain. For more information, go to www.trager.com or call 216-896-9383.

Other classes and techniques that can benefit you

This has just been an overview of physical approaches to the pain and muscle stiffness that plague our lives. There are many other things that you can try that might suit you better, which you can explore on your own. Some people like group classes such as water aerobics at a local YMCA; others prefer to try self-hypnosis, meditation, and a gentle exercise tape. One of the best sources for videotapes for all fitness levels, including one for "fibromyalgia patients who don't want to get started in an exercise program," is the Oregon Fibromyalgia Foundation. Visit their Web site at www.nfra.net. Keep trying to find a discipline to help strengthen and relax your body—there is one out there for every level and every personality.

IN A SENTENCE.

> *Don't give up if you are in pain and immobile—there are many helpful therapies you can try.*

living

Putting Your Health House in Order

IT'S BEEN said that the best way to live a long life is to get a chronic illness, because it will force you to pay attention to your health. When you learn to control your stress levels and when you start to exercise, you've made two giant steps toward not just controlling your fibromyalgia but improving your overall health as well. The fact is that anything you do to make yourself healthier will help you to feel better despite your fibromyalgia. It's important for you to realize that your general health status has a great deal of influence on how you feel, and how well you will cope with your fibromyalgia flares. It's time now to look at the rest of your body and make sure you're doing everything you can to be as healthy as possible. In other words, it's time to put your health house in order.

Fibromyalgia doesn't make you more likely to develop another illness

I'm asked every day if fibromyalgia causes thyroid problems, obesity, or osteoporosis, just to mention a few. Luckily, fibromyalgia hasn't been shown to increase your risk for any other illness. Countless studies of the demographics of fibromyalgia bear this out. Fibromyalgia's connection with almost every other illness has been extensively explored. However, since your body is struggling with the energy drain that occurs from the symptoms of fibromyalgia, other problems can be an indirect result.

If you're a woman, you're more at risk for autoimmune conditions such as **Hashimoto's thyroiditis, rheumatoid arthritis,** and **lupus**. If you're a man, you're more at risk for conditions such as **gout** or heart disease. If you're a premenopausal woman, you're more likely to be anemic, and if you're approaching menopause you may already be experiencing some symptoms from your changing hormones. Circulatory ailments from illnesses like diabetes and the huge bodily stress caused by obesity carry many additional risk factors. What this means is you need to keep close tabs on your health, cut out your bad habits, and develop some new good ones. It's also important not to ignore any new symptoms you may develop. It isn't safe to chalk everything up to fibromyalgia.

Routine checkups are good for your health

Although most health plans these days won't cover routine physicals, fibromyalgics have plenty of complaints, so there should be no problem with getting a fairly complete exam. Before you see your physician, take a moment to list the symptoms that you need to have evaluated. You want to make sure nothing is overlooked.

Make sure to have regular blood tests

Even if you had a complete battery of blood tests done when you were diagnosed, you should have your blood tested annually. Not only can your fibromyalgia symptoms obscure other conditions, but the medications you take can have side effects. No matter whether you're taking prescription medications, over-the-counter pain relievers, or supplements, you'll need to have blood tests at least once a year. Be sure that you have kidney and liver tests as well as a complete blood count. If you belong to an HMO, don't assume that your physician will order all the blood tests you should have. It's important that you read up on your medications and know tests you should ask for. The package insert that comes with your medications will give you the information you need. For example, if you are taking a medication to lower your cholesterol, or over-the-counter Advil to relieve pain, make sure your doctor orders liver tests. Many problems can be averted by early diagnosis, and if a medication is damaging you in any way your blood tests can show it before you can feel it. The earlier an abnormality is detected, the easier it is to correct it.

Don't forget to tell your doctor about your risk factors

You should also make sure that you and your doctor have discussed your family history and risk factors. Many illnesses, like diabetes, heart disease, and blood pressure problems, run in families and there are things you can do to improve your chances of avoiding them. Maintaining a normal weight, exercising regularly, and even some medications can stack the deck strongly in your favor. It's a lot easier to stay healthy than it is to get healthy, so don't avoid this step. Thyroid problems often run in families as do certain cancers that your doctor can easily screen for. For example, if you're a male who has prostate cancer in your family, it wouldn't be wise to wait until age fifty to have your first screening.

Don't look for trouble

When you get your test results, trust your doctor, or if you need to, get a second opinion from a specialist. The Internet or a clerk at your local health food store are not always reliable places to get information. This is not to say that those sources can't be correct. It just means that anything you glean from places like that should be discussed and evaluated by a physician who knows you, and confirmed by standard and accepted medical testing. These days there are all sorts of companies advertising conditions that "don't show up on conventional testing." Maybe you've heard that thyroid tests aren't accurate because of a condition called Wilson's Syndrome. Or perhaps you've heard that even if your liver tests are normal you need something fancy to "detox" it from the "rigors" of modern life. Do the research on these claims. Don't just embrace them because they sound convincing.

A few words of advice: Don't be led to believe you are hormone deficient if your doctor can't find any trace of this. Hormones are easily and accurately measured these days. Don't believe that there are diseases that no one has heard of except the person marketing the cure. Very few people have obscure, unheard of deficiencies or illnesses. Be leery of anyone, even if they have impressive-sounding credentials, who diagnoses an illness in a special laboratory and then sells you a special cure you can't purchase anywhere else.

Trust your physician to steer you in the right direction

If your examination or your blood tests turn up an abnormality, work with your doctor to correct the situation. Remember that even a minor-looking problem may be deep-seated. For example, if your blood work-up shows you to be just slightly anemic, you could certainly be feeling the effects. By the time your blood tests register a low iron reading, your muscles have already been depleted of their stores. For this reason, too, you need to stick with any corrections you've been given. Many women are poor iron absorbers and will always find it difficult to maintain healthy levels. You'll need to take an iron supplement for quite some time, at least until the end of your reproductive years if you tend to be anemic. Be sure to ask your physician when you can expect to feel the benefit of making the correction. For example, if you've been given thyroid medication, you should be retested in about two months because it takes that long for your levels to be accurate. It's up to you to mark your calendar and make an appointment to get any retesting that's required on schedule. Your doctor has many patients, but you have only one.

You must take charge of your own health

Once your doctor has completed your examination and you've been given the necessary corrective measures, his or her task is done. No doctor is going to follow you around to make sure you're taking your blood pressure medicine or avoiding salt. During your checkups, your doctor may stress to you that you haven't followed instructions, but let's face it, you're not a child and the doctor is not your parent. If you want to be in good health, you must look at it as a process and realize that you have to work at it. If you're given a medication, for example, for blood pressure, and you develop side effects, call your doctor. Don't decide to discontinue medication on your own, and don't assume that your doctor can't give you another solution if the first one isn't helping. Work with your doctor until you are happy with the results.

A healthy diet is necessary to good health

You'll need to learn a few basics about nutrition and metabolism if you're serious about looking at your habits to see what you can do to make yourself healthier. Dietary changes are a drug-free way to reinforce your body's own healing ability. The description that follows hardly scratches the surface, but it should make it clear what you must keep in mind when considering the food you eat and the supplements people are trying to sell you. Many pharmaceutical and supplement companies feed on people with chronic illness because they know there is no cure available in mainstream medicine. Their claims often sound logical when in fact they are physiologically unfeasible.

Your digestive system at work

Before you take a closer look at the kinds and amounts of foods you should eat, you should understand how your digestive system works. Your body's digestive tract is like a factory. Food goes in and is processed and packaged for use. After that, it is distributed to your whole body, each part taking what it needs. Finally, wastes from this process, as well as from the manufactured products themselves, are collected and flushed out of the body. What you eat is raw material, not a finished product. Fat doesn't enter your body and go to fat cells, any more than if you ate liver it would be carried to your liver. Eating something, or taking something in a supplemental form, does not necessarily get it into your cells.

Everything you consume enters your digestive system through the doorway of your mouth and the conveyer belt of your esophagus. There isn't a perfect correlation between what you eat and what becomes of it. The cells in your body don't directly use the food you've eaten for power, they use a manufactured fuel for energy. Certain fuels are more easily consumed, just as certain fuels burn better in your fireplace. The quality of the raw materials you supply has an effect on the quality of energy you produce. This is why eating right will help you to feel better.

The power of ATP

Your cells are powered by a chemical called ATP, or adenosine triphosphate. ATP is mostly created in special power stations inside cells called mitochondria. Rather like small generators, these stations push ions or charged particles back and forth across a membrane in a very complex series of events that results in the energy we need.

How effectively this system works depends on many things, including the quality of the raw material supplied to create the ATP and your general health. Many people feel that the defect causing fibromyalgia must occur at this very basic level because the whole body is so completely affected by the condition. Dr. R. Paul St. Amand, M.D., who works with the guaifenesin protocol, believes that energy production is compromised at this level by an intercellular buildup of phosphate and calcium. Other researchers feel that an enzyme involved in the production of ATP may be defective in fibromyalgia. It would take very, very little to throw off the delicate balance of this minute machinery. Indeed, muscle biopsies of fibomyalgics have shown ATP to be low, as have some other specialized studies involving a **magnetic spectroscope**. As fibromyalgics we agree that we can't make enough energy.

Raw materials are important

Our bodies were designed to run mostly on protein and fat, nuts, seeds, and a little plant food that might be in season. We need protein to be broken down into amino acids, raw material to build new cells, and plant fiber or roughage to keep our digestive tracts healthy. Our bodies can use fat for fuel, and we need fats because certain vitamins are fat-soluble so the only way to get them is to eat fat. You don't have to eat carbohydrates; your body can manufacture them. There are no essential carbohydrates, only essential fatty acids and essential amino acids that come from eating proteins and fats. In addition our bodies need minerals and thirteen vitamins that generally must be provided by the foods we eat.

Highly processed foods and sugars aren't very useful for the body in the long haul, and fill us up so that we can't eat enough of the healthy foods we need. It makes a great deal of sense that everyone would be healthier if they went back to a more basic way of eating. The huge epidemic of digestive disorders, heart disease, obesity, and diabetes is a new phenomena clearly linked to our modern diet. If it makes sense for everyone to change their eating habits, then it makes it doubly important for those of us with chronic, energy-stealing illnesses to do it.

Improving the way you eat is a powerful way to feel better. Most people are really astounded at how much better they feel when they eliminate excess sugar, caffeine, and refined carbohydrates from their diets. Changing our diets can have long range benefits as well. Let's not forget that 60 percent of cancers in women are diet related. A high-carbohydrate diet contributes indirectly to increased levels of circulating estrogens. High triglyceride levels are known to displace estrogens from steroid-binding globulins. High fiber intake from unprocessed foods can reduce these levels and decrease the risk of breast cancer, among other things.

Diabetes and FMS

IF YOU have diabetes and fibromyalgia it is extra important for you to keep your blood sugar levels under control. Diabetes causes the nerves to be more sensitive, and is a common cause of neuropathy, or damage to the small nerves. This is a painful condition that is even worse when you add fibromyalgia to the equation. Diabetes can also lead to a host of circulatory problems that cause people to be increasingly immobile.

Eat more vegetables and protein and less processed foods

A healthier diet consists of more protein and vegetables than we usually eat. The recommended daily requirement for protein is 0.36 grams per pound of body weight. Using this calculation, a 150-pound person should eat 54 grams of protein a day. Animal sources (egg, meat, milk) are complete proteins, meaning that they contain all the essential amino acids, while plant sources are usually low in protein or missing some of the needed amino acids. The proper combination of vegetable proteins can do the trick, however. Your body can convert protein to glucose—this is why you do not need to eat any carbohydrates or sugars.

Very fresh vegetables or frozen ones, lightly cooked, provide the best vitamins and fiber—heavy cooking can destroy both. Frozen vegetables usually contain more nutrients than the fresh stock you buy at the supermarket because transit time dramatically reduces them. For example, within twenty-four hours of being picked, green beans lose 40 percent of their vitamin C content.

Fruit should be reserved as an occasional treat or pick-me-up, because it is mostly water and **fructose**, or fruit sugar. This form of sugar is certainly easier on the body than white processed sugar, but it isn't much of an improvement. Any vitamins that occur in fruit are much more plentiful in vegetables.

Learn to avoid added sugars that exist in processed food. You don't need sugar in your cereal or breads. You don't need sugar in your tomato sauce, peanut butter, or in your condiments. You don't need corn syrup in salad dressings, either. With just a little extra effort you can find products without them or make your own. Reading labels for sugar, corn syrup, honey, dextrose, and other sweeteners will demonstrate to you how much hidden sugar you are being served every day.

Carbohydrates can cause weight gain and other problems

Carbohydrate consumption causes insulin release by raising the blood sugar. High insulin levels eventually cause excessive insulin resistance, which is responsible for many problems, including heart disease, type 2 diabetes, and high blood pressure. Insulin is the only hormone that puts fat into fat cells, causing us to gain weight. Without insulin release you cannot get fat. A high-carbohydrate diet, even in otherwise healthy people, can be responsible for **constipation**, irritable bowel, high cholesterol and triglyceride levels, yeast overgrowth, fatigue, mood swings, and headaches.

Carbohydrates can depress the immune system, to which allergies have also been linked. A recent study showed that after ingesting sugars including starch, honey, orange juice, or glucose, the effectiveness of neutrophils at destroying bacteria and other microorganisms in the blood is depressed for more than five hours. (Neutrophils are cells that circulate in the blood whose function is to destroy any foreign bodies that they encounter.) If you've had recurrent yeast infections of any kind, chances are that you've already been told to restrict your intake of sugar and starch. If your blood sugars are running high or if your triglyceride levels are high, you've probably heard the same thing.

Avoid high-glycemic foods

The **glycemic index** is a ranking of foods that measures how fast the carbohydrate in a given food raises your blood sugar. Fiber and fat slow down the rate at which carbohydrates raise your blood sugar, so foods ranked lower on this index are much easier for most of us to tolerate. This scale is not designed to tell you exactly what you should eat, but it is another tool to help you get a proper balance into your diet. It will help you choose the right amount of carbohydrate and the right kind for good health. This balance is the basis, for example, of the popular Protein Power and Zone diet plans. Unless you are hypoglycemic and these programs are too liberal for you, you will certainly feel better if you eat a higher percentage of protein and a lower percentage of carbohydrates. When you have found a balance or diet that is right for you, your extreme hunger and dramatic food cravings will stop. You may have to learn this for yourself, but those feelings are not normal and instead are a sign that something is wrong.

Get to your ideal weight

You may need to lose some weight to feel better. Many fibromyalgics end up gaining weight—studies show that more than half of us have put on a considerable amount. Hauling around extra weight is no joke when you have fibromyalgia, not to mention the long-term dangers of obesity to your health. You've come this far, so you know that it's essential for you to stay active and to feel good about yourself. It's hard to do this when you're overweight, and as you get older and sicker it's more difficult to lose the weight.

Control your metabolism

It is much easier to drop weight if you increase your metabolism through exercise. Muscle burns more calories than fat even when we're asleep. You

The Approximate Glycemic Index Values of a Few Selected Foods:

Glucose	100
Potatoes	98
Honey	90
White Rice	72
White Bread	69
Bananas	62
Tomatoes	38
Strawberries	32
Whole Milk	27
Broccoli	10
Lettuce	10
Green beans	10

Note: A complete list of glycemic index values can be found online at www.mendosa.com

also need to increase your body's insulin sensitivity, because excess body fat is both a cause and a result of **insulin resistance**. To do this you'll have to give up once and for all the concept of calorie counting. While it's true that you can lose weight by eating 1,000 calories a day of sugar and starch, you won't be able to build up the lean muscle mass you need to maintain it. And you won't be able to lose weight at 1,000 calories a day for long. If you restrict calories to that degree, your body will slow down your metabolism in response. Our bodies' primal fear of starvation overrides our conscious thought that we need to look better for our high school reunion.

Restricting carbohydrates

To drop weight and keep it off, you'll need to limit the carbohydrates that cause your body to produce extra insulin and thus to gain weight. These include potatoes, wheat products, rice, rice cakes, corn, bread, bananas, dried fruits, and all candy and desserts. The amount of carbohydrates you can eventually consume without gaining weight varies greatly. Some people are extremely sensitive to carbohydrates and will gain weight quickly by consuming any amount over about 50 grams a day. The average range to maintain weight is between 55 and 150 grams a day. The average on a low-carbohydrate weight loss diet is about 35 grams a day. A pure protein (or zero carbohydrate) diet is extremely effective in causing rapid weight loss, but it's impractical and unhealthy for any sustained period. It also causes severe diarrhea in most people.

Learn about healthy fats

Another important factor in a healthy diet is the kind of fat you eat. Simply put, there are good fats and there are bad fats. A mounting body of evidence suggests that the level of heart disease, which has risen dramatically in the past century, is due to the increase of **partially hydrogenated fats** in our diet, not to all fats in general. At the same time, **essential fatty acids** are often lacking in the foods we eat because we've grown paranoid about the word *fat*. The word *essential* should catch your attention—you need to consume certain fatty acids (alpha linolenic acid and linoleic acid) because our bodies cannot manufacture them. You need them as building blocks for prostaglandins, cell membrane layers, and to increase your metabolic rate.

On the other hand, a diet high in **partially hydrogenated fats** can cause damage to our arteries through unstable molecules called **free radicals**. These fats are also associated with higher cancer rates than the fats we have been taught to fear, saturated or animal fats, which newer studies show don't deserve the bad rap they've been getting all these years. Partially hydrogenated fats are artificial products produced by adding hydrogen to a naturally occurring fat at extremely high temperatures. This makes this fat solid at room temperature. The result is a fat that has a longer shelf life, but that our bodies cannot handle. Partially hydrogenated fats form the basis of solid margarine, and are often present in foods such as crackers and baked goods like cookies. Hydrogenated fats have also been shown to inhibit our own normal fatty acid metabolism and decrease our good cholesterol, or HDL. Safer forms of fat for human bodies are the natural ones that occur in nuts, many vegetables, and grains.

So the bottom line here is to avoid overly processed foods and stick with natural products that require refrigeration and aren't loaded with chemicals or preservatives.

Food sensitivities

Examine your diet for other things that might be causing symptoms. Some people don't react well to artificial sweeteners such as aspartame and should use **stevia**, an herbal sweetener, or **sucralose** (Splenda), which is actually made from sugar. Others can't tolerate decaffeinated coffee because of the chemicals used to remove the caffeine. Some adults, especially Hispanics and African Americans, may be lactose intolerant. If eating dairy products that contain **lactose**, or milk sugar, makes you gassy, bloated, or gives you diarrhea, avoid them (heavy cream, sour cream, and natural cheeses should be tolerable). There are alternatives such as soy and medications like Lactaid that contain the missing enzyme you need in order to digest the lactose present in milk, cottage cheese, and yogurt. You don't have to submit to expensive and extensive testing for food allergies and sensitivities, the results of which may not even be very accurate. Instead, keep a diary and through observation learn which foods don't agree with you. Many foods that cause a positive reaction when tested for allergies on the skin won't bother you when you eat them.

DON'T FORGET that some medications have weight gain as a side effect:

O   Antidepressants such as Elavil
O   Flexeril
O   Estrogen

Limit your caffeine consumption

Although weight and nutrition are the most important issues to gain control over, there are other factors that might be preventing you from being as healthy as you can be. Caffeine is a stimulant, and one to which you can build up a tolerance. When you use it habitually as a drug to enable you to push yourself farther than you should, you are abusing caffeine and wearing down your body. As we've seen over and over, you will pay for this kind of overexertion in spades.

Most fibromyalgics feel much better when they discontinue caffeine, which is a fairly powerful stimulant in the amounts most of us habitually consume. Caffeine can make it more difficult to sleep, increase your blood pressure and heart rate, and irritate your bladder. Withdrawal from caffeine only takes two or three days, but the symptoms can be pretty intense in some people. If you've decided to take the plunge, it might be best to attempt it over a long weekend. Drink plenty of fluids, and be prepared for a headache and fatigue, both of which can be severe. Be careful not to use anything that contains caffeine (as does Excedrin) for your headache.

Quit smoking

Nicotine is also a stimulant, and it also causes blood vessels to constrict, which decreases blood flow. When this happens oxygen and nutrient delivery to muscles is limited, which can increase spasms and pain. Nicotine may make it more difficult to sleep at night, and studies have shown that it also may lower your pain threshold. Carbon monoxide in a smoker's blood binds to hemoglobin, which carries oxygen around the body, making it less available to your muscles. Some doctors have gone as far as saying that anyone in chronic pain who continues to smoke is making a huge contribution to that pain level. Of course, you also know that in the end, smoking will have other detrimental effects on your health, and will make it more difficult for you to exercise in the years when you may need it the most. More than four thousand chemicals are present in tobacco, including poisons such as DDT, arsenic, and carbon monoxide. If you are at all sensitive to chemicals, imagine what this combination is doing to your body. Obviously you should also avoid secondhand smoke and other airborne pollutants as much as you can.

Everyone knows that smoking increases your risk of lung cancer—when you breathe in smoke the chemicals in it gradually change the cells in the lung. But there are other effects, too. These same chemicals are absorbed into your bloodstream and injure the arteries that transport them. Compromised circulation is not something you want to have as a fibromyalgic. For example, less oxygenated blood reaching the brain won't help fibrofog. Smoking also depletes the body of certain vitamins and minerals, including vitamin C.

You can quit if you're committed

Nicotine is an addictive drug, and some sources say that the addiction is as powerful as one to heroin or cocaine. When you quit, withdrawal symptoms include anxiety, headaches, irritability, and restlessness. But if you do quit there are benefits to your body right from the very beginning, starting with your endurance. Ten years after quitting your risk of heart disease will be reduced to that of a nonsmoker. Even after a year your risk will fall by 50 percent.

There are now products on the market that can help you quit. These include nicotine gums and patches as well as the use of some antidepressants. It's definitely important to find a modality that will work for you, because it's really hard to stop. If you can't do it by yourself, ask your doctor to prescribe something to help you. It's time. You'll never be sorry you quit.

Other negative effects

Caffeine, alcohol, and tobacco also have a proven negative effect on bone growth and contribute to osteoporosis. It is likely that they have other negative effects that are much harder to measure than bone density. Cigarette smoking increases your risk of stroke by 300 percent. Imagine how hard it would be to battle back from a stroke with fibromyalgia.

Alcohol in moderation is not bad for people with fibromyalgia. However, it is contraindicated with many of the medications prescribed for fibromyalgia, so be cautious. Alcohol can certainly increase fatigue and reduce your sense of equilibrium, which are more difficult to manage when you're ill.

Your mental health plays a role in your physical health

Fibromyalgia is not a mental disorder. You didn't get fibromyalgia because you were abused as a child or because you're in a bad marriage. But if you have unresolved problems that are weighing you down, do ask for help. If you need to talk to someone about past issues or present problems, ask for a referral to a professional who understands a bit about fibromyalgia or chronic illnesses. Personal issues can weigh you down. Bad relationships are heavy burdens. Problems you can't solve by yourself are somewhere in your mind using up your energy. So don't be afraid to make changes and to deal with your issues. Check to see if your health insurance will cover the help you need. Ask your physician to make some suggestions. Do not assume that the help you need is beyond your reach. There are many centers with sliding scales and volunteer help if your medical plan won't cover the help you need. If you're unhappy or depressed, it *does* have an effect on your physical health. Everything will feel worse than it already does.

IN A SENTENCE:

> *Maintaining good overall health and putting the right kinds of things into your body are important steps for improving the way that you feel.*

learning

Taking Charge of Your Overall Health

NDW YDU need to look hard at yourself and decide what you need to do to improve your health. For most of us, losing the extra weight is the biggest obstacle to better health, so the first step is to find a healthy diet that works for you. When you've reached your ideal weight, it's up to you to create a healthy eating plan that you can stick to for the rest of your life.

The key is to find what works best for you

Which diet works the best? That, of course, is a multimillion-dollar question raised by a multibillion-dollar industry. Generally speaking, any diet works if you do it the way you're supposed to. I have friends who have lost weight on Jenny Craig, with Weight Watchers, with Overeaters Anonymous, with Sugar Busters, and with low-carbohydrate diets such as Atkins, Protein Power, or The Zone. Liquid diets, very low-calorie diets, and other food restrictions also work. The point is that any of these systems will work more or less if you stick with them. Since "sticking with" is the operative phrase for most of us, you should choose your diet carefully. But it's very important to always remember that a weight loss diet is temporary. *You should only use these diets to lose the extra weight.*

Some diets (like Jenny Craig) may not be for you because you can't afford to pay for their special meals. Others that require weighing food or counting numeric values on special lists may be too time-consuming and difficult. A lot of fibromyalgics crave sweets, and tasting the tiny portions offered by Weight Watchers might make your cravings impossible to control. Not having any sweet foods may suit you better than having a tempting bite. Only you know whether or not you can stop after one brownie.

Certain medical conditions play a role

If you're hypoglycemic and overweight, or if you have early diabetes and you need to lose weight, you don't have a choice. You'll have to go on a low-carbohydrate diet plan, which is the only diet that will allow you to control blood sugar levels. No other diet will work for you. But if controlling your blood sugar levels in not necessary for you and you have a small amount of weight to lose to get to your optimum weight, almost any diet will work pretty well. If you have a lot of weight to loose, you'll have to choose more carefully, of course because you have to pick a diet you can live on for a long period. You might even elect to have one of the newer surgeries, like gastric bypass, if your weight is seriously endangering your health.

Diet is just the first step

No matter which one you pick, you'll have to give up some of the things you like. Let's face it, the things you like so much and think you can't do without are usually the foods that got you into your predicament. Diets are not fun. If diets were easy, everyone would be thin. Diet pills, which work by raising the body's metabolism, are a true double-edged sword for fibromyalgics. This extra demand for energy will eventually backfire, and you will collapse. Bear in mind you have an urgent reason to feel your best, you have fibromyalgia. So it's important to stop throwing up roadblocks and get to work. Yes, I know you feel lousy. Yes, I know when you feel awful food is one of your few comforts. So eat something—just make sure it's the right something.

Although I'm not much of a meat eater, I do best on a low-carbohydrate diet. I find if there's no limit on portions or on how often I eat, I can make do. There are a lot of products out there made with Splenda (or sucralose), which is a no-calorie, no-carbohydrate sweetener made from sugar itself. The taste fools me, and satisfies my cravings for sweets.

A low-carbohydrate diet

If you elect to try a low-carbohydrate diet and you're not hypoglycemic, there are lots to choose from. Dr. Robert Atkins, M.D., has a series of books that even cover the science behind his diet. Suzanne Somers, Diana Schwartzbein, Fran McCullough, Barry Sears, and many others have best-selling diet and cookbooks. If you are hypoglycemic, though, you'll have to look at the recipes carefully to make sure there are no forbidden sugars or caffeine in them. Some of these diets are very complicated and include food combining and timing (Suzanne Somers) or percentages (Zone), and some are very straightforward and simple. On the Atkins diet you can eat as much of the acceptable foods as you want in any combination that appeals to you.

Limiting carbohydrates will boost your energy

Low-carbohydrate diets help boost energy levels in fibromyalgics. As you're probably aware, a low-calorie diet eventually slows down your metabolism. Your body doesn't know that you are purposely restricting your food intake; it senses on a primal level that a period of famine has arrived, and slows down to preserve its fat stores—the opposite of what you are trying to accomplish! If you've noticed on a low-calorie diet that eventually your weight loss slows dramatically even with heavy restrictions—this is what you've experienced. But on a low-carbohydrate diet, since you are still loading your body with calories of fat, protein, and even some sugars from vegetables, this effect doesn't occur, and it actually boosts your energy levels.

Low-carbohydrate diets are very easy to do

A basic low carbohydrate diet is simple. You can eat all the protein you want: meat, fish, eggs, and poultry. You can have any dairy product that doesn't contain lactose or milk sugar, including cheese, heavy cream, and sour cream. (You have to avoid milk, and limit milk-containing cheeses like cottage and ricotta to a half a cup a day.) There's also a long list of vegetables to choose from, but you have to avoid legumes (lima beans, peas, garbanzo beans, lentils) as well as starches. You can't have grains, rice, potatoes, corn, or bananas because they are mostly carbohydrates. Fruit is extremely limited on this diet because fruit contains fructose or fruit sugar, which translates to carbohydrates.

Don't cheat!

This diet will work very effectively as long as you don't cheat and eat foods you don't see listed. If you eat any form of the forbidden carbohydrates you will not lose weight. This diet is not as forgiving as a low-calorie diet. Any of the nonlisted carbohydrates will cause your body to release

Basic Low-Carbohydrate Diet
for Weight Loss Only

O No limit on proteins: beef, chicken, duck, eggs, all fish, all shellfish, tofu, all cheeses (except those that contain milk like processed cheese foods or slices, cottage, or ricotta cheese. Those are limited to ½ cup a day)

O No limit on the following dairy products: butter, cream (sweet and/or sour)

O All salad greens are acceptable

O No limit on low-carbohydrate vegetables: alfalfa sprouts, asparagus, bean sprouts, bok choy, broccoli, Brussels sprouts, cabbage (limit of 1 cup per day), celery, celery root, cauliflower, cucumber, endive, eggplant, escarole, daikon radish, jicama, kale, kohlrabi, leeks, lettuce (all types mushrooms, okra, olives, peppers (all types), radishes, rhubarb sauerkraut, scallions, snow peas, spinach, string or green beans, summer squash (zucchini/yellow/patty pan), tomatoes, water chestnuts, zucchini

O All herbs and spices

O One handful of the following nuts per day: almonds, Brazil nuts, hazel nuts, macadamia nuts, pecans, pine nuts, pumpkin seeds, sunflower seeds, walnuts

O No limit on fats and oils

O One small serving of 6 strawberries or ¼ cantaloupe melon

O Fresh coconut

O One half an avocado a day

O Two tablespoons of lemon/lime juice

insulin. Once you've done that the high-calorie foods you're eating will be quickly and efficiently escorted to your fat cells for storage.

Learning to read labels carefully is essential

Perhaps especially with a low-carbohydrate diet, but in reality with any diet, you need to read labels carefully, especially on processed foods. Even if you're on a calorie-counting diet it will make sense to choose foods with no added sugar. And you'll want to watch for the undesirable fats—the hydrogenated ones. On a low-carbohydrate diet you'll need to check labels for all forms of sugar and starch.

Get started now

If you need to lose weight, this is the month to select your diet and start. Remember that you can take breaks as you go along; for example, you can

LACKING ENERGY to shop for healthy food and then for proper food preparation is something we must fight on a daily basis. Changing your dietary habits may be the real test of your commitment to feeling better. Consider a Saturday morning trip to a farmer's market in good weather to combine exercise with shopping for food that's good for you.

reward yourself by easing up on the restrictions for a weekend every time you've lost ten pounds. You don't want to go whole hog on these breaks because you don't want to undo all the progress you've made. Just stop for a moment and pat yourself on the back.

Don't wait for the perfect time to start your diet. There's no perfect time. In fact, I've discovered that I do better if I don't set myself up in a big way. If I just slide into the necessary restrictions, I find it a pretty simple undertaking. Like everything else you do, sometimes it will be hard and sometimes it will be easy. Sometimes you will do very well at it, other times you will slip and backslide. It's a process, and it's time to get started.

Even if you're thin you may not be eating right

Even if you don't need to lose weight, you still need to be concerned with good nutrition. I know perfectly well that if your weight is normal or you are thin, most doctors will assume that you have good eating habits. Most of us realize that this is a joke on them. What's working to keep you thin may not be good solid nutrition—eating too little, or using stimulants such as caffeine or nicotine. At each age group there are specific long-term risks in not getting proper vitamins and minerals and not eating well. Preventive medicine and health maintenance begin with what you put into your body. No matter what size you are, if you're living on sweets or coffee and cigarettes you're not going to be the best that you can be.

Eating well if you don't need to lose weight usually means avoiding fast food and prepackaged foods. With a little effort, you will be able to find plenty of meals you can prepare quickly, or in advance. If you work, or are out of the house all day, consider buying a slow-cooker or Crock-Pot. If you are serious about wanting to feel better, you'll have to be serious about the food you eat.

* * *

Steps to Getting Healthy

○ Eat two or three healthy meals a day

○ Avoid caffeine, sugar, alcohol, and junk food such as prepackaged snacks

○ Drink enough water or fluids

○ Do fifteen minutes of light stretching in the morning and evening

○ Take a moderately paced walk during daylight hours, thirty minutes per day

○ If you are exhausted, or frazzled, lie down for at least half an hour and practice relaxation or take a short nap

○ Have regular medical checkups

IN A SENTENCE:

Because fibromyalgia is such a challenging illness, you must consider all the factors involved in maintaining the total health of your body.

HALF-YEAR MILESTONE

Now that you are halfway through your first year with fibromyalgia:

O YOU HAVE DETERMINED WHETHER YOU
   HAVE HYPOGLYCEMIA AND, IF YOU DO,
   HAVE ADJUSTED YOUR DIET
   ACCORDINGLY.

O YOU KNOW ABOUT ALL THE DIFFERENT
   TYPES OF MEDICATIONS FOR
   FIBROMYALIGA, HAVE REVIEWED ANY
   MEDICATIONS YOU MAY HAVE ALREADY
   BEEN TAKING, AND RETHOUGHT OR
   ELIMINATED THOSE THAT DO NOT AID IN
   YOUR RECOVERY.

O YOU'VE LEARNED ABOUT A NEW
   EXPERIMENTAL TREATMENT OPTION CALLED
   THE GUAIFENSIN PROTOCOL AND
   CONSIDERED WHETHER YOU WANT TO TRY IT.

O YOU ARE AWARE OF THE ALTERNATIVE
   THERAPIES AVAILABLE TO YOU.

O YOU HAVE TAKEN CONTROL OF YOUR
   HEALTH BY EXAMINING YOUR HEALTH
   SITUATION AND MAKING LONG-TERM
   CHOICES.

Fibromyalgia and the Workplace

NO MATTER who you are or what you do, it's likely that people rely on you. So whether you work in your home or in an office, you may have found that your work situation is greatly affected by your fibromyalgia. How you manage this situation is very important, not only for your own well-being, but for those who work or live with you.

Your challenges remain the same

Some of us have no choice but to remain at work full-time to support our families. Others of us may be able to work part-time, take some time off, or retire. Or we may be full-time homemakers with a whole different set of obligations. Whether you're bringing home the bacon, cooking it in a pan, or doing both, you'll need to be strong and remain realistic. Only you can know what's best for you, and what your options are.

Your work may be important to you

The decision whether to remain at your job or not is full of wide-ranging emotions. Many of us are deeply attached to what we do. It's a part of our identity and we can't imagine ourselves without that all-important job. To a certain extent, society defines us by what we do. Being unemployed, for any reason, can be depressing and isolating. Fighting for disability is a long, difficult ordeal, and requires that you concentrate not on what is positive in your life, but on your symptoms and limitations. (Imagine how hard it is to feel better when you're constantly regurgitating your complaints.) You'll have to write journals, letters, and provide other documents proving how sick you are when all you want to do is get better. So it's essential for you to examine all of your feelings when you approach this subject. Here's some basic information that will help you as you explore this topic and how it relates to you.

Working outside your home

We all need to feel useful; it's really a crucial part of all of our lives. Interaction with other people outside the home is also important, whether you get it through a paid job or volunteer work, full-time or only a few hours a week.

For those of you who have a growing and viable career, living with fibromyalgia presents a unique challenge. Quitting what you love doing is simply not an option, so it's important to reevaluate your job situation to see how it can be modified for your current health situation. You may be one of those rare individuals who can keep it together. Chances are, however, that fibromyalgia will take its ugly toll. Remember that your health must come first: Whatever modifications you make now will only better prepare you to jump back on the career track down the road.

If you don't already have a job and need to find employment, there are many types of jobs available—and lots of jobs that you may enjoy. Full-time, part-time, fixed or flexible hours are all options, depending on your health, circumstances, and training. Regardless of your illness, we are all entitled to a certain amount of protection under a law called the Americans with Disability Act. It is illegal for prospective employers to discriminate against you because you have a disability. The Equal Opportunity Employment Office has information about this issue.

Work is a good thing and a normal part of life. Work will get you out of bed, challenge you mentally and physically, and doing your job well will give you the positive feedback—which is such a good thing for all of us. If there's something you want to do, or love to do, you should absolutely find a way to do it. The key is doing it in an environment that is comfortable and does not exacerbate your condition.

Making adjustments

What you'll need to do to accommodate your fibromyalgia, of course, largely depends on the kind of work you do. If you work at a desk you'll have one set of challenges, and if you work on your feet and are constantly moving around, you'll have others. Only you can properly evaluate the challenges facing you and find the solutions. There are various ways to accomplish this. First, you can make a list of all your regular activities and try to establish which component of which task is painful or especially fatiguing. You can also look at ways to get the most use out of your break times—scheduled or unscheduled. That might be as simple for you as finding a place to lie down and stretch out your back and neck muscles. And many of us have at least enough flexibility in our jobs to assign certain tasks to days when we might have more energy or feel better, perhaps on a Monday, or after a light day.

When you start a new job or begin to reassess your current work environment, there are actually a lot of things you can do to make yourself more comfortable. Many things around you can be easily made less stressful for your body if you look at them carefully and experiment until you find a solution that works for you.

You may be able to plug in a fan, special light, or heating pad at your work station. I have also used an old-fashioned hot water bottle where there's no outlet. A job that requires a lot of time on the telephone can be especially rough on the neck and shoulders, especially if you're like me and you scrunch the side of your neck down to hold the phone while you're writing. Most telephones can be made more comfortable by using a head set instead of the standard receiver, and the cost is quite reasonable. It's worth the search to find comfortable keyboards, copy holders, and arm rests. A foot rest under your desk is another thing that can take strain off your legs and lower back. If you work on a computer with a monitor, try to find a monitor stand to raise it up a few inches higher. If all else fails, you can use a phone book or two to get it to the right height.

Modify, modify, modify

Generally you'll find that overly repetitive work can be painful if you don't take precautions, things requiring heavy lifting or force shouldn't be attempted, and stress will make things worse than usual. Dampness and sitting in one position too long can aggravate stiffness. You might even want to change the height or position of your computer monitor or keyboard at various times during the day to reduce strain on your neck from sitting in the same position. Don't forget that you can do research on your own. The Arthritis Foundation has several excellent pamphlets that can be requested by phone at 800-283-7800 or from their Web site: www.arthritis.org. There's also an outfit called the Job Accommodation Network, which you can contact at 800-526-7234 or www.jan.wvu.edu, that has useful information.

Telling your employer and/or supervisor

The decision to inform your employer about your fibromyalgia is entirely up to you. My suggestion is that candor is your best bet and will stave off future complications. This, however, may not be the solution that's best for you. If you've carefully chosen a job that you can do, and you're not creating a liability for the company, you may think it unnecessary to inform your employer. It's natural, if you're working toward a promotion, to feel that if you let on that you have limitations you'll be passed over out of ignorance or fear. You may be afraid to have an illness put into your work records in case you need to look for another job because it may make it more difficult to get hired. (Of course it's illegal for employers to discriminate against hiring you if you're qualified, but the reality is that it's difficult to prove and you may never know the real reason you didn't get a job.) Some small employers are frightened, for good reasons, of hiring a person with a potential disability, or that will be costly on a health insurance policy.

There are also some positive reasons to tell your employer about your fibromyalgia. First of all, I think most people feel better being honest and open. Most of us feel that if we do our best, and work as hard as we can, telling the truth about our condition won't be held against us. Second, if you need to ask for any special help like flexible hours, scheduled break times, or more comfortable equipment, you'll have to reveal the reason for your request. And if you ever need to file a grievance because you've been let go or harassed due to your illness, you'll need to have it in your records that you've told your employer about your limitations. Lastly, if you ever do need to file for disability, either long- or short-term, you'll need documentation.

AMY HARTH'S STORY

To disclose or not disclose . . . always a tricky question, and I think each person has his/her comfort level and risk-tolerance, and each situation is different. With each job experience I've become bolder about disclosing. In fact, I disclosed at the end of a job interview on Friday that I really want and will be crushed if I don't get.

Why? Why jeopardize a chance over something I could hide until later? Simple. I've learned that the people who discriminate against me for my limitations rather than valuing me for my contributions are in poisonous environments I don't want to be in anyway.

I've learned that ending up in a job that isn't good for me is a disaster for everyone. I end up miserable. I want to ask the questions I need up front to make sure I'm considering a job I'll be able to do and be happy in.

I've learned that I love the open relationship I have with my current employer, and that I'm never going back to the stress of having a secret.

I've learned that if I do incredibly good work and make myself valuable, a good employer isn't going to ditch me just because I have a medical problem and need some flexibility. Because guess what . . . Other people have children, spouses, get divorced, have sick family members, and need flexibility too.

I've learned that in the absence of information, people tend to imagine the worst. For example, they might be thinking you have some horrible, awful, unimaginable problem that makes you push deadlines. But if you disclose, you have the opportunity to define the problem for them so their imaginations don't go into overdrive. You don't need to tell them the gory details. Just that you have a medical condition and you have your ups and downs.

Before you have this conversation with your employer though, think about what you can do for them and what you would need in order to be able to do it. And then consider whether it's something they can reasonably give to you. Keep it positive.

Talking to your co-workers

If you have co-workers in close proximity, you should share your situation with them if you've been given any special attention or equipment. Here again, you don't have to discuss fibromyalgia by name if you'd rather not. You can just say "I have arthritis" or "soft tissue arthritis"—and let them know that it's nothing serious, just an inconvenience, and you need to be comfortable to do your best. Generally, if you're a hard worker and try to keep a cheerful attitude, you won't run into much resentment. Most people have good hearts and are willing to help if they can as long as they see you working hard.

Strategies for good communication

The best way to approach any situation with your employer is to be ready to present the problem and a solution. If you walk in with an issue and drop it in his or her lap, you can expect that it will be treated as a hassle. On the other hand, if you can spell out both what you need—for example, a chair with more support—and the solution—where to get this better chair and what it will cost—you'll have an easier time of it. Don't expect your employer

---

The Americans with Disabilities Act (ADA)

THE AMERICANS with Disabilities Act was passed in 1992 to protect employees with certain limitations. The first thing you need to know is that it doesn't apply in every situation. If you work for a company that has less than fifteen employees, the ADA doesn't offer you any protection, even though you obviously face the same physical challenges that employees who work for larger companies do.

To qualify under the ADA, you have to be able document that you have "physical or mental impairment that *substantially* limits one or more of your major life activities." The law also clearly states that any request that you make must be considered reasonable, which basically means that it can't cause your employer undue financial hardship. You are also protected from being fired because you've asked for special consideration. Accepting a job in a larger company may be something to consider because you'll have more protection under the law. Family leave and certain kinds of medical leave may also be more easily granted by larger companies. For more information about the ADA, free booklets are available from the Office of Equal Employment Opportunity (EEOC), which has offices all around the U.S. For the location of the office nearest you call 800-669-4000 or log onto their Web site at www.ojp.usdoj.gov/eeo/.

---

act on vague complaints because the more nebulous they are the less serious they will seem, and the longer it will take to properly address them. Remember that they're running a business, and you are just one element of that business. If you need some ideas about the kinds of chairs and workspace assistance available, Adaptability is a company that can help you. You can reach them at 800-288-9941 or online at www.adaptability.com.

When addressing your concerns, you should make sure that your requests are reasonable and not overwhelming in number. In other words, don't wear out your welcome in your supervisor's office. A lot of things can be handled on your own, and should be. Much will also depend on your job performance and your relationship with your employer. It's up to you to gauge the situation and work within the confines.

Taking time off

If you're going through a particularly bad period, you may have rights such as family leave, vacation time, and sick leave. You may be able to afford some unpaid time off, or you may qualify for some sort of short-term disability. If you have a human resources department available at work, you can take advantage of their knowledge. Short-term disability is much easier to get than long-term disability, and usually requires little more than a doctor's letter and a form to be filled out. It does not require any examinations or second opinions. If you qualify, you are usually eligible for three months, and it begins when your sick time and vacation time is used up. Since this is a temporary measure, it's not as difficult to get as long-term disability. Finally, if you are barely hanging on, don't cut back your hours before you quit. If you're trying to get permanent disability, your award will be based on your most recent earnings.

The Family and Medical Leave Act (FMLA)

THE FAMILY and Medical Leave Act (FMLA) is a recently enacted law that allows people to take time off to get treatment for an illness, or to help a family member who is sick. Employers of a certain size must grant eligible employees up to a total of twelve workweeks of unpaid leave during any twelve-month period for one or more of the following reasons:

- for the birth and care of the newborn child of the employee
- for placement with the employee of a son or daughter by adoption or foster care
- for the care of an immediate family member (spouse, child, or parent) with a serious health condition; or
- for medical leave when the employee (or a family member) is unable to work because of a serious health condition.

If you qualify, and if your employer has a certain number of employees, you can choose to pursue this option. Your physician must fill out forms to substantiate your claim. It may be difficult for you to see from looking at the form how fibromyalgia would qualify, but it falls under category 4, "conditions requiring treatment." You will be allowed to take time off as needed (from a day or two to a few months), or perhaps even to work part-time until your "condition stabilizes." This is an option that shouldn't be overlooked because you may be able to resolve your health issues during this time.

What If You just Can't Work?
—Long-term Disability

IF YOU just can't do it anymore or if you're too sick to hold down a job, you can apply for disability benefits. You may have long-term disability insurance through a private carrier such as UNUM, or you may be applying for state disability or Social Security disability—either way you'll have to file a claim. Expect a long and difficult road to win if you're going for long-term benefits. UNUM in particular is known to be extremely hostile to fibromyalgia—inevitably they try to make it a psychological condition ("you're depressed, aren't you?") so they don't have to pay. Several lawsuits have been filed against insurers because of this.

Eventually you'll need a lawyer, but many won't even take your case until you've been turned down several times. This means you'll need to be prepared to do much of the work on your own. A lifetime of benefits begun at age forty is a fair chunk of change to any insurance carrier, so expect them to fight you tooth and nail. Don't be surprised if they put you under surveillance, or appear unannounced at your door to see how you look, *and we all know most fibromyalgics don't look as sick as they feel.* Unfortunately, that's just the beginning of how ugly it can get. Fibromyalgics are in an especially difficult position because there are no objective data such as lab tests or X rays to prove that we're sick. You'll probably be told that "everyone's tired, everyone has pain."

It can't be denied that fibromyalgia is not without some controversy, even in the research institutions where it is studied. As you can imagine, this gives the enemy a certain amount of ammunition to use against us. But you're in good company. There are only a few conditions, such as terminal cancer, that qualify a person for disability right away.

Though you must prepare yourself for a long and protracted fight, there are still things you can do to help yourself while you wait. In any legal battle, the side with the best and most complete records has a definite advantage. Invest time and what energy you have into putting your paperwork in order. Letters and reports from doctors, from previous employers, and descriptions of what your last job entailed, are all necessary. Keep your files organized, and get copies of all pertinent information including any medical examinations or work files. Physicians are entitled to charge you a small copying fee, but your records are your property. If you discover an error in any of your medical records you have the right to have them amended. Make sure you do all of this in writing and keep copies of your correspondence. Staple responses to questionnaires and make sure everything has a date when it was received, and when it was answered. You'll also need copies of all your bills, bank statements, monthly payments, and other financial papers. If you borrow money from a family member or friend, document it with a copy of the check and of your bank statement. Everything needs to match up. If you can't keep up your filing, designate a file box to stash all this pertinent information until you have the energy to put it all in order.

While it's obvious you need a lawyer who understands disability claims, it's also crucial to see a physician who specializes in fibromyalgia and who has experience with disability cases and is able to fill out all the necessary reports. (An additional charge for reports is customary, by the way, and insurance companies won't pay for it.) The more experienced the doctor who fills out your forms, the better chance you have that they will be filled out in the way insurance companies demand. Where most physicians can easily handle the small amount of paperwork required for short-term claims, when it comes to long-term evaluations, most doctors aren't trained to assess the level of disability and have no idea how to go about determining what you can do. Assessing functional limitations in a person with no arms should be fairly easy. But can a fibromyalgic lift twenty-five pounds? And if so, what does it mean? If you can't work because most of the time you feel brain dead, how long you can sit in a chair is of no consequence, and in any case, it varies greatly from day to day. Many doctors are reduced to writing, "The patient states she is too tired to work for eight hours," on the form and mailing it back. This, of course, is not good enough to support your case, and is why you should find a doctor who knows just what to do. We all know that the system is set up poorly and is not easily adapted to our illness, with its lack of objective, irrefutable data. We can lament all we want to, but for the present time your only hope is to work within the system.

Look at your papers with a skeptical eye and if you have any doubts about any issues, discuss them with a lawyer. If you have any record of being treated for depression, or have had any workplace injuries, you may have an added burden of proof to meet. It's also been suggested that a long record of going to doctors for various complaints can work against you because it might be alleged that you've been making the rounds looking for someone to agree with you about how sick you are. Instead of giving you credit for searching for a solution, you'll be accused of trying to fabricate a problem.

Before you hire a lawyer, or take any steps at all, be sure to read up on disability benefits and decide whether or not you really qualify for them *as they are written*. In most cases you must be incapable of any type of work at all, not just your own. Requirements also vary slightly depending on your age. The Social Security Administration has free booklets, and their publications can also be accessed online at www.ssa.gov, or call them toll-free to locate the office nearest you at 800-772-1213. There is a lot of work to do if you have no choice but to file for disability. But you can start the process over the phone.

The initial steps don't take very long. You'll hear rather quickly about your first application. As I said before, you can count on being denied on this one—so don't be surprised. You have sixty days from the date your denial was mailed to file an appeal, so do it right away. You will be required to fill out more paperwork and be examined by one of the insurer's physicians, who will undoubtedly find nothing wrong with you. You have the right to bring your own doctor with you to this exam. If you go alone to any interviews or examinations, take a tape recorder. Expect this stage, including the testimony you'll make before the judge, to last about six more months.

If you're denied a second time, once again you have sixty days to appeal. This will start the next phase of your claim, which takes an average of eight months. Your evidence will be placed before a council that decides whether or not to support you and kick it back to the judge for reconsideration. If you lose this round, your final recourse is to file suit in U.S. District Court for a new hearing. As you can see, the process is long and difficult, and you have no guarantee that the final outcome will be in your favor.

Disability has become an industry, not just for fibromyalgics, but for everyone. You'll see advertisements everywhere for lawyers, physicians, and advice, so look carefully. Be aware that the customary fee is about 25 percent of your settlement. Ask your physician or support group for a recommendation if you aren't sure where to go. For more information there's a publication called "A Pocket Guide to Federal Help for Individuals with Disabilities" that has information about your rights, including educational and vocational, and about disability itself. You can send a written request to the Department of Education, Room 3132, Switzer Building, Washington, D.C. 20202, or call 800-949-9232.

In the event that you get better and want to go back to work, Social Security provides incentives and plans to help you to accomplish this goal. You can be granted a trial employment period before you jeopardize your status. If you were granted Medicare, you are allowed to work for approximately three years without losing those benefits. Later on, you can purchase Medicare coverage on your own. This is actually a very important consideration because once you've been disabled, it's awfully hard to get any medical insurance coverage, even at a highway robbery rate.

Managing Issues with Medical Insurance

MEDICAL INSURANCE is an issue for anyone with a chronic illness, and in dealing with it the overwhelming percentage of us will have a fight on our hands at one time or another. You always need to bear in mind that insurance is a *for*-profit industry, and routinely posts large ones. CEOs take home large bonuses each year and they can't expect to do this unless they control their spending (on you.) Insurance companies, despite their advertisements, are not a strong hand to hold you up when you need it. Instead, if you have fibromyalgia, your insurance company is a strong arm you'll have to wrestle with, often until you're sicker and more exhausted than when you started. There are many costly illnesses like diabetes, cancer, heart disease, and AIDS that have clear-cut methods of diagnosis and proven treatments. For this reason it's especially important for these companies to pick on chronic illnesses like fibromyalgia that are difficult to prove, and for which every single treatment is actually "experimental" or "unproven." It's easy for them to deny modalities under the umbrella term "not medically necessary," which means that you won't die or be forever deformed if you don't receive them. Insurance companies especially frown on massage, acupuncture, and physical therapy and limit the amount of services you can receive because your illness does not have a start and finish date that they can count on. They'll control the medications you're allowed to take and the amount you can get, as well as how long you can spend with your doctor. You'll soon discover that medical care in the United States is now controlled more by insurance companies than by physicians, who will often do all they can to support you to no avail. They resent, with great justification, having their every action scrutinized by case managers who are usually not even physicians, and if they are, are long-retired doctors from unrelated specialties.

As if this were not bad enough, many fibromyalgics have difficulty even getting medical insurance without horrendous expense. Laws differ from state to state, but even so, unless you plan to stay employed by a large company (or remain married to someone who is and who won't retire before you're old enough to qualify for Medicare) you will eventually face an underwriting nightmare. If an insurance company senses that they may spend anything close to what you pay in, they'll make it extremely expensive for you. Since most fibromyalgics, are, like myself, "women of a certain age," as the French charmingly put it, we are in real trouble. Menopausal women are considered an insurance risk because they often require hysterectomies or other surgeries, and are at risk for a number of expensive conditions like osteoporosis and reproductive cancers. Given all of this, what are your options?

The first option, which may be too late for you, is to pay cash for your fibromyalgia-related services. If no insurance company is ever billed using the

diagnosis code for fibromyalgia, there's no way for it to turn up in their computers. You'll have to make sure no mention of it is made in the records of your primary care doctor because the insurance company will read these carefully before
they issue you a policy. It's nearly impossible to pull off this feat, but it's something
you should definitely consider. If you're concerned that your kids may have inherited your illness, think long and hard before using insurance to cover their
expenses. For one thing, it's highly possible that younger ones, especially boys,
will outgrow their complaints. Despite this, it will be difficult for them to get insurance later on if they have records naming fibromyalgia, so you should try to protect them if possible.

Another option is to join an HMO, which is less stringent about whom they
cover because they ration services for everyone. If you have children, this may be
the best option cost-wise because all their illnesses and injuries will be covered
in full with no out-of-pocket expenses. X rays, mammograms, and annual examinations are all included in the price of coverage. (They are not free because you
have paid for them—they are built into the premiums you pay.) Your monthly premiums will be lower as well. However, you can count on having to pay for anything
you want to try that's different. But in certain cases you may be able to get them
to cover out-of-HMO consultations if you wish to see a certain specialist and you
have lots of free time to pursue and annoy them.

Whatever you end up doing about insurance, be sure you know your options
and rights under your policy. Understand the appeal process. You can expect to
have requests out of the norm, so you should check appeal procedures before you
purchase the policy. Almost every day I remark to someone: "Your insurance company is your friend until you sign on the dotted line below their name. Once you
do that, you're spending their money, not yours, and you can expect to be in an
adversarial position simply for that reason." For example, certain medications may
not be covered because they are not included in the formulary. This is a list of medications for which your insurance company gets a good deal, which is simply a
financial incentive to force you to use them. But an appeal process does exist, and
by having your doctor fill out a form detailing why you can't use a certain medication, you can usually get what you need *if your medical records support this
need*. Anytime that you speak to someone at your insurance company about an
issue, be sure to write down the date, time, *and the name of the person you spoke
to*. This little bit of information will help you win many battles.

If you are shopping on your own for a policy, I believe that an insurance broker is a good way to go. He or she can explain how policies work, the deductibles
and what's covered, compare premium prices, and you can weigh your options
with your own situation in mind. Also, if you are declined for coverage by a certain
company, he or she can help you appeal this decision. It can be done successfully,

but only if you have not run up a huge amount of bills with a previous insurance company. It will be impossible for you to convince a prospective insurance company to overlook something that has already been documented as costly. Don't expect to be able to hide anything—computers are all linked and have made getting away with it unlikely. In the event that you do run up a large bill your insurance company will not hesitate to go back through your records in an effort to turn it into a "preexisting condition." It is not worth the risk to try to get away with any deception because you may end up having your policy voided just when you need it the most.

MEDICARE

If you are declared disabled or are over sixty-five years of age, you are eligible for Medicare coverage, which is actually a very inexpensive type of insurance coverage. You will have an annual deductible, and you'll be responsible for 20 percent of the amount Medicare deems reasonable and customary as long as you see doctors who are providers. Laboratory work and certain procedures are covered at 100 percent with no deductible. The fees for seeing a physician who is not a Medicare provider is also limited by law, so you may be responsible for a slightly larger amount. Supplemental policies are available at a price: different fees for different levels of coverage. An insurance broker can help you with this as well.

There are other nuances involved in picking your Medicare coverage. For example, there are hospital deductibles and fees if you are admitted. Medicare has extensive regulations regarding what they consider medically necessary. The Balanced Budget Act of 1997 seriously limited modalities like physical therapy, among other things. Services may be denied after they have been performed, and your doctor may require you to sign a waiver making you responsible if this happens. As with any insurance policy, make it your business to understand what is covered and what it will cost you, so you can make the best decision based on your own personal situation.

As with private insurance, there's also an option called HMO Medicare. For your monthly premium many routine services will be covered, and probably the bulk of your medications. You may also get some vision and dental coverage. If you choose to see a doctor who is not a member of your HMO, you'll be responsible for the entire fee. You will be restricted to the specialists and services that your HMO ordains that you can have when it allows you to have them.

WORKERS' COMPENSATION

Some fibromyalgics are involved in workers' compensation cases, which means they can link their illness to an on-the-job injury of some kind. This will only work if you've had no documented complaints with any previous doctor that sound like fibromyalgia. If you complained about back pain to a doctor ten years before your accident, you can count on them to ferret it out and deny your claim. Since evidence is accumulating that fibromyalgia is not caused by an injury, but may be made worse by one, proving that it's job-related is getting increasingly difficult. If you file a claim, you will be eventually ordered to see an "independent medical examiner," who is paid by workers' compensation to perform your exam. The irony in this is obvious, since most of these physicians rely on workers' compensation for the bulk of their income and charge for reviewing records and writing reports. You should expect their statements to be accepted as gospel. Expect denial if your injury is nebulous or if it doesn't have an ending date. Remember that any sort of treatment you require must be authorized in advance to be covered.

Find other employment, if necessary

If you have done your best but you simply can't cope with your job, you may need to find a new one. If switching careers requires retraining, your doctor can help you contact a governmental program that can help you do this. The Rehabilitation Services Administration is a federal program that works in conjunction with each state. The RSA Web site (www.ed. gov/offices/OSERS/RSA) will direct you to the offices and Web addresses for the branch in your state. You can also visit www.votech. about.com for general information. If you don't have a computer, use the state government pages in the front of the phone book to find the office nearest you. The Office of Disability Employment Policy has lists of companies that are open to hiring workers with limitations. You can find them on the Internet at www.dol.gov/odep, or contact by mail c/o U.S. Department of Labor, Frances Perkins Building, 200 Constitution Ave, NW, Washington D.C. 20210, or by telephone at 202-693-7880.

Working from your home

Some lucky fibromyalgics have a job or a skill that allows them to work at home. Perhaps it's something you can explore if you are working on being retrained for a new job. Computers have made this a very workable solution for writers, artists, and people who specialize in any form of communication. There are also Web site designers and tech support people, and the need for trained workers in this area is growing. Career counselors may be able to point you in a new direction that you hadn't considered. Bookkeeping is something that you can learn online or by yourself rather easily with a tutorial. Newsletter publications or graphic design work might be something you could get paid for. If you have an advanced degree, you might be able to teach a class online or at the local college, while still doing the bulk of your work in the comfort of your own home. If you don't have the necessary degree, you can try a junior college, or a community college that has classes in special skills like gardening or making crafts. And, if you're good at crafts, you can make items to sell on eBay or at craft fairs. Whatever your skills, closely examine how they could be used in a different scenario to further support you in your healing process.

In this competitive work environment, many people with fibromyalgia fear that they simply can't keep up. This is a very real concern, and one you should be aware of. There's just no market for people who can't keep their commitments regardless of excuses. Here's a tip from Miryam Williamson's book on fibromyalgia, in which she shares a trick she uses to get her work done on time. She tells clients that she's booked six weeks in advance, which gives her longer without them realizing it. Realistic timelines and deadlines will be a huge factor in determining your success if you're self-employed.

IN A SENTENCE:

> *Keep an open mind and explore all your options if you find that your work life needs adjustment to accommodate your fibromyalgia.*

learning

Housework Is Real Work, Too

WHETHER OR not your housework is a full-time job, it has several advantages and disadvantages. It's tougher to get fired, but then again, you can't ask the law to provide for your comfort. You'll have to do that for yourself.

The first rule about housework, whether it's your full-time job or one that's heaped on top of a job outside of the home, is simple. "If you can't live up to your standards, lower your standards." No one has ever died because the windows weren't washed, or because there's dust behind a refrigerator. But children and marriages *can* suffer when there's not enough attention being paid to them. Your family should come first in your home. Any energy you have left over after you've nurtured the people you love can be used for housework, not the other way around. Your kids will leave home before long, and no matter how many times you've cleaned out your garage it will still be dirty.

Ask for help

If you can hire help weekly to do the heavier work, don't hesitate, just do it. If you have someone who can change the sheets on all the beds, vacuum thoroughly, and clean the refrigerator and stove, you'll really be halfway there. If you can't afford weekly, try to find someone to come less frequently, even once a month. If you're in a support group, maybe you can share the cost of a cleaning person to come in—splitting the time and the cost but guaranteeing her the income she needs.

Downscale and simplify

For the rest of your chores, closely study your obligations and simplify your tasks. Vacuuming is always nasty, but less so if you get a very lightweight vacuum cleaner, like an electric broom or dust buster. I have two: a heavy one that I use when I feel up to it to do thorough cleaning, and a light one for frequent cleanings. It's well worth the investment and the light one doesn't cost much. You can keep it handy so you don't use up all your energy dragging the heavy vacuum out of a back closet.

If you don't have a dishwasher, use paper plates. Get a stool for the kitchen so you can reach things easily without jumping (OK, I'm on the shorter side!), or to sit on when you do chopping, slicing, or dishwashing. Buy one of those nozzles you attach to the hose to clean your windows. If you have one of these, your kids will jump to help you, especially if you have boys. Too bad you can't clean house with fire, because they'd help with that, too! You can buy wipes premoistened with glass cleaner and furniture polish that will do for quick cleaning. Then you won't have to dig the heavy bottles of cleaners out from under the sink and then put them back. Appliances and walls with texture (or wrinkle finish) won't show fingerprints the way flat ones will.

Laundry is another nasty job (I've almost survived four teenagers), but it's a lot easier if you do small loads frequently. It's a lot less strenuous that way, lifting, carrying, folding, and putting away. If you have a big family you can use a laundry bin that's divided with separate laundry bags so that your laundry is already sorted when you get to it. You may also be able to locate a "Wash and Fold" Laundromat near your house and drop laundry off when you take kids to school and pick it up on your way home. Even if you only take in sheets, jeans, and kids' playclothes, it will make a noticeable dent in your wash loads. Buy as many clothes as you can that don't wrinkle and only require a quick turn in the drier so you don't have to iron too often. (Keep loads small when you dry clothes: less wrinkling). Cotton blends, for example, are a lot less work than pure cotton. Make sure you buy a light iron, for the times you can't avoid doing some ironing.

The single greatest piece of equipment I have (not counting my dishwasher) is one of those new mops that is light and has a swiveling base to which you attach a pre-moistened wipe. Some come with a squirt bottle of bleachy liquid attached, but you can always use your own cleaner instead. (Just use folded paper towels with whichever cleaner you want squirted on to them.) You can use this tool for many tasks: walls and cobwebs in corners, ceilings (if you're really ambitious), shower stalls, bathroom floors all around the toilets, kitchen cabinets, kitchen floors of any kind—tile, wood, or linoleum—doors (to wipe off fingerprints), and for full-length mirrors if you have them. Just squirt glass cleaner on a piece of paper towel, and attach it to the bottom and you can clean glass-windows and mirrors—with very little effort. I have found many, many uses for this extremely light, easy to maneuver gizmo.

You can also buy those little plastic plate things to put under the legs of your furniture that allow you to slide the furniture around without scratching the floors. Unlike most of the gimmicks I've seen on television, these really work and will make cleaning behind things easy—if you're inclined to clean behind things, that is. I only have to do this when my mother or mother-in-law visit, and they don't come very often. But if yours lives in the neighborhood, these are a worthwhile investment. Save coupons for carpet cleaning and if you find someone who's reasonably priced and does a reasonable job, make a new friend.

Another thing that's handy is to have pull-out shelves in lower cabinets so you can access them easily. Bending over and reaching way back for pots, pans, plastic storage containers, or cleaning supplies can really get to you. Look carefully around your house and study things that are a stress on your body. Again, the Arthritis Foundation and other organizations have publications that go into much more detail. There are rails for showers, kitchen tools that will not be so stressful on your hands or arms, grippers to extend your reach, and so on.

Managing the day-to-day

While you may be able to put off the housecleaning, there are some things that can't be delayed. Paying bills is another bear of a job for fibromyalgics. By the time I feel up to the task, the due date always seems to be past, the envelope is missing, or sometimes the bill is. You can avoid this by throwing away all the excess paper when you open the mail and slipping the payment stub in place in the envelope. Then take a pen and write in big letters on the back the due date so you can't miss it, and put the envelopes in chronological order by this date. Another problem is having no idea what you've paid and when you paid it. You can solve this problem by getting those checks with the carbon copy duplicates. Another big problem for you might be your ATM/Debit card. If you find that you often have not recorded debits you've made and this turns into a problem each month when you balance your account, seriously consider giving up debit cards. Bouncing checks has become expensive, as have the service charges on overdrawn accounts. Consider using your credit card instead, and paying it off monthly. Even if you do end up paying a bit of interest in the long run this amount could be considerably less than accumulated bank charges. You can do without an ATM, despite its convenience.

Most utility companies now give you the option of allowing them to debit the amount due every month directly from your bank account, paying them on the Internet through services like PayPal, or you can just enter your credit card number on most of them. You'll find that nearly all monthly bills can be charged these days. If you do this, you can get bill paying down to writing one or two checks a month. If you can afford to get a little bit ahead on your payments you can also just pay everything on the first of each month. You're paying some things a few weeks early, but the stress it relieves is worth it.

Maintenance issues

If you have a spouse or significant other, hopefully you can rely on them to help with ongoing maintenance issues such as caring for the yard (if you're fortunate enough to have one), or maintaining your car or your home. While these are tasks that most relatively healthy people can easily handle, for a fibromyalgic these basic day-to-day chores can be overwhelming. As I've mentioned above, the key is scheduling as well as asking for help.

If you live alone, don't think that you have to spend a lot of money to get someone to help with chores. As with many other things, you can always find someone to help you out as long as you plan in advance.

Do you have a close friend or family member who can occasionally volunteer? Most people are glad to do so as long as it's infrequent and doesn't impose on their time too much. Or perhaps a colleague or neighbor has a teenager who would be glad to rake your yard or take your car for an oil change in exchange for a small amount of spending money. You need to know in advance what needs to be done so you're not left in a crisis state (which is physically hard on your fibromyalgia, anyway).

IN A SENTENCE:

> *Taking care of your domestic life is essential, but there are ways to get things accomplished without overdoing it.*

living

Juggling Fibromyalgia and Your Personal Life

YOU KNOW already that fibromyalgia has an affect on every part of your life—from your public life at work to your most private life at home. This month we're going to look at some of the ways you can better manage your personal life while juggling your symptoms and your obligations.

Your sex life

Phew, this is an unpleasant topic, isn't it? Sex and fibromyalgia, sex and chronic illnesses, sex when you don't feel up to tying your shoelace or washing your face . . . what a cheery thought. Sex when your back hurts and you've got leg cramps. Sex when you're waking up in pain and falling into bed at night exhausted and haunted by the pile of laundry you haven't done. When on earth are you supposed to feel like having sex?

Sexual activity is a normal part of human life. If you're sexually active and/or in a relationship, then sex is part of the picture—for both you and your partner. Figuring out how to maintain some sort of healthy sex life is essential to keeping your identity as a normal, healthy individual, even if you don't feel so normal right now.

• • •

It doesn't have to be a marathon

When it comes to enjoyable sex, common sense should be the order of the day. A warm bath or shower can help relax muscles, and setting aside time to be together is a reasonable suggestion for all couples these days. Open communication is essential, no matter how difficult it may be for you. Remember that silence will sometimes give your partner the impression that you no longer find him or her attractive, when you may instead be just too tired or in too much pain. If you have the added stress of small children, you'll have to work even harder to make the time between you special. Remember that small kids make it a difficult time for all couples, and that's magnified when one of you is chronically ill. Please don't close down: Even if you are too tired for sex, physical contact of a comforting nature is essential. Lots of fibromyalgics refrain from touching because they're afraid to "lead on" their healthy spouse when they feel unable to have intercourse.

There are health benefits, too!

Sexual activity provides other benefits. Endorphins are released during sex at a high level that can last up to three hours. In both sexes the hormone **oxytocin**, the bonding hormone that makes us feel loving, is released with orgasm—up to five times the normal amount. When administered experimentally to people who had sexual side effects from taking antidepressants, oxytocin was strong enough to override the drugs. It also may play a role in REM sleep and it's been found that people with high levels of stress have low levels of it. Oxytocin release increases libido in both sexes, which is helpful if fibromyalgia and/or your medications are suppressing your sex drive. In men, sex encourages the flow of testosterone, which strengthens bones and muscles and helps transport oxygen. Sex also appears to raise DHEA levels in both sexes. Although experiments with some of these hormones are limited and difficult to accomplish for various reasons, there's enough circumstantial evidence to support the benefits of a healthy sex life.

Make sure your medications aren't exacerbating the issue

While diminished libido is part of fibromyalgia for many reasons, if it's constant, be sure to review all your medications to make sure they are not the problem—especially since "sexual side effects" is found in the small print of many medications. Antidepressants are notorious for causing problems in both men and women, as are some of the muscle relaxants. You can talk to your doctor about this, or do some research on your own to find both the culprit and a solution. For example, if you take an antidepressant that's helping you but is lowering your libido, you may elect to skip your dose on weekends if your doctor agrees to it. You'll still get the benefits of the drug (because they last a long time in your system) but lose some of the bothersome side effects for a few days. Again, your doctor is your best resource for this information. You should never stop a prescription medication on your own.

Getting pregnant

Before you even think about getting pregnant, you'll have to do some legwork and look at the medications that you take. Many of the commonly prescribed drugs for fibromyalgia are not safe to take during pregnancy. You'll have to check with your doctor(s) to discuss this issue. Some medications need to be discontinued gradually, but others can just be stopped with no ill effects. You should make sure medications are completely out of your system before you even attempt to become pregnant. Some of the antidepressants, for example, can stay in your system for a week or two. Don't forget to discuss any vitamins or over-the-counter medications and supplements with your doctor. Herbal compounds in particular have been implicated in miscarriages. Men should also check with a physician before the process begins. Although it's much less likely that any damage is caused to a fetus via sperm, there are some medications (especially hormones) that are known to be risky.

Challenges in pregnancy

For women who routinely use pain medications, the early part of pregnancy can be difficult, especially when you're battling morning sickness, fatigue, and mood swings in addition to your fibromyalgia. Your doctor may allow you to take an occasional Tylenol, but other than that it's unlikely that you'll be allowed more. You'll have to make do with heat packs, ice packs, exercise, and meditation. Acupuncture, acupressure, and massage may help you as well. Trigger point injections and even nerve blocks may be helpful in extreme cases. I imagine Botox injections will soon be an option as well. Gentle stretching throughout pregnancy, including prenatal yoga, will be very helpful. There are some stretching videos for pregnant women for sale (and probably for rent) if you are in the mood to do something structured.

One last word on the subject of medications: If you are having extreme difficulty with the thought of coping without your medications, schedule a conference with your physician. You might even consider a special consultation with a fibromyalgia specialist. For example, Dr. Daniel Wallace, M.D., a Clinical Professor of Medicine at UCLA/Cedars-Sinai, who has a large practice in Los Angeles, feels that there are safe options for you, and this may be true. While the *Physicians' Desk Reference* routinely states that the safety of drugs is not known during pregnancy, many excellent studies have been done that refute this. I have seen one that followed children of mothers who had taken antidepressants all the way up into their school years and saw no problems with them. The tricylics, such as Elavil and Flexeril, and the SSRIs, such as Zoloft, have several good studies under their belts. It will be up to you and your physician to look at these studies and decide for yourselves whether you should resume your medications or stay on them.[1] If your regular physician feels this is beyond his or her expertise, see a specialist.

Changes to your body

During the first three months of pregnancy, called the first trimester, your hormone levels change dramatically. Estrogen and progesterone levels are very high, which can cause you to feel worse, just as you did premenstrually. Sensitivity to smell gets much worse, so if you already have this as a symptom of your fibromyalgia, be prepared. Nausea and morning sickness can be difficult to deal with. The usual ways to deal with these are fine for fibromyalgia. Symptoms can be somewhat mitigated by the happiness and anticipation of your pregnancy, which, by the way, increases endorphin production and add to your sense of well-being.

As pregnancy progresses, several things happen. The obvious change in the shape of your body means that muscles are being stretched and there's added pressure on certain areas, such as the lower back. Your body will helpfully release hormones such as **relaxin** that helps allow your pelvic girdle to expand. Relaxin promotes a dramatic remodeling of the connective tissue and reduces the number and density of collagen fibers and the length of elastin fibers. The result is that the ligaments in the back and pelvic girdle relax, as do ligaments all over the body.

Generally the middle part of pregnancy is a good time for fibromyalgics. Often they report that they feel better than they ever have, with less pain, more energy, and a feeling of happiness and contentment. This is due to the powerful effect of hormones, which can actually mask your symptoms. This lasts until near the end, when your increased size limits your mobility, the positions you can sleep in, and so on. If you suffer from heartburn or reflux normally, this will get worse as your pregnancy pushes your stomach upward. During the last month of pregnancy when **Braxton Hicks contractions** increase, your body will respond with some endorphins, but you can count on being physically uncomfortable to some degree.

Delivery and postpartum

One of the first things you should do as you get into the middle part of your pregnancy is to make arrangements for help after delivery. You can count on the aftermath to be tough, and since it's a crucial time for you to bond with your baby and stay close to your partner, it's important for you to handle things in advance. Physically and mentally, fibromyalgics crash and spiral downward after the birth. If you have a friend or a family member who is committed to helping you, that's great. If you can afford some household help such as a cleaning lady, maid, or a **doula**—who will help with the process of caring for the baby and help setting up your personalized routine—you should do it. Some insurance companies are even paying for this service now because it is less expensive than a longer hospital stay.

If you don't have the option of hiring someone, be careful to do as much as you can ahead of time. You can cook and freeze meals, arrange for older children to spend some time with friends if they aren't in school, and so on. Make sure you have plenty of supplies like food and other staples on hand. Have groceries or hot meals delivered. Consider asking a family member for a diaper service as a gift. Anticipate things you often have to run out and buy, like school supplies for older kinds, and stock up. Warn your partner in advance that you expect to be down for the count and will need extra understanding and help. If there's family leave time available for your partner, ask him or her to consider using it! If you have family members willing to pitch in, make a list of the things you need help with and have them volunteer for specific tasks.

Sleep presents an added challenge

A major problem for all new parents is disturbed sleep patterns, which are worse for fibromyalgics, whose sleep is disturbed anyway. Obviously, you'll be up and down all night feeding and caring for your new baby. You may be so exhausted that you can actually fall asleep and nap when before it was impossible. Or you may have to rely on breast pumps or bottle feedings at least on weekends so that someone else can feed the baby and allow you a longer period of uninterrupted sleep.

Don't be rigidly opposed to bottle-feeding if it's necessary. While it's natural and important for you to want the best for your baby, having an exhausted, emotional mother who eventually collapses is not best. Plenty of babies are bottle-fed. Just find a balance that will work for you, and don't listen to anyone else. Remember that at the beginning, everything will seem like a huge issue, and you can fall into the trap of thinking that if you do the wrong thing your child will suffer for life. Do not allow this to happen. You have to learn how to choose your battles. Stay away from all forms of advice that are extreme. If you have a friend who tells you awful things will happen if you use plastic diapers, *don't listen*. Your friend doesn't have fibromyalgia or she would understand.

Managing your symptoms and a new baby

You may have been lucky enough to get a break during pregnancy, but your pains and other symptoms will return with a vengeance. If you breast-feed you'll still be limited as to what medications you can take for relief. Again, a heating pad, gentle massage, and warm showers may be the most helpful modalities of all. About a week after the baby is born you can also begin very gentle stretching again. (You will have to be much more careful if you've had a cesarean. In that case, adhere strictly to your doctor's advice.)

If you have a history of depression, be especially careful and see a doctor right away if you feel like you're having problems coping. Multiple studies have been done about the use of antidepressants while breast-feeding. Tricylic drugs such as Elavil have not been found in any measurable amounts in nursing babies, and sertraline (or Zoloft) has been detected in small amounts without any adverse effects on children studied for many years. Prozac (floxetine) has been implicated in colicky symptoms in nursing babies. Postpartum depression can be dangerous, so talk to your doctor if you have symptoms you feel you cannot control. It's now been suggested that women with a history of any depressive illness accept prophylactic measures. There are safe options for you, even if you choose to breast-feed. Also keep in mind that women who have just given birth are more sensitive to medications, so if you do elect to take an antidepressant postpartum, ask your doctor to start you with the lowest possible dose and titrate up.[2]

Puberty

Male or female, as we age, our hormones change. At certain points in our lives—puberty for both sexes (it occurs earlier in females than in males) and at menopause for women—these changes are dramatic.

Puberty itself causes kids to be moody, indifferent, tired, and unpredictable. Thus it's hard to tell how it's affecting fibromyalgia, except that puberty isn't physically painful. This should help you differentiate. Normally the problems come to a head just before puberty itself. Through a mechanism we don't quite understand, most children feel better and lose their symptoms during puberty. The majority of boys will not get them back, but in girls, menstrual migraines or headaches as well as old familiar symptoms will begin again in earnest once it's over.

Menopause is a time of great fluctuations

Menopause is defined as the period that begins one year after the last menstrual period. For this reason, it's clear that there is substantial lead-in time, or a gray zone, during which cycles are irregular; bleeding is heavy or light, with sweats, hot flashes, loss of libido, and vaginal dryness. While this is not related to fibromyalgia, it does add to your general stress level and makes symptoms like emotional mood swings much worse. Just when you think you may not be able to stand one more thing, you may be hit by a day of fifty hot flashes. Until recently, hot flashes and other unpleasant symptoms were easily controlled with hormone replacement, but now for many women the risks may well outweigh any benefits. For vaginal dryness, hormone creams are still considered safe and you should pursue this with your doctor. Fibromyalgic women, with their acidy vaginal secretions, can be in for a load of unpleasantness if they don't work to keep this delicate skin strong and healthy, so don't delay this. Hormone creams function to thicken skin, and they are a good solution. For hot flashes, an antidepressant may help, and you will know within twenty-four hours if it does. It takes several weeks for these to work for depression, but not for hot flashes. If you derive benefits you may wish to continue for a while because these will also help with your mood swings. Gabapentin or Neurontin showed an 87 percent reduction of hot flashes in one study but has significantly more side effects. If neither of these works, do, please keep in mind that in the short term (five years) hormone treatment does not appear to be risky. If you have no uterus, and you only need estrogen, it has not yet been shown to be dangerous. Exercise will help to regulate your moods and thermostat, and you'll need it to protect your bones as well. If you haven't started an exercise program menopause is yet another reason to do it.

Andropause

There's a new field of research that deals with "male menopause" or **andropause**, as it is generally called in medical circles. It's true that male hormones decrease with age, though in the vast majority of the cases, it happens very gradually over many years and is not symptomatic. In cases where this hormone decrease is sudden or profound, the signs might be lethargy, depression, hot flashes, and decreased libido, symptoms consistent with fibromyalgia. In suspected andropause, a serum FAT, or free available testosterone, is the blood test you need. TRT, or testosterone replacement therapy, should not be done without excellent reason. As with hormone replacement in women, it can increase the risk of certain cancers. Prostate tests are an absolute necessity with TRT unless you are very young, and some doctors also demand prostate biopsies. If no benefit is seen from treatment no matter what your blood tests say, it should be discontinued because of the possible risks.

IN A SENTENCE:

> *Fibromyalgia will affect your sexual and reproductive life, but if you manage the symptoms effectively you can reclaim your sexual vitality and maintain stability throughout the cycle of your life.*

learning

Tips for Guys

AS A man with fibromyalgia, you will have unique challenges, too. While everything in this book applies to you (except vulvodynia and, of course, pregnancy!), the reality is that women suffer from fibromyalgia in greater numbers. This means that some of the generalizations might not be exactly right for you.

If women think that losing a job or having to ask for job modifications is difficult, talk to a man with an invisible chronic illness. And if that man is married and/or the head of a family, that stress level is much higher. Men are conditioned to see themselves as the primary breadwinners (whether they are or not), and fibromyalgia, with all of its debilitating symptoms, can present a hard blow to the ego. To top it off, men are usually advised to just "suck it up," and get on with things. Yet fibromyalgia remains one of those illnesses where the symptoms, despite your best efforts, are impossible to ignore.

If you're responsible for supporting a family, very real fears may accompany your physical suffering. How will you keep your family going? Figuring out how to balance your health with your responsibilities will involve a great deal of soul searching. Don't react to this very real illness with denial. You may very well have to seek out other employment and secondary options to support your family and manage this illness. This does not make you a failure—you are simply doing what needs to be done.

Communication, even if you hate it, is the key to relationships

It's important to enlist your spouse or partner in this process, because you both will be affected. In addition, men usually have a harder time talking to others, and don't usually have the warm, nurturing, "say-anything" friendships that women are accustomed to. Support groups are a good outlet, but are largely populated by women. Don't dismiss them though; many women today face the same grim realities of supporting families as men do.

Fibromyalgia is just as real as a heart attack is, but you probably wouldn't feel as ashamed if your heart acted up. Again, it's that stigma associated with fibromyalgia. If you have a computer, there are support groups specifically for men on the Internet where you can correspond with other men who feel like you do. Check out www.menwithfibro.com or www.plaidrabbit.com/fms/menspage. Also, Yahoo has a group for men with fibromyalgia and their partners that will help both of you understand that all your feelings are normal. Just go to Yahoo.com and look up "Fibro Men Support Group."

BOB HALL'S STORY

Sometimes I get so irritable I just know that hitting something would help. Hey, I am a man, the center of my universe; I am supposed to be able to do anything, the head of my family, the warrior, the hunter, and the king of the hill. People used to respect me, and now, how can anyone respect what I have become? Weak, frail, in pain night and day, tired all of the time, and without enough energy to do anything. Who could respect anything like that? Who could love anyone like that? The pain it never goes away . . . I thought at one time I could take anything, I could fight anything, but how can you fight something that's inside your head? Sometimes when the pain is so great I lash out in anger, and almost hate the very people that are left to care about me. This is not me. What happened? I used to have friends but now I seems like I have said "Well, I don't feel good today so I am going to stay home" one time too many. Everyone assumes I am "sick" so they don't call anymore. I feel so alone and yet I don't want anyone around me. Afraid? Yes, I am afraid. It is a word I never thought I would use, but I am afraid. I am terrified that I will never be needed again for anything. I have learned volumes about compassion. I still feel that you have to have

*fibromyalgia to understand the pain, but I am compassionate
towards anyone's illness now, regardless of what they have.*

*Several years ago someone asked me what it was like to be a man
and have fibromyalgia. I said "Well, it is like Samson when Delilah
cut off his hair."*

Parenting is a mixed bag

Being a parent is stressful for both women and men, and you may also
have the challenges of doing double duty around the house or caring for
older children if your family grows. It's important for you to pace yourself
and help eliminate unnecessary worries and tasks from your agenda. It's
very important to come to terms with your emotions and express them,
because it will be more stressful if you bottle up your feelings inside. Take
time to enjoy your children, because that more than anything will make you
feel better. If you work for a company that allows family leave, by all means,
use it whenever you can. You're luckier than many, and you should take
advantage of the time to work on your own health and help to take care of
your family.

There are other things to think about and work on. You may have physically active kids who participate in sports that are beyond your stamina,
and you know that a day's work can leave fibromyalgics incapacitated. If
you try to tough out the exhaustion you feel, you may crash and burn at a
crucial time. Though it may not come naturally to you to do it, try to think
of things you can do with your family that won't leave you struggling. You
may not be able to be a Little League coach, but you could still help with
small tasks during the games if they're on a weekend, or ferry the kids out
for pizza afterward. Don't neglect to look for other ways to make a connection with your kids—that's what truly matters.

There are activities you can do
that don't require strength

You may have no idea about puzzles, coloring, and art projects, but these
are things you can learn to enjoy, too. You can get a book about origami or
two thousand things to do with paper or something like that, and start with
paper airplanes. After all, it's about the reward of spending time with your
children and not the activity. Reading to your kids or (even better) letting
them read to you is another activity you can explore. Trips to the library on
a Saturday afternoon can be fun: Some libraries have story programs and
reading rooms that are quite nice places. It would both give you something
to do, and get you out of the house so that your partner can rest.

Outings are a great way to spend time with your kids

If you're not sensitive to noise, and lots of men are not, arcades and places like Chuck E. Cheese can be used to get kids out of the house and are not terribly strenuous. Be sensible if you go to places like the park, and explain beforehand what you feel up to. One of the concerns often voiced by men with fibromyalgia is that they are poor role models for their children because they are ill. You certainly don't need to be a professional athlete to embody the most important human traits. Trust me—what your kids will value is the time you spent with them, whether it's super-active time or a more passive experience.

Men like to do big things

I've noticed than men naturally seem to think in terms of the big gestures, like digging up the whole garden, or cleaning out the entire attic or doing something huge and noticeable. While this is certainly a lovely part of maleness, you should scale down your projects and helping hand a bit. Any job you finish is better than a huge job started and abandoned because of fatigue. If you set out to help, pick something you can manage, or examine the larger task and break it down into smaller, more workable stages. That way, the project won't get out of hand and you won't get frustrated or upset if you can't complete it.

Men also seem to think in terms of action, of needing to do *something*. Just as we women fibromyalgics have had to learn, you need to come to terms with the fact that sometimes you can't *do* anything because you're too tired physically or mentally. Luckily that doesn't make it impossible for you to still do something helpful and wonderful, something that's even constructive. You can listen. You can open up your ears and heart and let your children or your partner tell you about what's going on. What her or his fears and frustrations are, and what was hard today and what was wonderful. And then you can talk, too. You can laugh and you can share, and you can save your strength to step over the pile of laundry in the hallway that has to wait for another day. Because it *can* wait. Laundry won't go anywhere by itself, but time will, and time with those you love will be gone before you know it.

Even though you are newly diagnosed with fibromyalgia you know that pain and fatigue can cause one day to blur into the next and seasons to change before you've had time to experience them. Don't put your family plans on hold indefinitely. Simplify, and remind your partner to do the same. Even for a healthy person with abundant energy there are too few carefree, happy days before children are grown and gone. The greatest gift you can give your partner and your family is to be well enough to be there for that special soccer game or school play. Ask your wife if you don't believe me: Which would she rather have, you with her, spending quality time, or lying in bed because you tried to do too much the day before and didn't finish it anyway?

IN A SENTENCE:

Fibromyalgic men have a different set of issues to deal with, but if you anticipate problems and plan ahead the effect can be minimized.

Take a Vacation

WHAT? TAKE a vacation? I know what you're thinking. "I wish. How can I take a vacation when I can't even get to the supermarket?" Fibromyalgia is bad enough when you're at home and have easy access to everything that you need. The idea of leaving home is probably frightening or may seem like too much trouble to arrange. Let's face it; travel is stressful-from the trip itself to disrupted sleep to climate changes to security delays and crowds at airports. However, everyone needs a break, and a change in surroundings from time to time is essential and restorative for both you and your family.

Don't despair. You don't have to schedule a hiking trip. There are vacation plans and destinations that fit almost every body and lifestyle. Just because you have fibromyalgia does not mean you have to be left out.

There are vacation plans to suit everyone

Think small. If you haven't taken a trip since you got sick, don't be too ambitious. It certainly doesn't make sense to schedule a walking tour of the English Lake District if you are exhausted after you take the garbage out. Guided tours of the National Parks or European capital cities sound glamorous and, sure, they're a lot of fun, but they require that you keep up with a group. On many tours you can't select your own meals or make time to rest when you need to. This makes them inappropriate for someone with fibromyalgia.

Yet even if you feel lousy there are things that you can enjoy. Hot springs or spas may have midweek packages that aren't expensive, and you can relax and treat yourself to a massage or facial or any treatment that strikes your fancy. You might have to search a bit for a place near you, but you'll be surprised at what you can find with a little effort—especially now that the spa trend has caught on throughout the Americas. There are a lot of reasonably priced places that don't get a lot of publicity. In Southern California, for example, there's a place called Glen Ivy Hot Springs just a few hours away from where I live. There are mineral baths, steam rooms, mud baths, and warm soaking pools. They don't allow small children (except on certain days), and everyone there looks the same way you do in a bathing suit. A place like this is ideal for a short vacation and I promise that you'll feel comfortable walking around no matter what shape or size you are.

Do the research

You probably haven't heard of Glen Ivy (which calls itself Club Mud), even if you live in California, and that's exactly my point. It's not a world-famous resort, or a glamorous destination. But it's a place where you can relax, be pampered if you want to treat yourself to a massage or a facial, fit in, and have a wonderful, relaxing time. There are other places like this, and probably some near you that you've never heard of.

Unless you look carefully you'll never know about places like these. So do a little research. The Evergreen Hotel chain in the United States is a special option for people who are chemically sensitive. They can be reached at 800-929-2626. I also know of a woman who has a bed and breakfast especially for people with fibromyalgia and hypoglycemia. Her name is Jane Baxter and you can reach Road's End at Poso Creek at 661-536-8668. She will care for you, and let you set your own pace. She has fibromyalgia, and she understands.

Finding a perfect destination

The Internet, of course, is an ideal place to do a search. You can also ask support groups and friends for suggestions. Travel agents can help you, too. If you work with an agent, be sure he or she understands your limitations and what kind of experience you are looking for. A good travel agent is used to helping people with disabilities, and can certainly make suggestions and ask for special accommodations with your reservations. Resources like the Arthritis Foundation also might be able to help you.

There are lots of Web sites for disabled people or travelers that need a little extra help. Information is available for a variety of special needs. Some groups have message boards with vacation ideas you may not have heard of, as well as access guides, transportation options, and wheelchair or scooter rental information. If you can get onto the Internet you'll be able to collect a lot of useful information, so consider a trip to the library if you don't have a computer at home.

Some companies are dedicated to helping people with illnesses

There is a company called Accessible Journeys that specializes in helping people with special needs. They make travel arrangements and have advice on every kind of travel need. These are located in a state-by-state database at www.projectaction/org, or you can call 800-846-4537. If your travel agent doesn't know about this treasure trove of information you are invited to pass it on. Accessible Journeys works hard to help. "We use no magic formulas, quote books, or computer programs to slap together a quick tour quote for an independent itinerary. The end product of our effort is an individual customized itinerary." Accessible Journeys does not charge the traveler, although they do require a deposit to begin work, which is credited toward your purchase.

Think about what you really need to be comfortable

If you're going to make a longer trip, you can look for houses, apartments, or bed and breakfasts where you might be a little more comfortable. Many of these can be rented for a few days or a single week. You'll have a bit more space, and if you need to rest you'll be in surroundings where you can take care of yourself. Even a small refrigerator and a microwave will make a huge difference if you're too tired to go out. If you have a hotel room with a mini bar, there's usually a lot of stuff you can take out that doesn't require refrigeration and you can replace them with things you've brought along. You can also buy collapsible or folding coolers to carry your food or drinks.

Buy travel insurance

Once you make plans, you might be worried that you'll be too sick to travel as scheduled. Travel insurance is a good idea if you think this is a possibility. Obviously if you have a family looking forward to an adventure, you'll find yourself going anyway. But if you're traveling by yourself or with a partner, traveler's insurance is a reasonable idea. Do *not* expect the airlines to waive fees for cancellations with a letter from your doctor, even if your doctor is willing to write one. Like many other outfits, the airlines have cracked down on doctor's letters and medical excuses and they probably won't accept one. You may be able to swing a credit voucher for future travel, but these days you're more likely to get a presidential pardon than an actual cash refund.

Make a list and check it twice

With your first vacation, less is probably more. Make a few trial runs to places near home if you're nervous about taking a longer trip. Traveling in the middle of the week when fewer people are on the road is a good idea if you can mange it. Start working with a packing list, review it periodically, and add things as you go along. As you review it, cross off things that you never use, or that seem too bulky. You'll find that you need less than you think you do. When you're confident that you have a list that works, type it up and keep it in a file. That way you won't need to spend the days before you leave running in circles and getting crazy because you weren't organized. Keeping it on file is important, so that if you ever have to make a sudden trip for a family emergency you'll have an easy time getting ready and won't have to struggle with forgetting your contact lens case or favorite pillow.

Pack early and don't bring the kitchen sink

Allow yourself plenty of time to get organized. JoAnn's husband laughs at her because she packs her suitcase a week before she leaves. "But it's not my final packing," she says. "I work with what I've put in, look at it several times to be sure I'm not carrying too much or too little. I know that if I start early, I can finish early and rest the day before we leave. Having fibromyalgia means I can't always predict how I'll feel tomorrow. It's better to get it done early than not being able to get it done at all."

No matter where you are going there's only one rule to observe when packing: Pack light. The more you have to haul around, the harder your trip will be. Most of the time you don't use half of what you bring—and if you forget something you can always buy it. Put toiletries in small containers that seal tightly. When you select clothes, pack some that can be rinsed out in a sink and hung up to dry. If you make a few outfits out of clothes that go together and can be layered and take a small bottle of laundry detergent, you will have a lot less to deal with. I like to pick a couple of complementary colors and take only those items that work with one another. Be sure your clothing choices and your shoes are comfortable. Don't travel with new shoes; wear them at least a few times first. You may think that the more you bring, the more comfortable you will be because you will be prepared for anything, but I promise that's not the case, especially if fibrofog hits you on the road. You'll be more apt to leave something behind when you have too many bags to keep track of.

Choose the right kind of luggage

Buy suitcases with wheels and a long, comfortable handle. Some companies sell padded attachments to handles if yours is the bare-bones type. Take a trial run and if you find that the handle digs into your hand, buy one of these. When you're tired and sore, even one more pain can be too much and ruin your day. Heavy travel bags can be impossible to manage, and it isn't always possible to find a luggage cart when the airport is crowded. Do yourself a favor and buy the right luggage to begin with. Don't try to adapt the wrong kind. Removable wheels are a hassle and hard to figure out when you don't feel well.

Consider replacing your purse with a backpack

You've probably noticed how uncomfortable it is to carry a purse when you're in a flare. Instead of a purse, consider a small backpack. You can manage a little more weight that way, and not be weighted on one side when you're trying to walk. You may want to carry your money and identification in a fanny pack that you keep around your waist at all times. If you have fibrofog, and it gets worse when you're tired or overstimulated, you don't want to take a chance with losing a purse.

Have everything you need to get by with you on the plane

If you're going by plane you should always take a small carry-on bag with your medication, a change of clothes, your toiletries, and a heating pad or hot water bottle if you use one. Airlines do lose luggage and flights are delayed. If your medication is packed away you won't be able to get to it if you end up sitting in the airport because your flight isn't on time. You might also slip an inflatable pillow into your carry-on, in case you are stuck waiting in a terminal. Remember that security is tight these days so be careful what you pack in your carry-on. You don't want to be delayed because you've mistakenly packed a sharp nail file.

Get ready early so you can rest before you leave

If you haven't learned by now not to procrastinate when you have fibromyalgia—here's your chance. You want to be extra ready, extra early. Nothing will help you more than relaxing and getting as much sleep as you can the day and night before you leave. There's nothing worse than starting a vacation exhausted because you tried to do too much at the last minute.

IN A SENTENCE:

> *A vacation or short trip may require some extra planning, but you need a break and you should not limit your activities because of your fibromyalgia.*

learning

Practical Travel Advice

ONE THING that is changing for the better in the world around us is handicap awareness. Suddenly the world is an easier place if you need a little help. Airlines, hotels, car services, buses, and trains all have new rules in place to accommodate people with limited mobility. With the basic information here and your telephone or computer, you should be able to ensure that your trip will go smoothly.

Airline travel gets you to your destination faster

Traveling by air has the decided advantage of getting you to your destination quickly. If you make reservations on airlines well in advance you'll have a better choice of flight times and seating. If you have trouble being this organized, you can book your flight through a travel agent or online and still get a seat selection that suits you. Many airlines have seating charts on their Web sites that show which seats are taken. You can look through the flights until you find one where you can get an aisle seat or a bulkhead seat. If you use a cane or have asked for a wheelchair, don't expect the airlines to seat you by an emergency exit. Instead, you'll be able to preboard and get settled in before everyone else.

Carefully check the timetables

Check connecting flight information carefully. Some layovers are unnecessarily long, but others are not long enough for you to stretch, relax, and get something to eat. Keep looking, or have your travel agent keep looking until you find a suitable option.

Ask the travel agent or the airlines when the airports are likely to be the least crowded. You'll probably find that the best time to fly is midweek, in the middle of the day. There's usually a morning rush, after which the airport is almost deserted, and then the end-of-the-day travel crush begins around four P.M.

A little planning will make you more comfortable in transit

For a long trip, one of those inflatable neck pillows is a real help. You can sleep in a more comfortable position, not all scrunched up on one side. If you put your carry-on luggage under the seat in front of you, it can be used as a little footrest. For a longer flight consider a muscle relaxant, melatonin, or a short-acting sleeping pill to make the trip easier. Many flights now hand out little earplugs to muffle the noise, but you might want to take a pair of your own just in case. If you prefer, carry a CD, tape, or MP3 player with comfortable earphones with the music of your choice to help you relax.

Choosing your airplane meal

You'll need to be careful about what you eat on the airplane, especially if you have bowel or bladder symptoms. Check to see if your airline offers a selection of meals. Sometimes a vegetarian meal is a good choice if you're worried about the effects of mystery meat in a strange sauce. Be sure not to drink soft drinks that contain caffeine. The air is very dry on a plane and the combination of caffeine and sitting in a tight position will quite often stir up an attack of irritable bladder. If your problem is irritable bowel or hypoglycemia, or if your stomach is easily upset, seriously consider packing your own meal. You will never regret the extra time it took to pack some edible food. You will also have something to eat if your flight is delayed.

Be sure to plan for time spent in airports

Airlines will provide you with a wheelchair if you ask them. Be sure to request this about forty-eight hours in advance. It also doesn't hurt to confirm your request. Most airports have motorized skycaps who will ferry you from gate to gate for a tip. Carry small bills in an outside pocket for tips and for a skycap if you have enough luggage to need help.

It stands to reason that if you travel by air you'll need to spend time at the airport. Always have a pair of sunglasses in your purse. Make sure that if you are sensitive to noise, you have a small pair of rubber earplugs. They muffle the noise of other travelers and loudspeakers so you won't crawl out of your skin. Since September 11, lines are longer, although they seem to move fairly quickly. The trade-off is that people in airports, despite the delays and searches, are much friendlier and more helpful.

Car travel has advantages

If you're driving, it will take longer to get there, but you'll have the advantage of stopping whenever you need to. One thing that will help is to plan to stop regularly every two hours to stretch. Truck stops, rest stops, and just pulling off the road are options. If you pull of the road into small towns you can usually find a place to park where you can walk around and find a restroom. If you're traveling with kids or pets you can let them out to run around and burn off some energy. When you figure the time it will take you to travel, figure in an extra half an hour for every two hours on the road just to be safe. Vacation driving is different than running errands. You really can slow down and smell the roses if you feel like it.

Make sure you have what you need for a comfortable ride

Be sure to take along some extra pillows to keep yourself comfortable in the car. Bucket seats can be a big problem for backs. They are *not* comfortable for fibromyalgics. If you bring a pillow to sit on, you'll be surprised at how much it helps. Some people like to bring neck pillows to keep their neck relaxed and comfortable. Take a moment to stick a hot water bottle under your seat. You can always stop at a restroom or even a restaurant and put some hot water into it.

If you're the driver

If you are the driver, there are several ways to be more comfortable. A steering wheel cover can make the wheel more pleasant to grip. You can also get wide-angle side mirrors and rearview mirrors that will make it easier for you to see. These will increase your field of vision and you won't have to crane your neck and twist around. When your neck and shoulders are stiff, these will be a godsend. There are also seat belt covers or cushions that can make driving more bearable.

Most fibromyalgics can only take long trips by car if they are not the driver. The combination of fibrofog and fatigue can make the idea of a trip into the unknown daunting, to say the least. When you don't feel well you can get very, very lost. Be sure you have a compass, map, and cell phone if you decide to make a car trip (or, if you're fortunate enough to have one of those GPS systems, you're set).

Educate yourself on car comfort

If you're planning a long car trip, or if that's how you take your vacations, there's an excellent resource for you. Frank Wildman, Ph.D., a Feldenkrais expert, has a videotape for sale that educates people on how to help their bodies survive these adventures. Some people think it helps to start practicing his techniques before you leave. This tape is available from www.movementstudies.com or by calling the Movement Studies Institute in Berkeley, California, at 800-342-3424.

Train travel is another option

Travel by train is a wonderful option that most people have forgotten all about. Although trains are notorious for running late, they are a very comfortable and sane alternative for fibromyalgics—and can be quite an adventure.

Train accommodations can be comfortable and restful

On a long trip, pay the extra cost for a sleeper car: You'll be able to move around, sleep comfortably, and you won't get jet lag. The sleeper prices also include free meals, with your choice of anything off the menu. You'll have privacy and can doze when you like, or read quietly without being disturbed by other people. You can see the country but you don't have to worry about getting lost, and you can rest when you're tired. You can bring a cooler with snacks or eat in the dining car. Trains also have club cars that serve snacks, sightseeing cars, and even show the latest movies at night for free. If you are traveling with children they don't have to stay in their seats and can walk around and explore. Train stations are generally not crowded, and you can use a cart to get your luggage all the way onto the train. (If you live in a major metropolitan area, consider getting on the train at the nearest suburb. You can generally park your car for much less than it would cost to park in town, if not for free, and walk right out to the tracks.)

Train Travel by Amtrak

AMTRAK IS "wholly dedicated not only to the letter of the Americans with Disabilities Act, but its spirit as well."

○ Amtrak asks that you use the toll-free telephone number rather than their Web site to book travel if you wish special accommodations. You can ask for special help in the station for arrival and departure. Call 800-872-7245 for general information and 877-268-7272 for information about special services.

○ Amtrak offers a 25 percent discount to disabled passengers. A letter from your doctor is one of the things they'll accept as proof of a disability. However, since the discount is based on their highest fare, discount fares such as excursion rates may actually turn out to be cheaper. Also ask about their frequent "2 for 1" rates.

○ With seventy two hour advance notice some trains can provide you with special meals. They will also bring meals to you in your compartment or seat if you need that service.

○ Amtrak says they will make every effort to refund or reschedule due to illness. A letter from your doctor is acceptable to them to start the process.

If you have a compartment be sure to pack a small overnight bag. If you have a suitcase, you'll want to leave it in the special luggage compartment. You'll have access to it, but you won't have to lug it in and out of your compartment. On a longer trip you'll be able to get out at some of the larger stations and walk around. Some trains even have entertaining tour guides who board and give narration as you pass through special areas.

Bus is another way to go

Bus trips are generally not the best option for fibromyalgics. They combine the worst things about plane travel—you're stuck in a small seat—with the worst part of car traveling—it takes a long time to get there. If you go by bus you have to stop when they stop and eat in bus terminals on their schedule.

Greyhound and Trailways are trying hard to help

The obvious negatives of bus travel aside, there are some good things to say as well. It's usually inexpensive and serves smaller towns and more places than airplanes or trains. You won't have to deal with the waiting and lines you see at airports, and both Greyhound and Trailways have programs for travelers with disabilities. You'll find that they go out of their way to be helpful.

Greyhound has a special telephone number just for disabled travelers (800-752-4841), which you should call forty-eight hours prior to departure. They say that even if you just show up they will make "every reasonable effort" to accommodate you. Proof of disability is not required, and they save special seats up front. Greyhound will provide luggage assistance and help you board, exit, or changes buses.

Cruise ships are a real getaway

Cruise vacations are very popular. They combine the conveniences of an all-in-one resort with a chance to do some sightseeing. There are cruises of many lengths, to many destinations, and also those that have themes or are educational. As with land resorts, the price range varies dramatically from line to line, as do the accommodations and the service.

Cruise lines still have a ways to go

The bad news is that the official position of the international cruise ship industry is that the American Disabilities Act does not apply to them. Helpfulness will vary from line to line and ship to ship. It is important to get written confirmation of any promises that they've made to you. (Bear in mind that cruise ships consider advanced pregnancy as a disability and won't allow women in their third trimester aboard.)

This said, some of the newer ships and lines are bending over backward to accommodate passengers with less than perfect mobility and various levels of handicap. Princess Cruise Lines, Holland America, and Royal Caribbean are some of the most helpful, and Celebrity and Carnival are also reportedly working on accessibility. Carnival ships have gym equipment if this is important to you. To provide special services, Radisson requires a doctor's letter documenting your disability. The brand-new American Queen (run by Delta Queen) paddlewheel steamboat will even take wheelchairs now. Travel agents say it's important to check that the ship you want to take was built in the last five years. You can also ask the cruise line for a "Special Needs" brochure that will detail their services.

Things to find out before you book your cruise

The first thing to ask about is the size of the cabin where you'll be staying. Some of them are very small and if you have a hard time maneuvering you might want to ask if they have something larger. Many cabins also have small refrigerators, which will be important if you're bringing some of your own food, or if want to keep something handy in case you don't feel up to dining. Ask about room service; many lines have it now.

Another important thing to check out is shore excursions and how they're handled. If they're primarily guided tours, you'll need to decide if you feel well enough to keep up, although you can do this on a day-to-day basis. If the group tours don't work for you, another option is to rent a taxi and take a tour by yourself, or with your companion. If you see other people with limited mobility consider talking to them and banding together. Check with the crew to see what time you need to rejoin the group and where.

Accessible Journeys, which was mentioned earlier, is also the largest group cruise operator in the world, and specializes in cruises for "slow walkers, wheelchair travelers, their friends, and their families." They work with all the major lines, including those listed above and Crystal Cruises, Disney Cruise line, and Radisson Seven Seas.

Jet lag and time changes can be rough on you

Since most people don't have all the time in the world to take vacations, you'll want to do a few simple things to help you get the most out of yours. Once you arrive at your destination, you need to make sure things are right before you settle in.

If you're taking a longer trip and are prone to jet lag, you should pack a small bottle of melatonin. (Make a trial run with this at home to make sure that it agrees with you. It should help you sleep.) Melatonin has been scientifically proven to reset the pineal gland and help you get adjusted to your new time zone. You'll probably only need it for a night or two, but don't forget to save some for when you get home. Usually 2 or 3 mg at bedtime does the trick.

Another tip is to get some sunlight in the late afternoon when you arrive. Daylight also has an effect on the pineal gland and helps to reset it, but it takes about three hours for this to occur, and you'll need to take your sunglasses off, or wear very lightly tinted ones. If you can take a short walk, or sit outdoors when you arrive, this may be all you need to do.

Make your hotel room reservations carefully

Make sure you talk directly with the hotel where you're going to stay. Don't talk to centralized offices that are reached by 800 numbers. Chances are, if you call the main office you'll speak to an operator who has never seen the hotel you're inquiring about. Make sure that you have a

---

Important Advice for
Booking Your Hotel Room

○ Get special arrangements confirmed in writing by fax or e-mail.

○ Confirm your room with a credit card so it will be held for you if you are delayed. Always recheck your reservations two days before you're scheduled to arrive.

○ If you have your confirmed arrangements and arrive to find what you're expecting isn't available, the hotel must put you up somewhere else that meets your requirements. If this happens, be aware of your rights and ask to speak to the manager. Arguing with the desk clerk will get you nowhere.

○ If you are traveling without a reservation stop early for a better selection of rooms. Always ask to see the room before you pay for it.

---

non-smoking room if you are sensitive to smells. Make sure that you are on the ground floor if there's no elevator and stairs bother you. It's also nice if you can find a hotel with a Jacuzzi and a gym. It may not seem important, but if exercise is part of your routine and it helps to make you feel your best, it's worthwhile to check.

A little strategy can pay off

While it might be a nice idea to get a room near the elevator so you don't have to walk too far, remember that these rooms can be noisy because everyone will be walking by your door, day and night. It might seem tempting to be near stairs, shops, and the lobby but these rooms will also be noisier. Whether or not a hotel has room service might be another consideration in case you don't feel well enough to go out after a difficult day.

Make sure your hotel room is comfortable before you unpack

Once you get to the place you're staying, do some reconnoitering immediately. Check the bed where you'll be sleeping because the wrong bed can ruin your stay. If it isn't satisfactory, speak up. If you need more pillows or more blankets call housekeeping right away before the hotel fills up. Check the thermostat and heating/air-conditioning to make sure they are operative. Make sure you have everything you need and everything works properly before you settle in. Changing accommodations will be more of a hassle the longer you wait.

Don't start your vacation with a hectic day

While it's important to get rest before you leave, you should also plan a light day the day you arrive. You very well may be tired from the trip, so don't expect too much from yourself. Make an agreement with your companions that if you need to rest they will not be held back but will feel free to do something without you. Make sure they understand that you are happier resting when you need to, so there's no need for them to change plans. Morgan M., a fibromyalgic who recently visited Venice, Italy, told me "I had some perfectly charming times sitting quietly by myself watching people, or resting in a new place. There's a certain kind of restfulness you can get when you're away from home—when there's nothing you need to be doing. When I'm at home I always see something that makes me feel like I should be doing it, but when I'm on vacation I am forced to slow down. Half the fun of traveling for me is relaxing and watching other people and taking in the ambience."

Local phone books are good resources

When you arrive, make sure you have a local telephone book with yellow pages. Having this handy will make your life easier. You can find take-out food places, stores, and taxi services. If you have a hotel with a concierge you may not need this, but if you're staying in a smaller place, or in an apartment, a telephone book can make looking for things a lot less frustrating.

The Internet's Yellow Pages will make it easy to locate things you need in the city where you'll be staying before you leave home. For example, if you need a car service from the airport to your hotel, just look up Car Services and Limousines in your destination area. If you're uncertain about categories and you don't know the name of any companies, use your own Yellow Pages at home as a guide. Many larger companies now have Web sites or toll-free numbers so you can arrange and prepay for numerous services before you even leave home. Remember that the more you do before you leave the less you will have to deal with when you get there.

Most of all, remember to take it easy

Keep your plans reasonable and be optimistic. Not every trip turns out as planned and not every day will be perfect. You will have to shake off the bad moments and concentrate on the good ones. As with every other aspect of fibromyalgia, a sense of humor will come in handy. Always remember that the more normal things you do, the happier and fuller your life will be. A vacation is a gift you can give yourself and share with those you love the most.

Now, get started, and bon voyage!

IN A SENTENCE:

> There are many ways to make your vacation more enjoyable and many resources to help you do this.

MONTH **10**

Finding a Support Group

EVEN IF the idea is unappealing to you, or you simply don't consider yourself a "joiner," there are many good reasons to join or start a support group. No matter how wonderful and supportive your family and friends are, in the end you still may feel a certain isolation about having an illness that others around you don't have. The responsibility for managing your symptoms is solely yours, and one from which you never really get a break.

Why a support group is important

Perhaps you don't have a lot of family members around you. Or maybe you don't see your old friends as often as you used to because you don't feel well most of the time—and when you *do* see them you don't want to talk about your health. Maybe you've lost a lot of friends because of your inability to keep your scheduled plans. By now you understand that this is an illness that you have to incorporate into your life instead of ignoring it. Sometimes it just comes down to needing some comfort and understanding from someone who's been there. What if you could spend quality time with people who have exactly the same problems that you do?

Well, you can. It's time for you to remember that there are millions of other people who have fibromyalgia, too. They have the same worries that you do, most of the same symptoms, and the same sense of isolation. You don't have to go through this alone; you can get to know these other people. You can pick their brains for suggestions, and comfort one another when things are rough. You might actually find that your involvement helps others! A fibromyalgia support group is one of the easiest ways to connect with fellow sufferers who are all navigating through a world where "no one understands." It's a wonderful place to make new and understanding friends as well as to voice your fears and frustrations in a safe and non-judgmental environment.

Don't rely solely on online support groups

If you haven't already discovered it, there are many online support groups for people with fibromyalgia and other chronic illnesses. These groups vary greatly in structure and size as well as in theme. Online support groups certainly have a place if you spend most of your time at home or if you enjoy writing or sitting behind your computer. In the beginning, when you were just learning about fibromyalgia, these online groups were probably a wealth of information and opinions. But now, well, let's face it, they don't get you out of your house and they don't help you move on with your life. It's time to find some real live people who can help you come out of your shell and get off your computer. I'm not saying at all that online groups aren't helpful, but the purpose of this book is to get up and running again—even if running is just a quick drive across town. It's time to realize that online friendships can only go so far and that personal interaction is vital to your recovery. Getting involved with a support group is one of the very best ways you can do this.

What to look for in a group, and where to look

If you have a computer or you can go down to the library and use one, there are some sites that can help you. The Fibromyalgia Network (www.fmnetnews) keeps a very long list of current groups, and fibromyalgiatreatment.com has a list of groups supporting the guaifenesin protocol, for example. You can also call your local chapter of the Arthritis Foundation and hospitals in your area. Hospitals often offer their conference room for groups and generally know what's in the area. Local newspapers carry support group listings in their community calendar section. Your physician or physical therapist might also know of one and may be acquainted with the leader.

Check out the groups in person

Once you've got a list of groups, you'll need to go and visit them. Some groups are just gripe sessions and you'll find that others are dominated by a few individuals who monopolize the whole session. Stay away from these because you won't get anything out of them, and listening to people complain for a couple of hours is only going to bring you down. I have a friend who once commented to me after visiting a group: "I don't know what those people had, but I can't believe it was fibromyalgia." This is an important point because when you find a good support group you should not feel skepticism, you should feel relief. You should feel that you have walked into a room full of people who understand you, and feel that you are believed, honored, and safe.

Try to evaluate the groups fairly

Lots of people with fibromyalgia find themselves visiting several support groups and then complaining that "they're all filled with sick people." Yes, it's true, they are. And if you've been a very active, healthy person for most of your life, the last thing you want to do is associate yourself with a bunch of people with a debilitating illness. Yet the sooner you come to terms with the fact that this illness is now part of you, and many of these individuals were once dynamic people themselves, the sooner you can fairly determine which group will work best for you. Self-loathing is an element of every illness and will bring you down faster than fibromyalgia itself. The primary purpose of support groups is to illustrate that there are folks out there who struggle with family, work, friendships, and energy levels just as you do.

Additionally, every group has its strengths and weaknesses, and each member brings something different to the meetings. The benefits you gain by helping another person are often just as satisfying as finding a supportive ear for yourself.

Strange dynamics do exist in support groups

I want to emphasize that you should carefully avoid a group that pulls you down. There are some that are just a collection of really sad cases complaining about their lives. They would be complaining even if they didn't have fibromyalgia. These encounters will not help you to build a positive attitude and will leave you feeling worse than when you went in. You want to find a group that will have a positive effect on your psyche. On the other hand, any group can have a "down" night, so you might consider going to more than one meeting if the group looks at all promising.

If you live in a rural area or in a small town and you don't want to start your own group, you can always look for chronic pain groups or chronic illness support groups. Although not all these people will have fibromyalgia, you will find that their loneliness and concerns are much like yours. So you needn't be constrained by the word fibromyalgia itself.

IN A SENTENCE:

> *Support groups come in all shapes and sizes and it may take a bit of shopping around to find one that works for you—but keep looking, it'll pay off.*

learning

Starting a Group That Works for You

IF YOU can't find a group that meets your needs, seriously consider starting your own group. Although I like groups, I'm much more a starter by nature than a follower, and you may be like me. First of all, if you start a group you can pick the time and place that it meets. If there's one in your area that doesn't suit your schedule, remember that there are certainly other people in your boat. If you have children with busy schedules, or need to have meetings when someone else can care for them, picking your own time is no small advantage. Also, if you are following a certain protocol, you might want to have members who are doing what you are. After you visit a few groups you should have a definite idea of what you want to do and what kinds of things you want to avoid.

Shop around for other members

The first thing you'll have to do is get together a few other people to help you start your group. Hopefully you have a friend or two who also have fibromyalgia, but if not, check with your doctor's office. The office may be willing to give your name and phone number to people they think might be interested. You might want to make cards with your information for them to keep handy. Understand that they will have to ask people to contact you due to confidentiality. They cannot release the names of their patients to anyone.

You can also give flyers to physicians. Most doctors feel frustrated treating fibromyalgia patients and are on the lookout for a resource. Some doctors or other medical professionals might be willing to help you with your group, but others may be hesitant because of negative experiences in the past. If this is the case, ask your doctor to be a guest speaker once your group gets going. If the meeting is informative and upbeat, your physician may change his or her mind and pitch in more often. For example, several physical therapy offices in my area have groups set up that meet there.

If you already have friends with fibromyalgia, you've got a core group. You can have them invite people that they know, and so on. Chiropractors and massage and physical therapists also may agree to pass out your flyers. If you are in an online group you might want to post a message to locate people who live in your area. I have to say that no one I know who has started a group has had a hard time finding members. Most of their groups get large quite quickly and often they end up having to limit membership.

Scheduling the meetings

You'll need to decide how often you want to meet. Less than once a month isn't a good idea because your group will lose momentum and focus. If you want to have different kinds of meetings you can devise a revolving schedule. You should always make sure you have a set pattern, though, and a printed schedule to hand out at your meetings. Every two weeks is the average for most support groups.

You can set up the schedule however you want. Some groups like to have periodic guest speakers who know about fibromyalgia or topics of concern to anyone with medical problems. You might invite physicians, massage therapists, or a hospital wellness coordinator who knows about community resources. An insurance specialist might be an informative speaker if your group has voiced problems with their coverage. Acupuncturists, hypnotists, and time-management specialists might be other interesting speakers. You might invite a pharmacist to talk about things such as storing medications and taking them properly, or you might invite a yoga or tai chi teacher.

Getting started—The nuts and bolts

First, of course, you need to find a location. If you intend to keep your group small, maybe you can do it in the comfort of your home if you have a den or a living room that's large enough. If you want to hold it somewhere else, check with local parks or community centers, hospitals, libraries, and hotels—anyplace with meeting rooms. If you have a small group you may want to alternate homes or locations to make it as accessible as possible for all members.

You'll also need to think about how long you want your meetings to be. You might want to hold them one Saturday a month for several hours, or have some meetings during the week and then every few months have a long Saturday afternoon meeting. Think carefully about what you want to do—how often and for how long the meetings should be—because consistency is important and people will lose focus if you keep changing the schedule.

Growing the group

Think seriously about what you plan to do with your group and how many people you want to include. Larger groups are harder to manage and activities are harder to arrange. You might want to try to hold the number at, say, ten or twenty. Or you might want as many people as you can find.

Local newspapers are a good resource. It's my experience that small newspapers need interesting stories. If you contact their health writer or the person in charge of local events they may be interested in writing a whole story about fibromyalgia. In any case, most of them do have a section that lists local meetings. Give your information to hospitals and post flyers in libraries or any place that has a board featuring local events. Local radio stations often have public service announcement segments. Make an effort to find the station that serves the group you want. It might be advisable to avoid sports stations or teenage audience stations. Local cable television also has community bulletin boards and local shows that might be interested in doing a story about you and your group.

Posters and flyers are easy to make if you have a computer. Just buy some brightly colored paper and keep the information simple. If you don't have a computer you can certainly make flyers by hand and have it copied inexpensively at a local office supply store. Have someone who doesn't have fibromyalgia read them over to make sure you've included all the necessary information before you take them out to be printed! Remember the basics: who, what, where, when—and keep the flyers easy to read.

Don't forget to be social

Allow for time for people to just hang out either before or after your meeting. Be sure to have a sign-in sheet and have everyone sign in with their address and telephone number. This will give you a mailing list if you plan to have a special event such as a guest speaker. If members agree, the list can be circulated so everyone can have a support group member to contact if things get bad between sessions.

Be realistic about your group and encourage the members to do so as well. It will take work in the beginning to get it going, and there may be times when it seems as if you are doing all the work yourself. If you feel this happening, be honest and appeal to your group members to pick up some slack. Be specific and spell out what you need clearly. Make a list of the tasks you need help with and ask your members each to pick one. Some of the responsibilities might be making flyers, arranging for refreshments, taking phone calls from interested people, or maintaining the mailing list.

The first meeting

Your first meeting should be simple. You want to have an informal time for people to talk, tell their story, and get acquainted. You might want to write up your own story and rehearse telling it a few times because you'll probably want to speak first to break the ice. After you have all introduced yourselves, be prepared bring up the subject of ground rules. After all, it's very important for you all to feel safe. The first subject to discuss at this time is privacy—you should all agree that whatever is talked about at meetings will never be mentioned outside formal meetings. You should discuss ways to be nonjudgmental and uncritical of each other. You might want to make resolutions about dedicating a certain amount of time to positive suggestions as well as to gripe sessions. Perhaps you could all agree to each bring one positive or uplifting thought written on a note card to every meeting and read and exchange them.

You and your group should agree on guidelines and perhaps write up a brief statement describing your group that you can use in future publicity. A sample statement might be:

> This group was formed to provide comfort and understanding for people with fibromyalgia. We invite our members to talk openly about their problems and frustrations, but also to share information, encouragement, and positive experiences. Our purpose is to add to the quality of our lives through friendship, support, and knowledge. Discussions should stress positive attitudes, and suggestions should be directed at solutions.

When you get your group set up you should make a small packet to hand to new members. These should contain basic information about your group, including the philosophy you've adopted. If each member is expected to volunteer to help in some capacity or take turns hosting meetings, say so in your brochure. You want things to be clear up front.

Expect attendance to be erratic

All groups have ups and downs in terms of attendance. Certain seasons, like the winter or summer holidays, will be more difficult. If your group members have children, the end of the school year might be a busy time for them. Enthusiasm, too, will normally wax and wane. If you notice that most sessions are just informal discussions, consider suggesting a project. A good one is putting together a simple cookbook with easy recipes. When you have fibromyalgia, cooking for a family is a big challenge and it's easy to get into a rut of having the same meals over and over. New ideas can be a great help. Or you could have each member bring a certain kind of dish, such as a favorite dessert, and swap them.

Your support group may have people who cannot attend every activity or meeting. It is important for members to feel that they can come as they please. You don't want to put pressure on them to come if they don't feel up to it. They should also feel safe to share or to be silent. Your support group needs to be open to allowing participation at any level.

Keep it lively

Some support groups sponsor a prominent public speaker once a year or so. This is an ambitious project, but if you feel up to it, you'll be rewarded by helping the entire community. You'll need to get a large hall and make the arrangements. Usually expert speakers require at least that their expenses be paid, and some expect an honorarium. If you charge a fee for the public to attend and have enough publicity you may even be able to raise extra funds to donate to research. Most experts these days are also authors, so if you are interested in someone like that you can contact their publisher for details on any book tours or seminars they may be doing in the area. You might even want to band together with another or several similar support groups who would all benefit from a major speaker. However, bear in mind that this is an ambitious project and should be saved until your group has been together for a while and has a strong structure and energetic members. For regular meetings, you might want to have only people with fibromyalgia, or invite those with other chronic conditions like lupus or rheumatoid arthritis. A few times a year you might want to include significant others for a different kind of get-together. You might want to plan family days at a local beach or park, or have potluck gatherings at each other's homes. Getting families together at least periodically can be a nice idea, and can demystify the support group for the family. You might want to schedule a regular combination of things: Every other month try to have a speaker and on alternate months have a roundtable discussion. You could have a family potluck, say, four times a year, or just one holiday party.

Other ideas for your group

Some smaller groups set up a treasury, so money is available if the group wants to hire a speaker or have an adventure. At each meeting a specified donation is made. At the end of the year this money could be used for a special outing such as a visit to a day spa or a weekend away together.

Other groups meet around the holidays to share craft ideas for gifts. Maybe one of your members has a special talent, or you could invite a teacher from a local college to teach you crafts. Learning to make bath salts or gift baskets is an easy way to solve some of the exhaustion caused by holiday shopping. One group I know had each person bring ten of an item for a holiday gift basket with a preselected theme. Then, at their meeting they each made a basket for a female family member or two. The ways to pool resources are endless once you start to think about it. You can share books, magazines, videos, and have one meeting every so often be a reading club where you discuss a book you've all read. If your group is small you could all meet to attend a weekend college class. Just remember that your goal should be to make supportive new friendships and keep active. You want your group to be a group of friends who have fibromyalgia, not fibromyalgics who get together to complain exclusively about their illness.

Your group can also have option activities like a Saturday morning walking group. If that time isn't convenient for everyone, consider choosing exercising buddies and get together regularly to motivate each other and offer companionship. A little company can make exercising more enjoyable and harder to beg off.

Revamping your membership will be necessary from time to time

If you need to periodically find new members you can always try putting out flyers again or asking your local paper to run a story. You'll be surprised at how active word of mouth is, and how many members will come to you, yet you must realistically expect some attrition when people move away or need to work or have family problems.

The key to a successful support group is to remember that everything changes. Whether you've started a group or joined an existing one, if it stops working for you, make a change. Even if you eventually drop out of attending meetings, if you've been involved with the right group, you will take away not only some good friendships, but a lot of wisdom and understanding as well. And hopefully, you will have shared some too.

IN A SENTENCE:

> *There are many kinds of support groups, and if you can't find one you like starting your own is certainly a rewarding option.*

MONTH **11**

living

Discovering Fibromyalgia in Other Family Members

WHEN YOU'VE learned a lot about fibromyalgia something funny happens. You start to see your symptoms in the people around you. Now that you've been living with fibromyalgia for nearly a year, it's only natural to look at your family and wonder if they, too, have the illness. And what about friends, and other people you come across in your everyday life? What can you or should you do to help them?

Looking at the people closest to you

It's hard not to be worried about your children. As we get older, the memory of some of our parents' struggles may touch a cord. Did your mother have headaches, too? Fatigue? Irritable bowel? Maybe your significant other has fibromyalgia, too? In my experience it's not uncommon to find a husband and wife who both have fibromyalgia.

You might ask yourself why this would happen. But when you think about it, you'll realize it's natural for people to nest with a partner who has the same energy level. So if you've had fibromyalgia all your life you may have chosen someone who is a lot like you when it comes to your daily activity level. Although opposites attract, when it comes to settling down it's hard for someone who is active all the time to make a life with someone who struggles to get out of bed. Although your partner may have a milder case than you do, you still may discover that you have a number of symptoms in common when you look closely.

On the other hand you obviously don't want to overreact to every complaint of the people around you. After all, many illnesses have similar symptoms. Over the course of a year it's normal for even healthy people to have various complaints. Children go through periods where they naturally need more sleep as they prepare to grow. Teenagers are moody and languid even when they're perfectly healthy. When it comes to older family members, memories of the past are imperfect, and not everyone you know is looking for your input about their aches and pains. What's the famous joke? *Denial isn't just a river in Egypt.* You'll need to keep it firmly in mind if you plan to offer unsolicited advice. Denial is something you'll run smack into sooner or later. And you'll learn it's a powerful emotion. The fact is that some people don't want to admit they have what you have, even though you think you're trying to help them. What should you say, and how should you say it? How do you go about making sense of your family tree? What should you share with your friends who complain to you about various familiar-sounding problems? And what symptoms should you be concerned about in your children?

Fibromyalgia and your family

We know that fibromyalgia runs in families. Though once this was an issue of debate, you'll find it's generally accepted now. It stands to reason that if you have it, probably at least one of your parents does too. If you have siblings or even cousins you're close to they may have symptoms that sound very much like your own. Flushed with enthusiasm and relief when you're finally diagnosed, and now, later in the process, armed with the knowledge you've acquired, you may be eager to help them and to share what you've learned.

When you learn more about fibromyalgia you realize that not everyone has every symptom. Knowing this, you can often be in the position to steer someone in the right direction. For example, if you have a relative with a history of bladder problems who also complains of pains all over her body, you may realize that she has fibromyalgia while she is still beating down the door of her doctor's office looking for answers. It's common for people to see a specialist when they have one horribly dominant symptom and miss seeing the overall picture. I ping-ponged between gynecologist and urologist for ten long and unproductive years, getting medications for symptoms while missing my underlying disease. It's hard to say who was more frustrated, my doctors or me. I know that if I'd had a friend, acquaintance, or family member who had pointed me in the direction of fibromyalgia I would have been not only less frightened and upset, but also eternally grateful. I could have found the help I needed a lot earlier. At the same time, years of being around this illness have taught me that you can't help everyone. Some people have very fixed and rigid ideas, or may have a doctor they adore who doesn't want to hear secondhand suggestions.

Why we want to help others so much

Especially if you've had a long, frustrating road to diagnosis, it becomes important to you to help others avoid your travails. Most of us have suffered a lot and continue to feel isolated and different to a certain degree. When we see others and think it's possible that we have something to offer them; it's hard to ignore the urge.

While it's natural to offer a helping hand, don't be pulled into any debates or arguments that can only drain your own energy and mire you down. The cardinal rule about helping people is that you can't help everyone. Believe it, and bear it in mind. Save your strength for the people that you can help—including yourself. It's not your job to persuade others that they have an illness that they aren't ready to accept they have. In many encounters all you can reasonably do is plant the seed and walk away. An occasional watering in the form of a gentle reminder is fine, but dragging the unwilling to the diagnosis of fibromyalgia will wear you out and not help a person who isn't ready to help himself or herself.

Who you're talking to will change what you say

If it's someone you don't know very well, you may just want to make a suggestion: "Have you asked your doctor about whether or not you could have fibromyalgia? That's what I have." But then what do you do when they answer, "Oh, no. My doctor says all my blood tests are normal"? How far should you go, and how involved can you get?

It depends a lot on your relationship with the person you're talking to. You might want to just casually suggest a second opinion and leave it at that if you don't know the person very well. To people you know better, you can share an article that you think is particularly descriptive. Many Web sites have good articles that can help people learn about the symptoms and how the diagnosis is made, or you might want to share this book or a magazine article. With your family members you may want to go into more personal detail about the reasons you think they should be interested in what you have to say.

* * *

I *never thought about my illness as a youngster. I was always more fatigued than others and had to struggle harder. I was just never good in sports, probably a huge disappointment to my father, who was a star athlete in school. When my pain began in earnest in my late teens my family did everything they could to get to the bottom of it. They took me from doctor to doctor, moved a couple of times seeking a better climate, and finally all I was offered was Darvon Compound, which I took steadily from age twenty-one to twenty-four. . . . I endured thirty years of undiagnosed pain that continued to worsen to the point where I couldn't function anymore. I'm sure I appeared somewhat unbalanced to my doctors. After all, I was fifty years old and felt worse than my eighty-six-year-old father and had no obvious reasons for pain*

Every person handles pain differently. After the first few years I figured I didn't have a life-threatening disease, just some abnormality so far undiagnosed that caused pain. People who knew me very well knew what I was going through. Others probably never knew because I always put on a happy face. I had known too many people who alienated everyone because they complained all the time. So I just endured it. I don't know whether it was a guy thing, or an American thing, or the stiff upper lip of my ancestors. I didn't let on to many people. After a while it was harder to keep a secret since it affected so many aspects of my life. Then people started saying to me, "I don't know how you manage." By then, I didn't know either.

As far as the other men I have known with fibromyalgia, most of them have struggled on like I have. The office I worked in had several. They were good friends, some of the best I've ever had. You know how it is when someone you know is going through the same things you are. But since none of us were diagnosed at the time, we could only commiserate with each other's trials. Most of us had been told by some wise older females that we had fibromyalgia. I never believed it for a minute and neither did most of the others. One by one we left our jobs because of our health, and only later did we learn what we had.

Your family is a more personal matter

Siblings and friends your own age may have about the same symptoms you have. For this reason, you'll probably find it relatively easy to identify people in your own age group who have fibromyalgia and it should be easy to relate to them and to answer questions if you're asked. It's possible, too, that you'll clearly see the symptoms in younger siblings who still may be in denial—struggling to be normal and blaming various activities or stress for physical problems. Here you can put a little bug in their ear, and expect that if and when symptoms get worse, you might get asked for advice. You may be passionate about the idea that you're saving them your agonies, and you may be able to see the road they're traveling from where you stand, but they must be able to see it for themselves before you can step in. It's hard enough to get some people to go to the doctor when they're sick! If people aren't yet ready to accept that they have a chronic illness with no cure and a strange name they've never heard of, forget it! Any doctor will tell you that the hardest thing to do is to treat people who aren't convinced they have a problem. Getting people to continue treatment for cholesterol, blood pressure, or anything they can't see or feel is a difficult task. You must abandon the idea of convincing people to seek help before they are ready, no matter how much you love them, and no matter how sure you are that they need your help.

Don't forget to include men

Men get fibromyalgia, too. Officially, about 15 percent of fibromyalgia patients are male, but it's easy to believe that it's underdiagnosed in men. To begin with, many men won't go to doctors, especially to complain about a lot of weird symptoms. It just doesn't seem right to a lot of them; it seems somehow weak. If you're a man, or have a husband, relative, or close male friend who has fibromyalgia, you'll quickly learn it's an especially difficult road. A man finds himself alone in a sea of female faces if he attends a support group meeting or a lecture to learn more. It may be harder to get a doctor or an employer to take him seriously. Quite often men don't feel comfortable listing the litany of symptoms of their illness. They may feel self-conscious, as if there's something wrong with men having as many complaints as they do.

Although most articles you come across are geared toward women, the major researchers doing work these days on fibromyalgia are all men. Dr. R. Paul St. Amand, M.D., and Dr. Mark Pellegrino, M.D., are two male physicians with fibromyalgia who have written books that men can read. Dr. Don Goldenberg's book (he's also a medical doctor) may offer some insight as he has some of the symptoms of fibromyalgia as well, and has a wife with the illness. None of these books speak specifically to the problems that a man faces, although an argument could be made for the fact that most of our struggles are universal, or at least variations on a theme.

These books and some online resources are listed in the For Further Information section of the back.

Men face different challenges than women

If a man is the main support of his family and faces the specter of disability he may need some special help from a counselor. If you are in a position to help a man make the decision to seek help, do it without hesitation. Remember that men are raised to believe that they must be strong and they must be providers, and that it is their instinct to want to fix things. Since there are no concrete ways to fix fibromyalgia and the symptoms fluctuate and vary in intensity, coping can be very difficult unless one learns to come to terms with all the emotions that accompany a chronic illness.

Parents and grandparents with fibromyalgia

The popularly published demographics of fibromyalgia state over and over that fibromyalgia affects predominately women between the ages of twenty-five and forty-five. If you're like me, you've read that phrase so many times you can say it in your sleep. In fact, you probably finished the sentence in your mind before you read the words. Why shouldn't you? You can't miss it. It's on the first page of every book about fibromyalgia, and is right at the top of every Web site. But what happens to all the women who were diagnosed at fifty-five? Don't they still have fibromyalgia when they're sixty-five if it's incurable?

Of course they still have it. It's just that if women or men are diagnosed later in life, quite often they're told that they have osteoarthritis because by that age an X ray shows some small changes in a painful joint. While it's logical that arthritis can cause some of their problems, it doesn't explain much except pain or stiffness. In many cases doctors don't get the rest of the litany from an older patient simply because it's been recited too many times to no avail. A lot of women especially get smart and realize that the doctor isn't going to take them seriously if they complain a lot, but instead will just assume they're lonely or unhappy if they launch into all their aches, pains, and ailments. Some give up and assume it's natural to feel bad all the time when they get older. But others never give up. Every day I get letters that read like this one, from an eighty-one-year-old woman in Kansas: "I have never been diagnosed but I am willing to bet money that I have lived with this for at least thirty years, fortified by various pain medications, gradually becoming more immobile."

Where does this leave you if you suspect one of your parents may be suffering with fibromyalgia? By now you probably have guessed that earlier generations of fibromyalgics were pretty badly treated. If your mother went to the doctor in the 1940s, '50s, or '60s or before, she probably didn't get much understanding or sympathy. Grandmothers and mothers may have been told that they were suffering from "empty-nest syndrome" or worse. They may have been diagnosed with a nervous disorder and given tranquillizers or "mother's little helpers." Symptoms were blamed on menopause, marriages that had become less than exciting, a need for attention, a weak character, or some kind of hysteria. *Neurotic* and *hypochondriac* were two other popular words.

How can you know a diagnosis will help?

A debate is raging in medical circles about what purpose making the diagnosis of fibromyalgia serves. There are physicians who feel that telling people they have fibromyalgia will make them sicker because it will give them the idea they're ill. These experts would argue that there's no reason to tell people who are coping with their problems the name of what causes them. But you have to think this issue through for yourself. Some people do have parents who won't embrace an illness they've never heard of, or that a trusted doctor has never told them they have. It may be sad to them that only now are they hearing of a condition they can't do much about. Others will feel vindicated, empowered, and relieved to have a name for their ill health, and a brotherhood of fellow sufferers. Some may have to learn, as some of us who are younger had to learn, that pain is not a normal part of aging, and that there is help for the pain and the other symptoms, too. Some of us wish our mother or grandmother had lived long enough to get a proper diagnosis. As one woman wrote to me, "I found out too late to help my mother who recently died after suffering for her entire life with fibromyalgia. I intend to do all I can to further the cause of research and getting the word out so that in the future no one else will suffer like she did."

While some of our parents may be happy with the status quo and not be interested in learning about another illness they may have, some will be empowered and feel redeemed that their various complaints over the years were not all in their heads. As with anyone else, it's important to respect your mother's or fathers' feelings. Offer information and assistance. If your offer is refused, you can repeat the offer gently as the occasion arises, but let the subject drop if your parent isn't receptive. You can only help those who are ready to be helped.

IN A SENTENCE:

> *If you believe a loved one may have fibromyalgia, it is essential to gently inform them of this possibility while being supportive of their choice to explore other options.*

learning

Should You Worry about Your Children?

"MY DAUGHTER has bladder problems and she's complaining about headaches. Should I be worried that she has fibromyalgia?" asks Cynthia C. "My son is having trouble in school and he's stopped playing volleyball because his legs hurt and he gets so tired. Should I take him to see the doctor or is this normal at his age?" asks Holly S. These are questions that you might be asking, too.

When should you worry about your children?

It's normal as a mother or father to worry about your children and to try to help them if they are suffering. When it gets to the point that complaints are interfering with their enjoyment of life, you should try to get them some help. While you can't force other adults to go to a doctor or admit that they are ill, your children are your responsibility.

Your children have no idea what it feels like to be normal

An important thing to bear in mind when talking to your children is that they have no idea what's normal—what other children feel like. I was thirty-five years old before I understood that it wasn't normal to wake up in pain every morning. I had always thought that people hurt on whatever part of their body they had slept. I thought my shoulder and backaches and stiff legs were something that everyone experienced. When I interviewed children for the pediatric book on fibromyalgia I coauthored, I was struck by their stories. Roughly 50 percent thought that something was different about them but didn't know what, and the other 50 percent thought that everyone hurt the way they did but that others were just braver and more competent. These kids generally described themselves as not having as much stamina as those around them, and having problems with concentration and mental recall in class that was frustrating and embarrassing. Some of them even thought they weren't as smart as their classmates. Pain was not one of their primary complaints probably because they simply did not know that pain isn't normal. I didn't think that I had headaches, though I had a headache every day by the time I was thirty. Why was this? It was because I came from a family where my mother and sister had blinding, completely debilitating, throbbing, aura-driven migraines. Since all I had was a dull ache and a stunned feeling, I didn't think what I had was a headache. It's all relative, and you must keep that in mind when assessing your children's symptoms. If their legs have always hurt when they run, they will think it's normal to feel that pain and they can't know that it's different for their friends. I also suffered from irritable bowel as a child. I did not know until I was an adult that the urgency I felt when I had to go wasn't normal. I knew where every bathroom was in town, and I still know. I can tell you which markets have public restrooms, and also which retail stores.

An early diagnosis for your child can be important

Remember the comfort you felt when you realized that you weren't crazy, or different, that you just had an illness that wasn't your fault? Once you knew what the problem was it was easier to devise ways to cope with your symptoms. This is a gift you can also give to your children. You want them to understand that they aren't stupid or weak, and that they can succeed despite their illness. Even though fibromyalgia is pretty nasty at times, there are certainly children with much more serious problems and disabilities. And that's something neither one of you should ever lose sight of.

Finding a doctor to diagnose your child may not be easy

It's not easy to find a doctor to examine children for fibromyalgia. There are still doctors who aren't really convinced that fibromyalgia is real, and

---

When to Suspect Your Child Has Fibromyalgia

○ Complaints of pains that may be called "growing pains" by your doctor
○ Headaches, backaches, and stiff neck that come and go
○ Fatigue even when your child has slept twelve hours
○ Insomnia, inability to sleep even when tired
○ Complaints of being too tired for enjoyable activities
○ Problems with homework in subjects that were previously easy to grasp
○ Falling grades even though the child is trying hard and was doing well before
○ Fatigues easily in sports, poor stamina
○ Constipation or diarrhea that come and go
○ Cramps, gas, and bloating or waves of nausea
○ Bladder infections, painful urination with no infection

---

others who don't believe that it occurs in children. There are a few really open, caring doctors, but chances are you're going to run into a problem. Many people have been accused of trying to make their children sick, or of projecting their symptoms onto them as part of some sort of agenda. (Some spouses and grandparents also make this accusation in perhaps kinder words.) However, there are many published studies about children who have fibromyalgia, and a Medline search can help locate these if you need them. In one study of 338 randomly selected children, it was revealed that 6.2 percent of them had fibromyalgia. If fibromyalgia runs in your family, the chance is much greater than that. It's also clearly more common than most doctors are aware. Most pediatricians don't read *The Journal of Rheumatology,* so don't be afraid to collect some articles for your child's doctor to review.

What to look for in your children

What exactly is it that you're looking for in your children? Children haven't been sick as long as adults, so they haven't had time to develop as many symptoms. You'll find, however, the same characteristic complaints, though most kids will not have all of them. Bouts of fatigue, irritable bowel, bladder problems, headaches, neck and back pain, and leg cramps are probably the predominant physical complaints. "Growing pains" or leg pains are generally recognized now as part of fibromyalgia. It's obvious that it doesn't hurt to grow. Babies triple their birth weight in the first year of life and they are not in pain. Problems with sleep include falling asleep or staying asleep, nonrestorative sleep, collapsing in exhaustion, sleeping for twelve hours but still feeling exhausted. Headaches are something else your child may complain of, especially on one side at a time. Neck muscle involvement is very common, so a stiff neck is something most children with fibromyalgia complain about.

Fibrofog hits kids just like adults

One of the things that fibromyalgics can recognize easily in their off-spring is fibrofog or a cluster of cognitive problems that vary in intensity from day to day. Especially when children are at an age where you help them with homework on a daily basis it's easy to notice if there's a huge variation in their capabilities. On a fibrofog day children will be weepy, tired, and struggle with tasks you know they know how to accomplish. Quizzing them or telling them that they should know answers usually provokes a highly emotional response.

It was this group of symptoms that led me to the inescapable conclusion that my son, Malcolm, had fibromyalgia. There was just too great a contrast between days when he could do his work and the days when he had no idea almost how to spell his name. His reactions to pressure from teachers and from me struck a cord deep inside me. I could remember the feeling so clearly of being told "You know the answer. You just did this yesterday." Often boys will be accused of having an attention deficit, and children of both sexes will be routinely called underachievers.

Watch carefully if you've been told that your child isn't trying. Some-times kids are; they just can't figure out how to complete the task that they were given. Know that if your child is dyslexic or has a learning disability these symptoms are consistent. Dyslexics don't read one day and then not the next. Their ability level remains constant from day to day. It's natural for a little boy to have more trouble than a little girl at tasks that require fine motor coordination and sitting still. It's also natural for there to be some variation in the attention spans of boys and girls. But hyperactive kids don't have days where they sleep fourteen hours straight and wake up tired. If your child is having trouble sitting still you might try asking, "What hurts?" or "What feels funny?" Remember that if your kids are young their phrasing might not be the best. "A headache all over my body" might sound like an amusing turn of phrase, but it's actually a really good description of how we feel some days, isn't it?

Irritable bowel is common in children with fibromyalgia

Irritable bowel is often the harbinger of full-blown fibromyalgia. Children will have bouts of diarrhea, constipation, abdominal pain, cramping, gas pains, stomach pain, and waves of nausea. Children will also pass gas excessively at times. Another of the common effects of irritable bowel is the need to use the bathroom—now. This is frustrating for kids and their parents, and it can also cause problems in school with teachers. Children are often embarrassed to tell you about these symptoms so if your child has bowel symptoms on the weekend you should consider broaching the topic to teachers. Since this cluster of symptoms is the most embarrassing, your child needs you to handle it firmly and in a matter-of-fact way. Remind your child that this is an illness; nothing is wrong with him or her.

Both boys and girls are at equal risk

For some reason, fibromyalgia in children seems to occur equally among the sexes. Dr. St. Amand and I tabulated the statistics of our patients before we wrote our book about pediatric fibromyalgia and we were stunned by this discovery. Since then, we've read a published study with the same results, and read that Mark Pellegrino, a physician who has treated thousands of fibromyalgics, sees about the same thing in his patients. No one seems to know what to make of these numbers because in adults the female preponderance is so well documented. For some reason it seems that boys outgrow the illness at puberty. Hormones or larger bones and muscles may play some role in this, and the answers will certainly become clearer when the genetic research is completed. For now what we should take away from these experts is that we should be as vigilant for symptoms in our sons as we are in our daughters.

Be vigilant

Any symptoms of fibromyalgia, alone or in combination, should alert you to keep an eye on your child. The most important clue you'll have is that if the symptoms are caused by fibromyalgia they will come and go with no rhyme or reason. If your child comes home from a week at camp and sleeps a lot for a few days—this is not a symptom of fibromyalgia. If your teenager becomes a night owl but makes up for this with regular naps, this is normal. But if suddenly, out of nowhere, your child's sleep is nonrestorative or disturbed, and the complaints go away just as mysteriously, you should be suspicious and watch for the pattern to repeat itself.

Teenagers are a special problem

Much of the above applies only to younger children because they are easier to observe than your teenagers. Unfortunately, even at the best of times, puberty is difficult, and it becomes even more so when accompanied by fibromyalgia. Girls may struggle with PMS and painful menstrual cycles, while many boys recover or at least go into remission during their growth spurt. Teenage girls can also suffer from premenstrual blood sugar symptoms. You may have success showing your daughter the proper way to eat at this time, especially because it doesn't involve an illness or medication. More than any other time of life, puberty is when it's the most stressful to be different than other kids. Remember this if you suspect that your teenager is developing the symptoms of fibromyalgia. Most teenagers will deny it because they don't want to be sick, or different, or like you. (Sorry, but this last phrase is true for teenagers! Most of them don't want anything their parents have.) You may find they'll attempt to explain away their symptoms—"I'm just tired because I've been up late at night on the computer" or "I hurt my legs from running in PE." You can't do much under these circumstances except to give them the information and wait for them to ask for help. Don't nag them every time they mention a symptom to you; just gently remind them now and then to keep the channels of communication open.

Practical ways to help your teen

Once you've determined that your child has symptoms, the best thing you can do is teach him or her a sense of pace. If you teach your child to start projects early, to rest when work is impossible, and catch up on better days, you will have taught him or her a valuable life lesson. Your teenager needs to listen and understand his or her body, to know when to continue and see a task through and when to stop and take a break.

Medications and your children

The double-edged sword of treating symptoms is even more pronounced when it comes to children. Few drug companies even test medications for pediatric use, and those that have been tested have only been used in the short term. For this reason, the effect of drugs on growing nerves, bones, and organs is not known except in the case of a small handful of drugs. You should be extra careful not to teach your children that drugs are a quick fix, the first thing to reach for when things aren't going well. The example you set of using other modalities first like rest, heat, and exercise will serve your children well.

If and when your child's doctor considers prescription medications for your child, take the responsibility of looking at the suggestion critically. Go on the Internet or ask your pharmacist for a package insert so you can educate yourself about side effects and possible risks. Remember that while the risk of any specific problem might be minuscule, when it comes to your child you should err on the side of caution. Be sure to know which medications can be used on an "as needed" basis, and which need to build up in the body to be effective. Always instruct your child on the proper way to take his or her medication and listen and observe carefully for any possible drug reactions. When your children are old enough, you will have to teach them about drug interactions and caution them about mixing alcohol and medications.

Pain medication for kids

For pain in children, Tylenol and Advil are appropriate and can be used together for maximum relief. Benadryl for sleep comes in a pediatric formula and can be used if needed. Experiment with small doses, even smaller than the package directs, and titrate up slowly. Children can catch up on sleep on weekends or go to bed early on nights when they have less homework, and are generally resilient if given support. Only a rare child can't manage with over-the-counter medications. You don't want to give your young child the notion that the answer to problems lies in a bottle of medication, or that he or she is not strong enough to work through a manageable amount of adversity.

If your child is having problems, be sure to see a qualified doctor who can advise you. Most doctors will agree that where children are concerned, less is more, but your physician may give you some advice or prescriptions for the most severe symptoms. Do not use herbals or other supplements on growing children. These have been tested even less than prescription drugs and many formulas have been found to be impure. Melatonin can be used to aid sleep, but it should never be used in teenagers, whose own level of that hormone is already high.

Communicating with your child's school is essential

School is for your child as your job is for you. A large portion of your children's life is spent there, and how well they do in school is very important now and in their future. Rarely do parents need to take advantage of home schooling, but there are laws to provide for children who need it. Meetings with your child's school can help to establish any special considerations you think will help. The most important thing to know about this process is to set up the meetings early in the school year, before your child has problems. Reversing a teacher's notions about a kid is tough, so don't let the situation get bad before you step in. Make it clear that you expect that your child will work hard and do everything he or she is capable of doing on a regular basis. You can bring a letter from the doctor if the school requests it, but don't overwhelm the teacher with medical records and articles about fibromyalgia. Respect the fact that teachers are busy and make your case simple for him or her to understand. Don't ask for impossible favors, but be sure that the teacher and the school feel free to contact you with concerns.

You can also send a simple letter to the school nurse explaining that fibromyalgia isn't anything that would cause an emergency but that you'd like to be notified if your child is sent to the nurse's office. Generally, unless your child asks to be sent home, the school won't notify you that your child has gone to the nurse. Investigating his absences, I discovered one year that my younger son had spent many hours in the nurse's office for various complaints. Luckily, it turned out he was not sick, but that the nurse was a beautiful young college student who fed him treats! If your child doesn't do well in regular classes, there are laws to protect you both, and to allow you to get the help you need. Don't be afraid to write letters and to make your voice heard at the school board if requests at your child's school yield no results. Individual educational needs can be met in various ways, and you should not stop until you are satisfied that you have what you need.

When to cut back on your child's activities

If your child is having severe symptoms, it makes sense to cut back on activities until his or her condition has improved. If your son's symptoms are mostly mental, for example, he might continue with sports, but take a break from his music lessons until he feels better. Most schools will let you leave standing orders for Tylenol or Advil to be administered by the school nurse if requested. Some parents try to get their children excused from gym class, but since exercise and stretching will help your child through the day this may not be the wisest course. You can instead ask that only certain activities be avoided if you can identify something that causes a flareup of symptoms.

Don't underestimate your child

Don't make a mistake, though, and underestimate your child. Overprotection is certainly motivated by love and the strong instinct to protect, but children are strong and may not be as sick as you are. Don't forget to give your child the chance to triumph over a setback. If he says that he can do something but you doubt it, it doesn't hurt to give him the benefit of the doubt. Always keep sight of the fact that your goal is for your child to have an independent and productive life.

Mommy birds have to nudge baby birds out of the nest, too, when the time comes. We all have limitations that have shaped us to some extent, but what's important is how we learn to handle ourselves in spite of them. Don't get me wrong—I know how hard it is to watch a child suffer, how the helplessness you feel can make you crazy. I know the desire to protect, to make everything easy to accomplish. More than anything else, my children steered me by telling me what they could do. I learned to listen to them and I have learned a lot about bravery and determination from them. Let your children lead you; they will know what they can do and what is impossible without you telling them.

Less help is often best when it comes to children

Most children don't need to see specialists. Family doctors and pediatricians can make suggestions for symptom management. Using small amounts of medications under supervision and teaching your child the lessons you are learning about the effects of stress and the benefits of eating correctly will work wonders. Most children become asymptomatic during the growth spurt of puberty and many remain so beyond that. With a little management and guidance from you, your children will do just fine. The lessons of compassion and triumph over adversity will help them all through their lives.

IN A SENTENCE:

> If you discover that your children have fibromyalgia, it is up to you to help them cope and understand their illness.

Staying Up to Date
with New Resources

YOU'VE LIVED through your first year with fibromyalgia, and you've come a long way. By now you understand your symptoms and have learned ways to manage them, and you've come to terms with being in charge of your illness. You've rejoined the world to the best of your ability and you are getting on with your life. You are in control of your diet, your exercise program, your relaxation techniques, and your medical needs. What's left?

Learning more every day

Part of being in charge of your life is keeping informed about developments in fibromyalgia. Medical research is progressing at a fantastic pace, and interesting observations and articles come out frequently. Of course, you shouldn't rock the boat for every single new idea; some of them may appeal to you and you'll want to make sure your physician has seen the material so he or she can review it with you.

Some studies offer insight using impractical therapies, like, for example, growth hormone studies. Dr. Robert Bennett, M.D., of Oregon Health Sciences University has spent many years studying growth hormone and fibromyalgia. Though in some respects it appears that in the short-term this hormone might help with some fibromyalgia symptoms, the cost and availability make it impractical as a treatment. But that won't be true of everything you read. Dr. Bennett just came out with a study showing that strength training helped fibromyalgics feel better than flexibility training did. Unlike his study on growth hormone, this article has a practical application that you can incorporate into your everyday life at no risk.

A computer will change your life

If you don't have a computer, my honest suggestion is that you do everything in your power to get one. Computers are a godsend for people with chronic illnesses. You can live anywhere and still learn or study anything, stay in touch with the world, access millions of resources, and join groups of people just like yourself. You can order books, groceries, housekeeping items, clothes, and even take classes. For these reasons, I can't suggest more strongly that you make this a top priority.

You also don't have to buy a brand-new top-of-the-line computer. Local newspapers list used computers for sale at reasonable prices, and you don't need anything fancy to use the Internet or write simple articles. As one fibromyalgic puts it, "I have found information, friends, entertainment, and solace on my computer. I am currently studying online—two classes. I don't have to drive over to campus, struggle with parking, or carry heavy books. I can do my assignments in my own spare time, sitting in my own home. If you need new skills, or want to start your own business, you'll need a computer to help you."

You don't have to own a computer to use one

If you can't buy a computer, or are waiting to get one, you can learn to use one at your local library. Actually, if you want to research anything about fibromyalgia, you'll have to. Despite the fact that there are more books out about fibromyalgia than ever before, most of them don't have the space to go into much depth about metabolism or physiology. If you live near a university with a medical school you can read books in the medical library, but

ACCORDING TO a study in the *American Journal of Psychology*, online support groups may have benefits. Ninety-five percent of those polled felt that communication in online support groups helped with symptoms of depression and isolation. Sixty-two percent received information from their support group that they took to their doctors.

you'll probably need permission to work there and you won't be able to borrow materials. But by computer, you can access medical journals and serious medical sites as well as find articles on coping and interesting stories written by others with fibromyalgia.

Check for breaking news

When you're using a computer, you can periodically check the recent news for any new articles about fibromyalgia. You can use a "search the news" option on various Web sites like www.cnn.com or www.yahoo.com. If you're on AOL you can go to the news channel and it will search all the major news sources for you when you enter the keyword *fibromyalgia*. You might find a favorite source of medical information like Jane Brody, a columnist for the *New York Times*, or one of the online experts. About.com and Webmd.com are two valuable sites that have both new and old information about health.

Newsletters and magazines are also good sources

Several organizations geared toward support, like the Fibromyalgia Network and the National Fibromyalgia Association, put out newsletters with some interesting articles. You can subscribe to them and read them carefully even if you don't have a computer.

You can also subscribe to various news services or newsletters that are generated by various Internet sites. Some of them will automatically send you any article that holds your keyword, and others are simply magazines that arrive via e-mail. If you are interested in certain subjects you will generally find that these will give you headline news stories about those subjects. There is rarely a charge for these Internet subscription newsletters, so you can try them for a while and if they don't seem to have information that interests you, just unsubscribe by following the instructions.

Carefully evaluate the information you find

It's important to separate advertising slogans from scientific material when you are looking for factual information. Finding the truth may take a little work, but when it comes to your health you need to do that work. The statement "scientifically proven" in most cases is about as accurate as "one size fits all."

When you look at a particular study, do so with a skeptical eye. Be sure to notice how many patients were studied, and who they were. Lots of people think growth hormone is a miracle cure that will bring back youth, but

Newsletters for fibromyalgia

Fibromyalgia Network Newsletter
Published quarterly
Cost: One year subscription $25.00 U.S. / $27.00 Canada
Covers new research and new medications and offers coping advice
To subscribe, contact:
    Fibromyalgia Network
    P.O. Box 31750
    Tucson, AZ 85751
    Telephone: 800-853-2929

Fibromyalgia Aware
Published three times a year
Glossy magazine
Cost: Donation of $35 or more
To subscribe, contact:
    National Fibromyalgia Association
    2238 N. Glassell Street, Suite D
    Orange, CA 92865
    Telephone: 714-921-0150

Healthwatch–Newsletter for CFIDS and Fibromyalgia
Published three times a year
Cost: This one is free, paid for by advertising
To subscribe, contact:
    The CFIDS and Fibromyalgia Health Resource
    1187 Coast Village Road #1-280
    Santa Barbara, CA 93108
    Telephone: 800-366-6056

the original cohort comprised a handful of elderly men. How does that translate to young women with fibromyalgia? Before you try expensive and possibly risky growth hormone, you should know the answer. You should also learn about long-term risks, so look at the length of the study for clues. Sadly we've all tried things that seemed to make us feel better for a few months, but then either stopped helping, or never helped at all. Looking carefully at data could keep you from rushing down a dead-end road.

Look before you leap

Many medications now on the market simply haven't been around long enough for us to know their long-term effects. Many supplements have never been studied at all. Expensive miracle mattresses or special blankets should have a return policy that can be verified in writing before you make the purchase. All fibromyalgics are different, and you won't know from reading about other people whether or not those modalities will be effective for you.

If a miracle cure for fibromyalgia is discovered, we will all know it very quickly. However, it's most likely that there will never be a "cure," because fibromyalgia appears to be genetic. So just as there's no cure for high blood pressure, there probably won't be any cure for fibromyalgia. This doesn't mean that we can't find things to help, however. Just remember that the more you learn about fibromyalgia the easier it will be to evaluate new information.

It's up to you how much you research

Somewhere in the time that lies ahead of you, you'll decide how much time you want to devote to reading more about fibromyalgia. I certainly don't expect that you'll be doing it more often than every couple of months or so. In the beginning, when you were first diagnosed, your life revolved around figuring out your illness, but the goal you were working toward was to free yourself from that burden. At a certain point you will have developed a routine that suits you, and your interest in every new miracle treatment should have waned to a healthy skepticism tempered by an open mind.

With any illness, especially a chronic one that you must largely manage by yourself, knowledge is power. Keep on looking for answers and using what you find. The future holds much more than we can imagine today.

IN A SENTENCE:

> *Staying up to date with resources and breaking information can help speed up your road to recovery by making you a more informed patient.*

learning

Searching the
Internet for Resources

Malcolm Potter

This section was written by my son, Malcolm Potter. He was diagnosed with fibromyalgia at the age of seven, when he uttered the oft-quoted description of his condition: "It feels like every muscle in my body wants to throw up." Malcolm is now twenty-one and works with computers.

THESE DAYS, if you have a question about most anything, chances are you'll hear the phrase, "Oh, just do a Web search . . . it's easy." Chances are also that the very same Web search will turn up very few pertinent results. You may be left wondering, "What good is the Internet if it doesn't have the information I need?" Well, much like a library, the Internet probably contains the information you're looking for (and a lot more)— provided you know where and how to look for it.

The Internet is a lot like a library— you have to learn how to use it

The first thing you need to learn is how to use the card catalog of the Internet, or more precisely, the card catalogs. Search engines are the main way that people find what they're looking for, but how many people know how to use them so that they get one hundred useful documents as opposed to the two or three that normally come up buried in a huge list of strange items? That is the question!

There are many search engines that you can use, and each is tailored for a specific market. For example, Medline and Pub Med are geared for searches of medical literature. I have found that the most useful for finding information is Google (www.google.com). While not necessarily more popular or widely known as its heavily advertised counterparts, Google offers far superior functionality. Google indexes far more Web sites than any other search engine. As of the beginning of 2003, Google says that it indexes over three billion Web sites. Google is also a true search engine and thus has real advantages.

You have probably heard of Yahoo (www.yahoo.com) from its many television advertisements and catchy theme song. Yahoo has been around almost as long as the Internet, and is one of a select few sites of its kind that actually manages to generate revenue. Yahoo, strictly speaking, is not a search engine in its true incarnation; Yahoo is simply a directory of sites, rather like the yellow pages of a telephone book. This has its pros and cons in relation to Google. Because Yahoo employs human editors to scour the Web-more human compilers than any other search engine—you will often find relevant sites in less time. This is especially true if you are looking for people-oriented topics such as support groups. What Yahoo lacks, however, is the sheer breadth of sites that a Google search can offer. In fact, if Yahoo cannot find a site in its directory that matches your search criteria, it will turn to Google to help return some relevant results.

Getting to the search engine you've selected is easy

To get to the search engine you've selected, you'll need to type in its URL (short for uniform resource locator), or address. In other words, before you can use the card catalog you've got to drive yourself to the library. Most computer browsers these days don't require that you type in the http:// anymore, so generally all you need to do is type in www.google.com, or www.yahoo.com, for example. If for some reason that doesn't work and you need to type in more, the address would look like this: http://www.google.com/. Whenever you're working with a Web address make sure you don't add or subtract any punctuation. For example: www.fibromyalgia-treatment.com comes up in German, but www.fibromyalgiatreatment.com is a Web site about fibromyalgia with a support group.

• • •

Understanding how a search engine works

Hopefully, by the time you've read this far, you've decided on which search engine is right for you. However, the fact is, it doesn't matter if you use Google, Yahoo, or any other of the dozens of search engines the Internet has to offer, the most important part of searching the Web is knowing how to search effectively. To search effectively, you must know how a search engine works.

Most search engines search a database of keywords from Web sites and match them to your search keywords to find relevant results. Generally, the more keywords you put in your search line, the more refined your results will be, but often it is better to carefully choose your keywords to get refined results. It's almost like the choice between a sledgehammer to break a boulder or a small jeweler's hammer hit in just the right spot; both get the job done, but if you know what you're doing, the latter takes far less effort.

If you are searching for a phrase, it's not as simple as just entering it into the search box. Say, for instance, you are searching for information on the subject of pediatric fibromyalgia. Entering those two words into the text box will show every Web page that contains those two words, but not necessarily together or even in the same paragraph. This can be frustrating when nine out of ten results are set up this way. A simple and easy way to refine your results is through the use of quotation marks. If you simply searched for *pediatric fibromyalgia*, then you might get a thousand results. A conservative estimate would be that around 90 percent of these sites would indeed contain both words, but they would not be connected in any sense. If, however, you searched with quotation marks around the words (as in *"pediatric fibromyalgia"*) then it would return every site that contained the phrase as it appears in the quotation marks. You may only get a hundred results, but they will probably all contain the information you're looking for. You can also mix phrases in quotations and keywords. So you could search for *"pediatric fibromyalgia" symptoms*, which would return results that contained the phrase and the keyword, but not necessarily together. You may also search using multiple phrases just like you would for multiple keywords. (It doesn't matter, by the way, to search engines whether or not you capitalize words.)

Understanding what a computer can't do will save you time

Another thing to pay attention to is words with the same spelling but multiple meanings. Let's say that you are searching for information on certain fish. In the search box, you might type *bass* to get a desired result. Unfortunately, you might then be treated to 60 percent of your results relating to a musical instrument or two. To solve this dilemma, you should make use of the common symbol for subtraction. Simply place a minus sign in front of the word you want to exclude from the results. *Bass -music* would yield all results that have bass, but it would exclude from those all that contain the word music. This would be a shame if you were trying to figure out whether fish like rock and roll or opera, but in most cases it's a helpful tool.

You can also perform broad or general searches for information

If you're not quite sure what you're looking for, the *OR* operator might come in handy. Simply type the letters "OR" between the two words you want to search for. Perhaps you want to search for your two favorite styles of music and, this day, you're in the mood for some slow music. You might use *slow rock OR opera*. This would yield all results that contain *slow rock* and all results that contain *slow opera*. Results would also come up for sites that contain all three words. It is important that you use an uppercase OR, otherwise the engine does not know that it is a logical operator designed to sift through the results.

Google (and some other engines) use a system called Page Rank, which means that the results they turn up are listed in the order of relevance. The lower you go on the list of Web sites they've turned up the less likely the site is to be useful to you.

You can start with user-friendly search engines

There are several search engines that will talk to you and answer your questions if Google seems too complicated for you to start with. While they may not be as detailed, they will help with most queries. Alta Vista (www.altavista.com) gives you a list of pages for your terms, and then a list of terms that have turned up frequently on those pages. These can help you narrow or expand your search and teach you about searching in the process.

Subjex.com actually holds a dialogue with you, and will help you find what you need by asking you questions. Askjeeves.com does a search in natural language—you can ask it a specific question. If the answer is simple, Jeeves will just give it to you. If you ask Jeeves who the President of the United States is, he will just tell you George W. Bush. But, if your question is more detailed, you'll get a list of Web sites.

How to find what you're looking for in articles

Google is a great way to find most things, but there is also material located on the so-called invisible Web also. This is a term that simply means resources that are stored inside databases. To use the library analogy again, if a library has a special collection, say, of old newspapers, there's often a special room for that body of information. Google can get you to the door of that room, but you'll need to search inside it for specific articles that might be of interest.

MEDLINE is probably the one most people use to search for information in journal articles. Researchers and physicians use this tool as well, simply because no one has the time to read every single medical journal. MEDLINE will search over four thousand medical publications for articles—more than eleven million of them. It is a service of the National Library of Medicine in Bethesda, Maryland, run by the U.S. government. While you usually cannot pull up the whole article, MEDLINE will show you an abstract—or a few paragraphs summing up the whole article. If you want to see the whole article you can order it for a small fee. Some Internet providers and Web sites offer free access to MEDLINE. The easiest to use is probably Medscape (www.medscape.com). There's a box at the top of the page that is the doorway to MEDLINE. If you're interested in reading new medical articles about fibromyalgia, you can check MEDLINE every few months or so.

The Internet uses a system of shortcuts designed to save you time

Another thing you should learn about is hyperlinks. These are little shortcuts that search engines themselves use to find subjects that are linked together. Many times when you come upon an interesting Web site it will have a resource page or even blue words in the text of a document. These, too, are little doorways, shortcuts to more information. If you choose to explore, click on them once, and you'll be taken to where they lead. To get back to where you started, you can push the back arrow on your browser.

Remember to carefully evaluate the material you find

The Internet is a great fountain of information, but as with anything, there is also a lot of misinformation. The greatest tool in searching the Internet is common sense. If something sounds too good to be true, chances are that most of the time it is. Just because one site says that something is so, that doesn't necessarily mean it is. It's the same in journalism-just because the *National Enquirer* says that something is true . . . well, you get the point. Credibility should not be assumed simply because someone has put up a Web page.

The Internet is estimated to grow at a rate of about 1.5 million documents per day. This means that every single day there is more information out there for you to find. It is important to keep searching to stay current. The information is out there. All you have to do is know where to look.

IN A SENTENCE:

> *There are many resources to help you to continue to learn about fibromyalgia, and a computer will make this task easier.*

Appendix 1: Medications

IT'S ALMOST a given that unless you are completely opposed to taking medications for fibromyalgia, you will be given many different compounds to try by your doctor. It will help you to keep a record of the things you've taken and what your response was. You should keep among your files a list detailing what you've taken, the dosage you took, the date you started, and the date you discontinued the medication, as well as a short note of your observations. If you had a bad reaction to the medication, be sure you've recorded what it was. You'll want this for your own information, as well as in the event that you change physicians.

USE THIS form to keep track of medications that you have tried. You can make a copy for each doctor that you see.

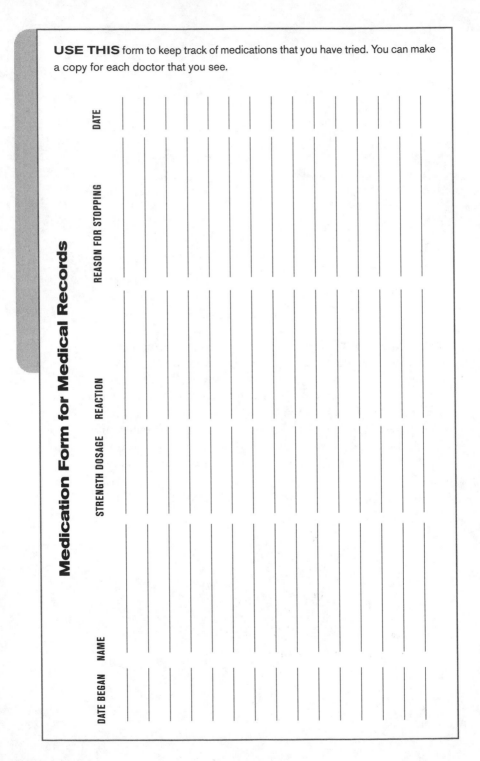

Medication Form for Medical Records

DATE BEGAN	NAME	STRENGTH DOSAGE	REACTION	REASON FOR STOPPING	DATE

Worksheet for New Medications

YOU SHOULD keep a record of all medications that you have been given. Use this list to get all the pertinent information from your doctor.

1.   Name of drug:_____

2.   Chemical name:_____

3.   Is there a generic available? (circle one)   YES   NO

4.   Strength of medication:_____

5.   Reason for medication:_____

6.   Dosing schedule:_____

7.   Take medication (circle one)   on schedule   as needed

8.   Taken with food (circle one)   YES   NO

9.   Taken with full glass of water (circle one)   YES   NO

10. Can I consume alcohol with this medication?   YES   NO

11. Drug interactions:_____

12. Any special instructions:_____

13. If I miss a dose I should:_____

14. Side effects I should watch for:_____

15. Warnings:_____

16. How long should I take this medication:_____

17. How long until it reaches full effectiveness:____

18. Do I need any special blood tests?_____

19. How often do I need to follow up?_____

Acetaminophen (Tylenol): Over-the-counter analgesic. It's a coal tar derivative and blocks pain impulses and reduces fevers. Considered one of the safest pain medications but large doses can affect the liver.

Adderal (dextroamphetamine sulphate): A potent stimulant generally used in attention deficit hyperactivity disorder. A controlled substance that side effects include tachycardia, insomnia, restlessness, headaches, diarrhea, dry mouth, bad taste in the mouth, and lowered libido. Should not be used with tricylic antidepressants, MAO inhibitors, or darvon/darvocet. Use with caution if you take blood pressure medications.

Ambien (zolpidem): A hypnotic, but one with low abuse potential, used for insomnia. Some patients do have to wean off of it slowly if they have been taking it regularly. Should be good for about six hours' sleep. Less sedating the following day than some older sleeping medications.

Armour thyroid: Animal thyroid extracts given by some physicians. These preparations contain a higher concentration of the thyroid hormone T-3 than humans produce and for this reason it acts as a stimulant. In low doses it suppresses the hormone gland, in higher doses can cause damage to the bones and heart. Low thyroid is not a cause of fibromyalgia, and this is not a legitimate treatment of the condition. Synthetic T-3 is marketed under the name Cytomel.

Aspirin (ASA or acetylsalicylic acid): Aspirin was invented in 1899, but natural salicylates have been used for pain in plant form for thousands of years. It is used as an anti-inflammatory, fever reducer, and blood thinner. It inhibits the body's production of prostaglandins. High doses are toxic, and any dose can cause gastrointestinal bleeding, although the lower the dose, the lower the risk.

Atarax (hydroxyzine HCL): Antihistamine and anti-anxiety drug usually used for itching, hives, or allergic skin problems. Side effects include drowsiness, morning fatigue, and dry mouth. Has some pain relieving effects.

Ativan (lorazepam): A benzodiazepine used as a tranquilizer and sometimes for sleep. Interacts with oral contraceptives. Side effects include fatigue, impaired mental agility, constipation, and listlessness. Should be tapered off slowly.

Baclofen (lioresal): A centrally-acting muscle relaxant used for spasms and tight muscles. Side effects include fatigue, drowsiness, dizziness, and headaches.

Benadryl (diphenhydramine): Over-the-counter antihistamine also used as a sleep aid in compounds such as Sominex and Tylenol PM. Generally effective in doses from 12 to 50 mg. Can be used by children. Side effects include daytime fatigue, dry mouth, and dry eyes. Can cause agitation in some patients.

Buspar (buspirone HCL): Anti-anxiety drug with very low abuse potential. May help with memory, and may be less sedating than some of the other anti-anxiety medications. Cannot be taken with alcohol or grapefruit juice. Side effects include drowsiness, dizziness, nausea, and very deep sleep.

Celebrex (celecoxib): A new anti-inflammatory, a Cox-2 inhibitor, that has less potential for stomach upset and other gastrointestinal problems. It is not stronger than prescription Motrin.

Celexa (citalopram hydrobromide): A newer antidepressant that should not be used with migraine medications such as sumatriptan and MAO inhibitors. Side effects are nausea, dizziness, and insomnia.

Codeine (codeine phosphate and codeine and sulfate): An analgesic that alters the perception and emotional response to pain through an unknown mechanism. It is a narcotic. Side effects include sedation, dizziness, lack of alertness, nausea, and irregular heartbeat.

COX-2 medications: This is a class of newer anti-inflammatories that are easier on the stomach than the older ones such as ibuprofen. Some new studies show that they may increase the risk of heart attacks and other cardiovascular events. This category includes the much advertised Vioxx and Celebrex. Insurance companies may balk at these alternatives if you don't have documented proof that the older NSAIDs gave you serious problems.

Dalmane (flurazepam): A benzodiazepine sleeping medication (and hypnotic.) Provides about eight hours of sleep. Side effects include morning fatigue, rebound fatigue, headaches, and anxiety.

Darvon, darvocet (propoxyphene): A mild narcotic pain medication, darvocet contains an addition of acetaminophen.

Depakote (divalproex sodium): An older medication used for migraines, sometimes prophylactically. Should not be used with amitriptyline, nortriptyline, diazepam, or clonazepam. Has many serious side effects including liver problems, pancreatitis, and fatigue.

Desyrel (trazodone): Antidepressant commonly used to help with sleep, unrelated to other antidepressant drugs. Must be taken with food. Side effects include dizziness and drowsiness.

Diflucan (fluconazole): Medications that end with "zole" are antifungals and are given for yeast infections. This 150 mg pill is taken once for a vaginal yeast infection, and is advertised as a "non-messy" alternative to vaginal creams. Long-term use requires frequent liver testing.

Dolorac (topical capsaicin): A topical cream made from chili peppers that is applied to stop local nerve pain.

Effexor (venlafaxine HCL): An antidepressant (serotonin and norepinephrine reuptake inhibitor). To discontinue this drug you must taper off slowly. Side effects include drowsiness, dizziness, headaches, insomnia, and sexual dysfunction.

Elavil (amitriptyline): The granddaddy of antidepressants known to help with sleep. It is inexpensive but often shunned because of the side effect of weight gain. May slow down the digestive process (constipation) and cause dry mouth.

Flexeril (cyclobenzaprine): Muscle relaxant related closely to tricylic antidepressants, touted because it may be more effective on small areas of contraction like the ones present in fibromyalgia. Also may help with twitches and nervousness. It is known to help with deep sleep, but side effects include drowsiness, dry mouth, and constipation.

Ibuprofen (Motrim, Advil, Aleve): A nonsteroidal anti-inflammatory medication that is marketed in both prescription and over-the-counter strength. Has some analgesic effect but works primarily on inflammation.

Imitrex (sumatriptan): The first of a new class of migraine medications that works as a selective agonist for vascular 5-hydroxytryptmaine. Should not be used if you have heart problems. Use with some antidepressants may cause weakness. Other side effects are fatigue, dizziness, and chest pain. Used as needed to relieve severe headaches.

Klonopin (klonazepam): Anti-anxiety drug that also is an antispasmodic and can help with digestive woes. Used also to treat seizures. Often given for sleep and for restless legs. Side effects include drowsiness, depression, and constipation. Must be discontinued gradually.

Lortab, Tylenol #3, Percocet: Codeine combinations used for pain when nonprescription medications like Tylenol and prescription medications like Ultram no longer work for pain. These are midstrength narcotics.

Marezine: An anti-motion sickness medication available over the counter.

Maxalt (rizatriptan): Medication for migraines. Side effects include chest and neck pressure and pain, dizziness, and fatigue.

Midrin (isomethepetene, dichloraphenazone, acetaminophen): A combination drug for migraines. A recent study showed it to be as effective as Imitex for preventing or aborting migraines, and it is much less expensive.

Motrin (ibuprofen): One of the older anti-inflammatory drugs. Has some analgesic effects and helps with menstrual cramps. Side effects include nausea, diarrhea, constipation, fatigue, or weakness. Over-the-counter forms of ibuprofen are Advil, Aleve, and Nuprin. Taken with milk may make it easier on the stomach.

Naprosyn (naproxen sulfate): A nonsteroidal anti-inflammatory medication that is marketed in both prescription and over-the-counter strength. Has some analgesic effect but works primarily on inflammation.

Neurontin (gabapentin): This is a medication designed to control convulsions. It is given for pain and for paresthesias, or funny sensations such as skin crawling. Side effects are fairly common and include fatigue and somnolence, dizziness, and nausea. This medication must be tapered off slowly, and has many drug interactions.

Norflex (orphenadrine citrate): Muscle relaxant used usually as a second choice for people who can't tolerate flexeril. Side effects are the same as the tryclic antidepressants: fatigue, constipation, weight gain, and dizziness. This medication is usually taken at bedtime.

Norgesic (orphenadrine, aspirin, caffeine): For moderate pain from muscle disorders. Contains both Tylenol and caffeine to help offset the drowsiness. Side effects include dizziness and constipation. Caffeine may cause palpitations and high blood pressure.

NSAIDS (nonsteroidal anti-inflammatory drugs): This class of drugs acts primarily on inflammation that is present in osteoarthritis and in muscle sprains, not fibromyalgia. They also have some analgesic effects and are frequently given for that reason. Common drugs in this category are aspirin, ibuprofen (or Motrin, Advil, Aleve, Naprosyn), Indocin, Volatern, Lodine, Daypro, Relafen, Celebrex, and Vioxx. These medications work best when they have been used consistently for at least a month.

Opioids: Narcotic pain relievers of various strengths that range from low dosages of codeine with acetaminophen to Percodan and the time-released Oxycontin. Also includes morphine and methadone. Side effects include fatigue, decreased mental agility and capacity, constipation, restlessness, vivid dreams, and nausea.

Pamelor (nortriptyline HCL): An older antidepressant of the tricylic class. Can help with restorative sleep, but can also be a stimulant. Has been used for hot flashes. Side effects include weight gain, constipation, anxiety, and blurred vision.

Parafon Forte (chlorzoxazone): Muscle relaxant that works at the spinal cord level. Can relieve morning stiffness and muscle spasm. Side effects include drowsiness, dizziness, lightheadedness, and fatigue. Should not be used with alcohol.

Paxil (paroxetine HCL): Antidepressant (serotonin reuptake inhibitor) medication that may help with sleep but also may be a stimulant for some patients. Can cut pain perception and may help with hot flashes. Side effects include headaches, nausea, constipation, dry mouth, and sedation or insomnia.

ProSom (Estazolam): A benzodiazepine sleeping medication that's a hypnotic. Provides about eight hours of sleep. Side effects include morning fatigue, rebound fatigue, headaches, and anxiety. Should not be used with alcohol or any other CNS depressant.

Provigil (modafinil): A stimulant used to increase energy. Can be taken as needed. Side effects include headache, nausea, diarrhea, dry eyes, and nervousness.

Prozac (fluoxetine HCL): Newer antidepressant that works by making more serotonin available to the brain. Has been shown to be effective in managing depression in fibromyalgia. Common side effects are weight loss, diarrhea, dry mouth, and nausea.

Relafen (nabumetone): One of the NSAIDs that may be easier on the stomach because it is broken down in the intestine, but still must be taken with food. Side effects include dizziness, headache, nausea, constipation, depression, fatigue, and weakness.

Remeron (mirtazapine): An antidepressant that is not related to other classes such as MAO inhibitors, SSRIs, or the older tricylics. Side effects include drowsiness, dizziness, dry mouth, and weight gain. Cannot be used with alcohol.

Restoril (temazepam): A sleeping medication (hypnotic) that may have less daytime hangover than others. It has been on the market longer than Ambien and many insurance companies will cover it. Side effects include fatigue and impaired mental function. Cannot be used with any other CNS depressants.

Robaxin (methocarbamal): A muscle relaxant. Can help with muscle pain and spasms, sleep, and morning stiffness. Side effects are fatigue, dry mouth, nausea, and blurred vision. Should not be used with alcohol.

Serozone (nefazodone HCL): Antidepressant unrelated to the others that helps with depression and sleep but does not cut pain perception as the others do. Has a significant number of drug interactions. Side effects include dizziness, drowsiness, upset stomach, and constipation.

Sinequan (doxepin HCL): A tricyclic antidepressant and antihistamine commonly prescribed to help with sleep. Fatigue is a side effect as well as weight gain, dry mouth, constipation, and anxiety. This has been tested on children and is available in pediatric drops.

Skelaxin (metaxolone): A mild muscle relaxant used for spasm and tight muscles. Side effects include fatigue.

Soma (carisprodol): Muscle relaxant also called a central nervous system muffler. Helps with sensitivities to light and sound, for example. Also relieves some pain, especially when used with acetaminophen. Fatigue is the major side effect, as well as dry mouth and weakness.

Sonata (zaleplon): A very short-acting hypnotic sleeping pill that lasts only about four hours so it can be taken if you wake up in the middle of the night and can't get back to sleep. Since it is so short-acting it doesn't cause daytime fatigue, but can have an effect on short-term memory like other hypnotics.

Tegretol (carbemezine): An anti-seizure medication used to treat nerve pain in fibromyalgia. It can reduce the effectiveness of birth control pills and other medications. Side effects include dizziness, unsteadiness, nausea, and problems with the thyroid, liver, and blood cells.

Topramax (topiramate): Anti-seizure drug used for nerve pain. Has many drug interactions and side effects including fatigue, dizziness, nausea, and nervousness.

Tramadol (Ultram): Pain medication in a new class that occupies opiate receptors in the brain. Originally marketed as being non-addictive, but this may not be true. Side effects include constipation and nausea, as well as fatigue. Tramodol is also marketed in combination with acetaminophen, as Ultracet.

Tricylic antidepressants: An older class of antidepressants used in fibromyalgia because they increase deep sleep, increase the availability of serotonin, and may help the body produce its own endorphins. Side effects include constipation, dry mouth, drowsiness, weight gain, dizziness, and anxiety. There is some evidence that they may lose their effectiveness over time for fibromyalgia. Examples include Elavil and Pamelor.

Ultram (tramadol HCL): Pain medication in a new class that occupies opiate receptors in the brain. Originally marketed as being non-addictive, but this may not be true. Side effects include constipation and nausea, as well as fatigue. Tramodol is also marketed in combination with acetaminophen, as **Ultracet**.

Vioxx: A new anti-inflammatory, a Cox-2 inhibitor, that has less potential for stomach upset and other gastrointestinal problems. It is not stronger than prescription Motrin.

Wellbutrin (bupropion HCL): Antidepressant that has an indication that it can help with weight loss. Also can lower the seizure threshold, so should not be used with Ultram and other medications that can do the same. Side effects include headaches, insomnia, anxiety, aching muscles, fatigue, and dry mouth.

Xanax (alprazolam): Anti-anxiety drug not used very frequently because of its addictive potential. Has some antidepressant activity as well. Must be discontinued very slowly. Side effects include fatigue, euphoria, constipation, nausea, and dry mouth.

Zanaflex (tizanidine HClL): Medication used to decrease spasticity of muscles. Can be given for restless legs and muscle spasm. Side effects include drowsiness and mental confusion and hallucinations.

Zoloft (sertraline HCL): A newer antidepressant used to help reach deep sleep. It is a selective serotonin reuptake inhibitor, which makes more serotonin available in the brain. Side effects include insomnia, dry mouth, diarrhea, and in some patients, sexual dysfunction.

Zomig (zolmatriptan): A newer migraine medication. Side effects include chest and neck pain and pressure, fatigue, and dizziness.

Zostrix (topical capsaicin): A drug derived from cayenne peppers. Used topically for nerve pain. Side effects include local redness and stinging.

Zyban (bupropion HCL): Antidepressant that can help with weight loss. Also can lower the seizure threshold, so should not be used with Ultram and other medications that can do the same. Side effects include headaches, insomnia, anxiety, aching muscles, fatigue, and dry mouth.

Some Safety Tips for Taking Medications

○ Call your physician right away if you have any unusual reaction to a medication. Do not try to handle the situation on your own. When you call be sure that you also have handy a list of the other medications you've taken, and the dosages.

○ If you take a number of medications, consider getting a compartmentalized pill box, the kind where you can put out your medications for the day or week. This way you can tell at a glance whether or not you've already taken your pills. If you only take one or two medications you can get in the habit of turning over the bottle with each dose so that if it's upside down you know you've taken your morning dose.

○ Get all your medications at the same pharmacy so that potential side effects can be called to your attention.

○ Check with your doctor or pharmacist to make sure that there are no foods or drinks that you need to avoid when you are taking your medication. Grapefruit juice and milk can interfere with the absorption of some compounds.

○ Check to make sure that the supplements or vitamins won't interfere with your medications. Iron is one over-the-counter medication that can't be taken with certain things. Calcium may be a problem with other compounds.

○ Know whether or not a medication should be taken with food. Put a sticker on your medication to remind you if you tend to forget whether or not you should eat.

○ If you need medications cut or split and you have problems doing this, ask your pharmacist for help.

○ Check your medications at the beginning of each week to make sure that you are not running out of anything that you need. Be sure to allow time for your doctor and pharmacy to refill what you need. If you have a vacation or there's a holiday weekend coming up this is especially important.

O Before any type of surgery (including dental work) be sure to check with your doctor about which medications you should discontinue, and when. Also be sure that you know when to resume each one.

O Keep medications in their original containers. If you find the labels hard to read, you can write the important information in bigger letters with a marking pen.

O Do not get up at night and take medications in the dark. Be sure that you have checked the label and the pill itself in the light.

O When traveling, carry your medication in your carry-on luggage. Never put it in a bag you've checked in case the airline loses your luggage. If you're delayed you'll have what you need with you.

O If you are going to be out in the sun more than usual on a vacation check the side effects of your medications to make sure that sun exposure is not a problem with anything that you're taking.

O Store your medications in one place, not in direct sunlight as on a kitchen shelf. Bathrooms may not be ideal either if your bathroom gets humid when you shower. Remove the cotton from a bottle you're using because it will draw in moisture.

O Clean out your medicine cabinet several times a year. Flush expired medications down the toilet so they can't be accidentally ingested or fall into the wrong hands.

O Don't leave medications in your car, where it may get too hot or cold for them.

O Stick to the dose that your doctor prescribed. Taking extra may not automatically increase the effectiveness but will increase your chances of side effects.

O Don't stop a medication because you don't think it is working. Some medications take time to build up in your system, and others (like thyroid medications) may not produce a sudden discernable change.

O Be very careful not to mix certain kinds of drugs such as sleeping pills, alcohol, and anti-anxiety medications. Effects on the brain can be multiplied and cause serious problems.

O Read the labels of medications carefully in case you need to avoid alcohol or certain activities.

O If any medication looks different or not quite right, check with the pharmacy. On over-the-counter medications, look carefully at the product to make sure that safety seals are in place.

O Last, but very surely not least, do not take anyone else's medications. No matter how badly you feel, how tempting it may sound, this is a very bad idea. If you have a friend who is taking something you think might help you, call your doctor's office and check it out. You may already be taking something similar and not know it.

Appendix 2: Supplements

WHILE THERE is no tried-and-true alternative protocol for fibromyalgia, many supplements and over-the-counter medications can relieve some of the symptoms. As time goes by more studies will be done on these substances, and more will be added to the list. Here are some of those that are successfully used by many fibromyalgics.

Commonly Used Vitamin and Mineral Supplements

Minerals such as calcium and magnesium have been shown to be of some help with symptoms of fibromyalgia.

B vitamins are often recommended for fibromyalgics who may be low in certain amino acids, and for other important health reasons as well. A simple, inexpensive B complex will do the trick.

Calcium can help you sleep, but it can also cause constipation. If that's the case, it should be taken with magnesium. The proper mixture is equal amounts of the two. If you are sensitive to dairy products you should be sure you get enough calcium.

What to Look for on the Label of a Supplement

○ **Expiration date**: Make sure the label has one of these. Herbs, especially, have a limited shelf life and need to have been cared for and stored properly

○ **Address and phone number of the manufacturer**: You want to be able to get in touch with the company if you have a problem or questions. Look for a physical address, not just a Web site. If there is a factory, you want to know where it's located.

○ **FDA seal**: This is present if the FDA has inspected the company and they have presented certain documentation.

○ **Independent laboratory testing**: This information may be found on the label, or by calling the manufacturer. Some companies voluntarily submit to testing for purity, and to verify the amount of active ingredient. Sometimes you'll see the phrase "GMP Compliance," which is a sign that the company adheres to the U.S. Food and Drug Administration's Good Manufacturing Practice regulations.

○ **Lot or batch number**: As with all products, you'll want to be able to identify the exact product you have taken in case of a recall or published warning

○ **Side effects**: You should check labels, and if possible, find a brand that lists potential adverse reactions on attached literature or on the label itself

○ **Warnings:** Most will warn against use by pregnant women and children as a matter of course, but look to see if you can find more contraindications.

○ **Interactions:** If you can find a product that lists possible drug interactions, it means that the manufacturer is willing to give you a little more information, which is good.

○ **Storage:** Herbal supplements should be stored in dark containers or bottles. This will preserve them from the effects of light.

Chromium picolinate in studies has helped with stabilizing blood sugar, although the research was not done on hypoglycemics or fibromyalgics. It may help to suppress carbohydrate cravings.

Vitamin D may slow the development of osteoarthritis, according to a large study, which could help fibromyalgics escape it.

Vitamin E (400 mg at bedtime) has been shown in a study to help with leg and foot cramps. It also may help with restless leg syndrome.

Calcium and magnesium added to this may make it more effective. Topical vitamin E will help with skin rashes, and can be used to relieve painful itching that may occur in vulvodynia. According to the Arthritis Foundation, vitamin E may also help with pain levels.

Folic acid taken usually with B vitamins has some beneficial effects on cell formation and repair. When energy is reduced in fibromyalgia this may be helpful.

Magnesium helps relax muscles, which can also help with sleep. Magnesium can also be helpful for constipation if taken alone.

Zinc has been shown in several studies to help fight a cold virus. It has not, however, been shown to help with the immune system.

WATCH VITAMIN C in excess as it may stimulate your appetite and also may acidify your urine. If you've ever experienced urinary tract burning, use vitamin C with caution and only gradually march up the dose. Also may cause flares of interstitial cystitis.

Commonly Used Chemical Supplements

Amino acids, like taurine, have been marketed with the suggestion that they may help with pain levels. Others are taken specifically for energy.

Chondroitin sulfate is a slow-acting supplement that is supposed to help rebuild cartilage to ease joint pain in osteoarthritis.

Coenzyme Q-10 (CoQ10) is a bioenzyme that may help control fibrofog during a flare. It is also known as ubiquinone because it is ubiquitous, or found everywhere in the body. It plays a role in energy production inside cells and for this reason it's usually taken in the morning as it may keep you awake.

Digestive enzymes are popular for people with various digestive woes and include papain, bromelain, and betaine. These are taken with meals. Sometimes they're marketed with hydrochloric acid, which would exacerbate acid stomachs.

Fish oil is oil from cold water fish that has been used for fatigue and stiffness. Several human studies have shown benefit in rheumatoid arthritis (not fibromyalgia).

Flaxseed oil is another omega-3 fatty acid used for pain and stiffness in rheumatoid arthritis.

GLA (gamma linoleic acid), an essential fatty acid that is supposed to ease pain and stiffness, has been used in rheumatoid arthritis. Sometimes it's used topically, but it has not been showed to have any benefit when used that way.

Glucosamine, which is made from the glucose molecule, is used for pain and for arthritis, as well as for vulvar pain by some practitioners. It may not be safe for people with diabetes or poor glucose tolerance. Often sold with chondroitin sulfate to help repair cartilage and ease joint pain and stiffness.

Malic acid is an acid that your body needs to make ATP. Experts seem to agree that it has "a modest effect on fatigue."

MSM (methysulfonyl methane) is a nontoxic sulfur compound that is used for pain and is supposed to help with inflammation.

NADH (Enada) is supposed to help your body make energy. In a study, 26 percent of patients thought it helped.

SAMe or S-adenosyl-methionine was originally imported from Europe, where it has been available for many years by prescription for depression, fibromyalgia, and arthritis. It is made from an amino acid and is supposed to make brain cells more responsive to serotonin. Since it is a prescription drug in other countries there are many studies you can review if you are interested. These studies show that it works about as well as prescription antidepressants, although because it is not covered by insurance it's a more expensive alternative for most people. Drug interactions are listed for this product and you should review these carefully.

5-HTP is often considered because some fibromyalgics have been shown to be low in the amino acid tryptophan, and in turn serotonin. A small number of studies have shown that 5-HTP may help with mood and better sleep. Taken before meals it may help prevent overeating and the craving for sweets. (Some diet pills raise serotonin levels.) It is a molecule that's small enough to enter the brain, where it provides the raw material to manufacture serotonin. Side effects include nausea, which is usually transient, and drowsiness.

YOU SHOULD NOT TAKE 5-HTP WITH ANTIDEPRESSANTS

CONSULT YOUR doctor before combining 5-HTP with muscle relaxants, narcotic pain medications, sedatives, Buspar (buspirone), or elodea.

Commonly Used Hormones

Armour thyroid: Called "natural" thyroid, but it is actually from the porcine or bovine gland and contains more T-3 than the human gland secretes. For this reason it will give more energy, which means it should be taken early in the day. No reputable study has ever shown a connection between low thyroid and fibromyalgia, though some symptoms are similar.

Colostrum: The first fluid produced by a lactating animal, a thin, clear "pre milk" that contains antibodies for any illnesses to which the animal may be exposed. The major reason it is being touted for fibromyalgics is that, taken orally, bovine colostrum has been shown to raise growth hormone levels in humans. This seems to provide more energy.

DHEA (dehydroepiandrosterone): A hormone excreted from the adrenal glands that is a precursor to sex hormones. Since it is a powerful hormone you should only consider supplementation when reliable blood tests shows that your own levels are low.

Melatonin: A neurotransmitter secreted by the pineal gland that helps set the body clock (helps with jet lag) and aids in sleep. Possibly makes Elavil more effective. (Side effect is depression). Melatonin levels fall as we age, and no risk has been seen in supplementation so far. It should not be used in teenagers or children because their normal levels are much higher.

T-3: Often associated with amour thyroid, T3 is an animal hormone containing 90 percent more T-3 than our human thyroids produce. This hormone can speed up your metabolism and give you more energy, so it should be taken early in the day, or in divided doses. You should always have your own blood levels checked to make sure that your TSH reading is normal. This level of the thyroid-stimulating hormone from the pituitary gives the most accurate available reading of your thyroid's function.

Whey Protein: Another supplement that is marketed with an eye toward fibromyalgics. Whey protein, unlike some vegetable proteins (such as soy), is called a complete protein because it contains all the essential amino acids. You'll recall that these are the amino acids that the body cannot manufacture but must acquire through dietary sources. (Other animal proteins such as egg proteins are also complete.) If you were relying on a powder for 100 percent of your daily protein requirement this would be very important, but as a supplement it's not as important. Whey protein is marketed to boost your immune system by raising glutathione levels.

Notes

Day 2

1. Buskila, D., Press, J., Gedalia, H., et al. "Assessment of nonarticular tenderness and prevalence of fibromyalgia in children," *Journal of Rheumatology*, 1993; 20:368–70.

Day 6

1. Interstitial Cystitis Supplement to May 1997, pp. 52-7.
2. Table Adapted from www.ic.help.com.

Day 7

1. *The Lancet* 360, August 3, 2002, by Marilynn Larkin.

Week 4

1. K. Hakkinen, et al. "Effects of Strength Training on Muscle Strength, Cross-Sectional Area, Maximal Electromyographic Activity and Serum Hormones in Premenopausal Women with Fibromyalgia," *Journal of Rheumatology*, June 2002.

Month 4

1. Devin Starlanyl and Mary Ellen Copeland. *Fibromyalgia and Chronic Myofascial Pain: A Survival Manual*, 2nd ed. New Harbinger Publishing, 2001, p. 270.

Month 5

1. James B. La Valle, et al. *Natural Therapeutics Pocket Guide 2000-2001*. Lexi Comp, 2002.

Month 8

1. Daniel J. Wallace, M.D., and Jean Brock Wallace. *All About Fibromyalgia*. Oxford University Press, 2002.
2. Katherine Wisner, M.D., et al. "Postpartum Depression," *New England Journal of Medicine* 347, no. 3, July 18, 2002, pp 194-8.

Glossary

ACETAMINOPHEN (TYLENOL): A mild over-the-counter analgesic pain reliever.

ACUPUNCTURE: Ancient Eastern healing technique that involves inserting needles into specific points to heal and relieve pain.

ACUPRESSURE: The use of pressure on specific areas of the body to relieve pain and promote healing

ACUTE: A process or pain that begins suddenly, and is sharp and severe.

AEROBIC: Exercise such as running or walking that creates increased oxygen consumption.

ADRENAL GLANDS: Small organs located on top of each kidney that produce many hormones.

ADRENALINE (EPINEPHRINE): The "fight or flight" hormone released by the adrenal glands that activates the sympathetic nervous system when the body senses danger. It raises blood pressure and heart rate, among other things. Designed to increase energy levels in emergencies.

AMBIEN (ZOLPIDEM TARTRATE): A hypnotic sleep medication commonly used for fibromyalgia that is relatively short acting.

AMITRIPTYLINE (ELAVIL): An older inexpensive tricyclic antidepressant that's been used for many years to help fibromyalgics, especially with sleep problems.

ANA ANTINUCLEAR ANTIBODIES: Proteins in the blood measured to confirm the diagnosis of lupus. Found in 96 percent of patients with lupus and 10 percent of those with fibromyalgia.

ANAEROBIC EXERCISE: Exercise done in the absence of oxygen for short periods. Examples are short sprints and weight lifting. The goal is to increase muscle strength

ANALGESIC DRUGS: Drugs that relieve pain. There are two basic groups: nonnarcotics like Tylenol, and narcotics, which are related to morphine.

ANDROPAUSE: A term used to describe male menopause, the period when sex hormones decline.

ANEMIA: A deficiency in the oxygen-carrying component of the blood, or red blood cells. Symptoms include fatigue, muscle stiffness, and stamina.

ANTIBODY: A protein that is made in the body and circulated in the blood in response to a foreign substance.

ANTI-CHOLINERGIC PROPERTIES: Drugs that work on the autonomic nervous system (involuntary) by impacting neurotransmitters.

ANTIDEPRESSANT: A medication designed to relieve depression. There are several classes that are used in fibromyalgia for relief of symptoms including pain, depression, and sleep problems. Some trigger the release of chemicals in the brain. Others prolong the active life of chemicals after their release.

ANTIHISTAMINE: A medication that inhibits or counteracts the release of histamines, which are chemicals produced in immune responses. Histamines dilate blood vessels and stimulate the secretion of stomach acid. Drowsiness is one of the main side effects of the older antihistamines.

ANTISPASMOTIC: A drug that relieves spasms.

ANUS: The last part of the gastrointestinal tract at the end of the rectum. It is a muscle that releases to allow the passage of fecal matter.

ATP (ADENOSINE TRIPHOSPHATE): A molecule that is the body's currency of energy used for nearly all functions. It has been found to be low in the muscles of fibromyalgics.

AUTOIMMUNE ILLNESS: An illness resulting from the body's immune system attacking the body's own tissue after mistaking it for a foreign substance. More common in women than in men.

AUTONOMIC NERVOUS SYSTEM: The system of nerves controlling the automatic functions of your body; like breathing or heart rate.

BACTERIUM: A single living cell that can replicate by itself. Some infections are bacterial infections and need to be killed with antibiotics (single form of bacteria).

BARBITUATE: A group of drugs derived from barbituric acid that act as central nervous system depressants. Used as tranquilizers to control seizures or as hypnotics.

BARIUM ENEMA: A diagnostic procedure where barium is inserted as a contrast material into the lower gastrointestinal system and X rays are taken to detect abnormalities.

BENADRYL (DIPHENHYDRAMINE): An inexpensive antihistamine that is also the active ingredient in over-the-counter sleep medications because it causes drowsiness in most people. It is safe and non–habit forming.

BENZODIAZAPINES: A class of drugs used for anxiety and sleep disorders.

BETA CAROTENE: A substance found in all plants and animals. Effects are identical to vitamin A. It is fat-soluble so it can build up in the body and cause carotenemia, a yellow orange skin pigmentation, when it is used in excess.

BIOFEEDBACK: A technique that teaches control over autonomic body functions.

BRAIN CYCLES: Collection of fibromyalgia symptoms that arise from the brain, such as problems with memory, concentration, cognitive skills, sometimes called fibrofog.

BRAXTON HICKS CONTRACTIONS: Early practice contractions of the uterus that ready the body for childbirth.

CA-125: A protein that can be measured in the blood. Used to detect ovarian cancer.

CALCIUM CHANNEL BLOCKER: A class of drugs that acts by the selective inhibition of calcium used in the treatment of certain heart conditions, high blood pressure, and stroke. Can also relax uterine spasms.

CALISTHENICS: Gymnastic exercises, like sit-ups and push-ups, used to develop muscle tone.

CANDIDA/CANDIDA ALBICANS: Yeast that can grow in the vagina and rectum. The cottage cheese-like discharge it causes is called candidiasis.

CARBOHYDRATE: A sugar or starch food made up of a string of sugar molecules. Fats and carbohydrates provide the body with its two main sources of energy.

CARBOHYDRATE INTOLERANCE: Symptoms that occur when a person has some of the symptoms of hypoglycemia and thus has problems metabolizing carbohydrates properly. Blood sugar readings will not drop to below 50 mg/dl in a carbohydrate intolerant person.

CARDIOVASCULAR SYSTEM: The organs and tissue involved in circulating the blood throughout the body.

CARISOPRODOL (SOMA): A central nervous system depressant that causes muscle relaxation and helps with the sensory overload of fibromyalgia.

CARTILAGE: A smooth, tough, fibrous substance that covers the ends of bones.

CELIAC DISEASE (COELIAC SPRUE): An inherited condition in which the intestinal lining is inflamed when the protein gluten is ingested.

CENTRAL NERVOUS SYSTEM: Nerve tissue in the brain and spinal cord.

CERVICAL STENOSIS: A tightening of the spinal canal that can lead to Magnetic spectroscope pinching of the spinal cord and result in pain and loss of motor coordination.

CHIARI SYNDROME: A malformation at the base of the brain that can be seen on an MRI.

CHONDROITIN: One of the most common chemicals in cartilage that is responsible for its resiliency.

CHRONIC FATIGUE SYNDROME: A syndrome that causes fatigue on a long-term basis. Thought to be part of fibromyalgia, it is a label given to patients with higher pain thresholds.

CHRONIC ILLNESS: An illness that lasts a long time, and comes on gradually.

CODEINE: A narcotic derived from opium or morphine and used as an analgesic, hypnotic, and cough suppressant.

COLON: Large intestine, about five feet long in the average adult. It is composed of six parts: cecum, ascending colon, transverse colon, descending colon, and sigmoid colon. Responsible for the formation, storing, and expelling of the body's waste matter.

COLONOSCOPY: A medical procedure that examines the colon via a small scope that is inserted rectally.

COMPLEX CARBOHYDRATES: Bread, pasta, rice, cereal, and beans are examples of complex carbohydrates. These are digested in the stomach and enter the bloodstream.

CONNECTIVE TISSUE: Long fiber tissue that supports and connects internal organs, forms the walls of blood vessels, attaches muscles to bones, and contributes to the formation of bones.

CONSTIPATION: Difficult or infrequent elimination of hard, dry stools.

CORTISOL: A hormone secreted by the adrenal gland during stress. Called a counterregulatory hormone, it helps to stop the fall of blood sugar.

CORTISONE: Adrenal hormone produced synthetically. The body converts it to cortisol.

CYSTITIS: Inflammation of the urinary bladder.

CYSTOSCOPY: A procedure that examines the bladder via a scope inserted via the urethra.

CYTOKINE: A protein released by the immune system that is a mediator in the immune response.

DERMATOGRAPHIA: A skin condition where one can use a sharp instrument to literally write on the patient's skin. This causes surface redness and renders the written inscription visible.

DESERYL (TRAZODONE): An antidepressant commonly used to help with sleep problems in fibromyalgics.

DETROL (TOLTERODINE TARTRATE): A medication used to decrease frequent urination.

DIGESTION: A process by which food is broken down and converted into substances that can be absorbed and assimilated by the body.

DIGESTIVE JUICES: Secretions that aid the digestive process.

DIURETIC: A drug that increases the elimination of fluid from the body.

DOULA: A woman who helps other women through childbirth and later to teach and help them with care of their babies.

DYSPAREUNIA: Difficult or painful sexual intercourse.

ELAVIL (AMITRIPTYLINE): A tricylic antidepressant used to improve sleep and suppress pain perception.

ELMIRON (PENTOSAN POLYSULFATE SODIUM): A drug used to control the pain and discomfort of interstitial cystitis.

ENDOCRINOLOGIST: A medical doctor who specializes in disorders of the hormone-releasing (endocrine) glands.

ENDOMETRIOSIS: A condition in which tissue resembling uterine mucous membrane occurs in various locations in the pelvic cavity.

ENDORPHINASE: An enzyme released by the body to destroy endorphins.

ENDORPHINS: Hormones that have a powerful pain-relieving effect on the body by raising the body's pain threshold.

ENDOSCOPY: A procedure done with a fiber-optic instrument inserted through the mouth to examine the esophagus, stomach, and duodenum, the first part of the small intestine. Can also be used for a similar procedure done on other parts of the body.

ENZYME: A protein that makes a chemical reaction go faster in the body.

EPILEPSY: A neurological disorder characterized by recurring seizures.

ESSENTIAL FATTY ACIDS: Lineoleic acid and alpha linoleic acids, which are necessary to the body but must be ingested because the body cannot manufacture them.

ESTRACE CREAM: A topical estrogen cream used locally to rebuild and nourish vaginal tissue.

ESTRADIOL: An estrogenic hormone produced by the ovaries, also used in hormone replacement therapy.

FELDENKRAIS: A therapy that involves teaching the body to move properly to lessen effort and pain.

FERRITIN: A protein that is the primary form of stored iron in the body.

FIBROFOG: A descriptive nickname for the cognitive symptoms of fibromyalgia. Impaired short-term memory that feels as if a fog exists between the patient and the rest of the world.

FIBROMYALGIA: A syndrome consisting of symptoms such as muscle pain and stiffness, fatigue, irritable bowel and bladder, as well as problems with memory and concentration, depression, anxiety, and insomnia. The cause is unknown, and there are treatments but no known cure.

FIBROSITIS: The former name of fibromyalgia, given to the syndrome by Dr. William Gowers at the beginning of the twentieth century. Inaccurate, since there is no inflammation in the illness, it was discarded in the 1990s.

FISSURE: A crack or split in tissue.

5HTTP: A precursor to tryptophan often taken as a dietary supplement by fibromyalgics to aid with sleep.

FLEXERIL (CYCLOBENZAPRINE): Medication similar to tricylic antidepressants that has been used as a muscle relaxant and to help with deep sleep.

FLUCONAZOLE (DIFLUCAN): An antifungal medication used to treat yeast infections.

FOLATE: A B vitamin that is necessary for cell growth and reproduction.

FREE RADICAL: A chemical with an unpaired electron that can cause damage to cells because it is reactive. Antioxidants can neutralize them, and these are found in vegetables and fruits.

FRUCTOSE: A sugar found in fruit that does not raise the blood sugar as fast as glucose but which the liver can convert to glucose.

GASTROENTEROLOGIST: A physician who diagnoses and treats disorders of the stomach, intestine, and associated organs.

GASTROESOPHAGEAL REFLUX: The disorder of the muscle that connects the esophagus to the stomach where stomach acid passes upward into the esophagus, where it can cause erosion. Can cause heartburn and acid indigestion.

GENITOURINARY SYNDROME: A cluster of symptoms that involve the urinary tract and the genitals. Includes irritable bladder, interstitial cystitis, vulvodynia, and vulvar vestibulitis.

GLUCAGON: A hormone secreted by the pancreas that stimulates the breakdown of glycogen, the stored form of carbohydrate, into glucose. Opposes the action of insulin by raising blood sugar.

GLUCOSE: The body's primary source of energy derived from ingested carbohydrates or produced in cells from fats and proteins. It is 100 on the glycemic index, the sugar against which others are measured.

GLUCOSE TOLERANCE TEST (GTT): A test that measures your body's ability to handle glucose, or a sugar load. Glucose is given on an empty stomach and blood is drawn at various intervals.

GLYCEMIC INDEX: A list that ranks foods by how they affect the blood sugar in comparison with pure glucose. In America you will also see a scale with white bread set as the 100 point. To convert the white bread scale to the classic glycemic index you multiply by 0.7.

GOUT: A disease caused by the excess production or renal retention of uric acid. More common in men than women.

GROWTH HORMONE (GH, SOMATOTROPIN): Hormone secreted by the pituitary. Affects metabolism and controls the rate of skeletal and visceral growth.

GUAIFENESIN PROTOCOL: A protocol designed by R. Paul St. Amand, M.D., whereby fibromyalgia is reversed using the medication guaifenesin.

HASHIMOTO'S THYROIDITIS: Autoimmune disease where the thyroid is destroyed by the body's own antibodies. More common in females.

HEMORRHOID: Itching or painful dilated, varicose veins in the rectum that can be external or internal.

HOMEOPATHY: A therapeutic approach based on the premise that very diluted substances can be effective in treating illnesses.

HORMONE: A chemical messenger produced in one organ that acts upon another by entering cells via receptors. Examples are thyroid, steroids, insulin, estrogen, and testosterone.

HUMIDIFIER: A device for increasing the humidity or water content of the air.

HYDRODISTENTION OF THE BLADDER: A procedure that fills the bladder with water under high pressure in order to see the abnormalities of interstitial cystitis in the bladder wall.

HYPNOTICS: A group of drugs that depress or slow down the body's function. Includes tranquilizers and sleeping pills. There are two kinds, benzodiazepines and barbituates.

HYPOGLYCEMIA: Low blood sugar, officially a blood sugar that falls below 50 mg/dl.

HYPOTHALAMIC-PITUITARY-ADRENAL AXIS: The balance between the hormones of these various endocrine glands. This axis controls stress response, immune system, thyroid and growth hormones. The hypothalamus also controls hunger, libido and to a large degree your autonomic nervous system.

HYPOTHALAMUS: The portion of the brain that produces the chemicals that release hormones.

INFLAMMATION: The body's response to injury or infection resulting from the infiltration of white blood cells into tissue caused by release of mast cells. Heat, swelling, redness, and pain can be signs of inflammation.

INSOMNIA: The chronic inability to fall or remain asleep.

INSULIN: Potent hormone that directs excess calories into storage. Released promptly when carbohydrates are eaten.

INSULIN RESISTANCE: A condition where insulin does not work properly. The cause is unknown at this time.

INTERSTITIAL CYSTITIS: Inflammation of the bladder wall, common in fibromyalgia. Symptoms include pain and frequent urination.

7 7

7 7 7

ity7777 77

IRRITABLE BOWEL SYNDROME: Symptoms of gas, bloating, constipation, and diarrhea without obvious cause.

KETOPROFEN (ORUDIS): A nonsteroidal anti-inflammatory often used in a topical form.

KLONOPIN (CLONAZEPAM): A benzodiazepine used for sleep and for anxiety.

L-TRYPTOPHAN: An essential amino acid and metabolic precursor to serotonin.

LABIA: Any of the four folds of tissue that make up the external female genitalia.

LACTOSE: Milk sugar consisting of glucose and galactose. It rates 48 on the glycemic index.

LACTOSE INTOLERANCE: A condition caused by the lack of the enzyme lactase making the digestion of lactose impossible. Symptoms include gas, bloating, and diarrhea when lactose is consumed.

LIGAMENT: A cordlike fiber that attaches to bones to keep them aligned properly.

LOTRONEX (ALOSETRON HYDROCHLORIDE): A drug marketed in 2000 for diarrhea predominant IBS. Withdrawn from the market due to serious side effects, but returned to the market for special use in 2002.

L-THERONINE: An amino acid taken as a supplement for energy and brain function.

LUMBAGO: Old-fashioned term for back pain.

LUPUS (SYSTEMIC LUPUS ERYTHEMATOSUS): Systemic disorder of connective tissue related to the production of various antibodies. It can affect multiple organs, and is distinguished by blood tests.

MAGNETIC SPECTROSCOPY: A non-invasive imaging that uses a magnetic field to detect hydrogen ions in the body. Uses radio frequency and magnetic fields but no radiation.

MAST CELLS: Cells that release histamines, heparin (an anticoagulant), and many other proteins. Found in the skin of fibromyalgics, bladder in interstitial cystitis, and the bronchial tree of asthmatics.

MELATONIN: A hormone secreted by the pineal gland involved in the sleep-wake cycle.

MIGRAINE: Severe headache that may be accompanied by visual disturbances and nausea. More common in women than in men.

MITOCHONDRIA: The power station of cells that convert ingested food to ATP.

MORPHINE: One of the strongest opiod analgesics, a derivative of heroin.

MRI: Magnetic resonance imaging technique that uses magnetic energy to create three-dimensional images of the body and the brain. More sensitive than X-rays.

MUSCLE CALLUSES: Name given by early German physicians to the areas of hardness they could palpate in the muscles of patients with fibrositis, or fibromyalgia.

MYCOSTATIN (NYSTATIN): An antifungal drug used to combat candida or yeast.

MYOFASCIA: Layers of fibrous tissue that lies under the skin that supports the muscles and holds the organs in place

MYOFASCIAL PAIN SYNDROME: A localized form of connective tissue disorder characterized by trigger points and referred pain.

NARCOTICS: Opiate-derived substances that depress pain and can cause euphoric feelings.

NSAIDs: Nonsteroidal anti-inflammatory drugs that work against inflammation and pain by inhibiting prostaglandin. This category includes aspirin, ibuprofen, naprosyn, and the newer Celebrex and Vioxx.

NERVE: A cordlike bundle of fibers through which sensory input passes in the body between the brain or other parts of the central nervous system. Conducts information throughout the body.

NEURONTIN (GABAPENTIN): An anti-seizure drug used to relieve nerve pain in fibromyalgiacs.

NEUROPATHY: An abnormal nerve sensation like burning or prickling.

NEUROTRANSMITTERS: Molecules released from nerve cells that transmit messages across the minute distance between two nerve cells by binding to a receptor on the second nerve.

OPIOID: An analgesic derived from opium.

OSTEOARTHRITIS: A degenerative disease of the joints caused by defects in cartilage either through use or by trauma.

OVA: Eggs that are the female reproductive cells.

OXALATE: A chemical absorbed from food, mostly those of plant origin, but also produced during energy production in the body. Excreted via the urine and known as a topical irritant.

OXYTOCIN: A pituitary hormone released during labor that causes the uterus to contract, also released during orgasm. Called "the bonding hormone" because it causes feelings of attachment.

PARASITE: An organism that grows, feeds, and is sheltered inside another organism.

PARESTHESIA: Altered sensation of the skin such as crawling, numbness, burning, or coldness.

PARTIALLY HYDROGENATED FATS (OR TRANS FATS): Fats that have been chemically altered so that they become solid at room temperature and have a longer shelf life. Research shows they increase the risk of heart disease.

PEPCID (FAMOTIDINE): A histamine-2 blocker that is taken to block the release of stomach acid.

PERINEUM: Region between the vulva junction and anus in females, between the scrotum and anus in males.

PERISTALSIS: The wavelike contractions of the digestive tract that forces the contents forward.

PHYSICAL THERAPIST: A person who has a degree in physical therapy.

PHYSICAL THERAPY: Any treatment using physical techniques such as movement or stretching.

PITUITARY GLAND: A gland in the brain that produces hormones such as the thyroid stimulating hormone and growth hormone.

POLYPHARMACY: The state of taking multiple medications with an unknown number of interactions.

POLYPS: A usually nonmalignant growth in the mucous lining of an organ.

PRELIEF: A supplement taken with food to neutralize its acidity. Used in interstial cystitis to reduce bladder burning.

PRION TRANSFER: Small particles that can carry infectious disease and transfer it from one species to another.

PROLOTHERAPY: A therapy for muscle pain where a sugar solution is injected into ligaments and tendons where the attach to the bone. Causes inflammation to which the body reacts.

PROPECIA (FINASTERIDE): A drug originally marketed for enlarged prostates used in a lower strength to reverse and inhibit male pattern baldness. Cannot be taken or handled by women of childbearing age due to the possibility of birth defects.

PROSTATITIS: Inflammation of the prostate gland.

PYRIDIUM (PHENAZOPYRIDINE HCL): A urinary tract analgesic available in both over-the-counter and prescription strength.

QUININE SULFATE: A natural alkaloid used to stop leg and food cramps. Available by prescription.

RAYNAUD'S PHENOMENON: A vascular spasm in the fingers and toes that causes them to blanch, or turn white, and can also go numb or tingle.

REGLAN (METOCLOPRAMIDE HYDROCLORIDE): A drug that increases the contractions of the stomach and small intestine, helping the passage of food. Also used short term for heartburn.

RELAXIN: A hormone released during pregnancy that increases the elasticity of muscles, tendons, and ligaments. Sometimes used as a treatment for fibromyalgia, but the effects on men and nonpregnant women is not known.

RESTLESS LEGS: Creepy-crawly sensations in the limbs, primary in the legs.

RHEUMATISM: Musculoskeletal aches and pains.

RHEUMATOID ARTHRITIS: The immunological form of arthritis that affects about 1 percent of the population. Untreated it can cause joint damage, especially in the fingers and toes. More common in women than men.

ROGAINE (MINOXODIL): A blood pressure medication that was found to stimulate hair growth. Marketed as a topical in two strengths for both women and men.

SALICYLATE: Salt of salicylic acid that occurs naturally in plants and is made synthetically. Used as an analgesic or topically for acne, dandruff, and in sunscreen and dentifrices.

SEDIMENTATION RATE: The rate of fall of red blood cells as indicated by the test of this name. High rates indicate inflammation or infection. An extremely high sedimentation rate indicates polymyalgia rheumtica.

SEROTONIN: A chemical found in the central nervous system and gastrointestinal tract, smooth muscle, and stored in blood platelets. Derived from tryptophan. In the GI tract it affects mobility, elsewhere mood, sleep, and pain.

SIGMOIDOSCOPY: Examination of the lower portion of the colon where most cancers occur done through a fiber optic instrument inserted via the rectum.

SIMPLE CARBOHYDRATES: Table sugar (sucrose), fructose, maltose, and lactose. These enter the body without being digested.

SOMA (CARISPRODOL): A muscle relaxant and central nervous system muffler.

SONATA (ZALEPLON): A mild sleeping pill that lasts only 4-6 hours, effective for night awakenings.

SORBITOL: A sugar alcohol often used in diet desserts. Can cause gas, bloating, and diarrhea.

STAMINA: Strength to endure illness, fatigue, or hardship.

STRESS HORMONE: A hormone released when the body is under stress such as cortisone and adrenaline.

STEVIA: An herbal extract used as a natural sweetener. Does not raise blood sugar.

SUBSTANCE P: A substance that is important in pain transmission especially at nerve endings.

SUCROSE (TABLE SUGAR): A mixture of glucose and fructose that raises blood sugar.

SUCRALOSE (SPLENDA): A sweetener made from sugar by rearranging the molecule. Does not contain carbohydrates and cannot raise blood sugar.

SYNCOPE: A brief loss of consciousness.

SYNDROME: A collection of associated symptoms.

TEMPOROMANDIBULAR JOINT: The jaw joint. Ninety-seven percent of fibromyalgics have pain in this area.

TENDER POINTS: Sites that are unusually tender when pressure is applied, usually where muscle attaches to bone.

TENDON: A band of connective tissue that connects muscle to bone.

TREMOR: A quivering or trembling of the muscles usually noticed in the hands or head.

TRICYLIC ANTIDEPRESSANTS: An older class of antidepressants, such as Elavil. The name refers to the three-ring structure of the basic chemical compound.

TRIGGER POINTS: A site in the connective tissue that is tender to pressure, associated with taut muscles, and creates referred pain, that is pain felt elsewhere.

TRIGLYCERIDE: One of the three blood fats known as lipids that is the principle constituent of body fat. Manufactured in the liver from sugars and starches and deposited in fat cells for storage.

ULCERATIVE COLITIS: Chronic, serious inflammation of the large intestine and rectum.

ULTRAM (TRAMADOL): One of a new class of pain medications that has a low potential for abuse.

UROLOGIST: A physician who specializes in diagnosis and treatment of disorders of the urinary tract.

VARICOSE VEIN: A vein that is permanently dilated that can protrude and cause painful symptoms.

VERTIGO: A sensation that everything around you is in motion.

VIRUS: Submicroscopic parasites that often cause disease and are unable to replicate without a host cell.

VULVAR VESTIBULITIS: Pain in the area of the vestibule or entrance to the vagina.

VULVODYNIA: A syndrome that includes raw, irritated, and burning sensations in the external female genital area that can also include vaginal spasms and painful intercourse.

YEAST: A type of fungus, also referred to as candida, or candiasis.

ZELNORM (TEGASEROD): A new drug for women with constipation-dominant IBS.

For Further Information

FOR MORE in-depth information, here are some helpful resources and recommended publications:

Days 1 and 2

R. Paul St. Amand and Claudia C. Marek. *What Your Doctor May Not Tell You About Fibromyalgia.* Warner Books, 1999.

Devin Starlanyl and Mary Ellen Copeland. *Fibromyalgia and Chronic Myofascial Pain: A Survival Advocate.* New Harbinger Publications, Inc., 2001.

Day 3

Chronic Pain Support Group
Web site: www.chronicpain.org

American Pain Society
4700 W. Lake Avenue
Glenview, IL 60025
Telephone: 847-734-8758
Web site: www.ampainsoc.org

Day 4

R. Paul St. Amand and Claudia C. Marek. *What Your Doctor May Not Tell You About Fibromyalgia Fatigue.* Warner Books, 2003.

Devin Starlanyl and Mary Ellen Copeland. *Fibromyalgia and Chronic Myofascial Pain: A Survival Advocate.* New Harbinger Publications, Inc., 2001.

Day 5

IBS Self Help and Support Group
1440 Whalley Avenue, #145
New Haven, CT 06515
Web site: www.ibsgroup.org

Day 6

Vulvodynia

National Vulvodynia Foundation
Phyllis Mate, Director
P.O. Box 4491
Silver Spring, MD 20914
Telephone: 301-299-0755
Web site: www.nva.org

The Vulvar Pain Foundation
203½ North Main Street, Suite 203
Graham, NC 27253
Telephone: 336-226-0704
Web site: www.vulvarpainfoundation.org

Howard Glazer and Gae Rodke. *The Vulvodynia Survival Guide.* New Harbinger Publications, Inc., 2002.
Joanne Yount and Meg Stolzfus (editors), *The Low Oxalate Cookbook.* The Vulvar Pain Foundation, 1997.
www.vulvarpainfoundation.org

Interstitial Cystitis

Interstitial Cystitis Association
110 N. Washington Street, #340
Rockville, MD 20850
Telephone: 800-HELP-ICA
www.ichelp.com

The Interstitial Cystitis Network
5636 Del Monte Court
Santa Rosa, CA 95409
Telephone: 707-538-9442
Web site: www.ic-network.com

Beverly Laumann. *A Taste of Good Life: A Cookbook for an Interstitial Cystitis Diet.* Freeman Family Trust Publications, 1998.
Robert Moldwin. *The Interstitial Cystitis Guide: Your Guide to the Latest Treatment Options and Coping Strategies.* New Harbinger Publications, Inc., 2000.

Day 7

National Headache Foundation
428 W. St. James Place
Chicago, IL 60614
Telephone: 888-643-5552
Web site: www.headaches.org

Restless Leg Syndrome
819 2nd St. SW
Rochester, MN 55902
Telephone: 507-287-6465
Web site: www.rls.org

Week 2

Original letter to Normals by Bek Oberin
Web site: www.tertius.net.au/foothold

Gregg Piburn. *Beyond Chaos: One Man's Journey Alongside His Chronically Ill Wife.* The Arthritis Foundation, 1999.
Miryam Erlich Williamson. *Fibromyalgia: A Comprehensive Approach.* Walker, 1996

Week 3

Relaxation Tapes
1 800-542-7782
Web site: www.relaxation-tapes-music.com

The Anxiety Bookstore
Telephone: 214-672-0564
Web site: www.anxietybookstore.com

Week 4

Exercise Videos for Fibromyalgia by Sharon Clark
National Fibromyalgia Research Organization
P.O. Box 500
Salem, OR 97302
Web site: www.nfra.net

Tai Chi for Seniors
30 Elaine Avenue
Mill Valley, CA 94941
Telephone: 800-497-4244
Web site: www.taichiforseniorsvideo.com

Stacie Bigelow. *Fibromyalgia: Simple Relief through Movement.*
John Wiley and Sons: 2000.

Month 2

Devin Starlanyl. *The Fibromyalgia Advocate.* New Harbinger
   Publications, Inc., 2000.

Month 3

The Hypoglycemia Support Foundation
   P.O. Box 451778
   Sunrise, FL 33345
   Web site: www.hypoglycemia.org

R. Paul St. Amand and Claudia C. Marek. *What Your Doctor May Not Tell You About
   Fibromyalgia.* Warner Books, 1999.
Devin Starlanyl and Mary Ellen Copeland. *Fibromyalgia and Chronic Myofascial Pain: A
   Survival Advocate.* New Harbinger Publications, Inc., 1998.
Mark Pellegrino. *Inside Fibromyalgia.* Anadem Publishing, 2001.
Fran McCullough. *Living Low Carb.* Little, Brown and Co., 2000.

Glycemic Index Online
   Web site: www.mendosa.com

Low Carbohydrate Products
   Web site: www.lowcarb.com

Low Carbohydrate Products
   Web site: www.86sugar.com

Atkins Center (recipes and products)
   Web site: www.atkinscenter.com

Month 4

Drug Data Base Online
   Web site: www.rxlist.com

Guaifenesin protocol

R. Paul St. Amand and Claudia C. Marek. *What Your Doctor May Not Tell You About
   Fibromyalgia.* Warner Books, 1999.

**Web site for update information, product list,
medical practitioners and support group**
   www.fibromyalgiatreatment.com

Month 5

Information about supplements and alternative treatments
   Web site: www.quackwatch.com

Potency and purity of dietary supplements
LLC
333 Mamaroneck Avenue
White Plains, NY 10605
Telephone: 914-722-9149
Web site: www.consumerslab.com

Mari Skelly and Andrea Helm. *Alternative Treatments for Fibromyalgia and Chronic Fatigue Syndrome.* Hunter House, 1999.

Month 6

General Information about various health topics:
Web site: www.about.com
Web site: www.webmd.com

Miryam Erlich Williamson. *Blood Sugar Blues: Overcoming the Hidden Dangers of Insulin Resistance.* Walker, 2001.
Ruth Winter. *The Anti-Aging Hormones.* Random House, 1997.

For low carb diet:
I recommend all books by Robert Atkins, M.D.
Web site: www.atkinscenter.com
You can find Atkins recipes, products, books on his site.

Month 7

U.S. Department of Justice
Civil Rights Division Disability Rights Section
950 Pennsylvania Avenue NW
Washington, D.C. 20530
Telephone: 202-307-1198
Web site: www.usdoj.gov/crt

Job Accommodation Network
West Virginia University
P.O. Box 6080
Morgantown, WV 26506-6080
Telephone: 800-526-7234
Web site: www.jan.wvu.edu/cigi-win/DisQuery

Miryam Erlich Williamson. *213 Ideas for Improving the Quality of Life with Fibromyalgia.* Walker, 1998.

Month 8

Fibromyalgia Resources for Men
Web site: www.menwithfibro.com

Month 9

Accessible Journeys
35 West Sellers Avenue
Ridley Park, PA 19078
Telephone: 800-846-4537
Web site: www.accessiblejourneys.com

**www.about.com has listings for environmentally
and chemically sensitive travelers all over the world.**

Glen Ivy Hot Springs Spa
25000 Glen Ivy Road
Glen Ivy, CA 92883
Telephone: 888-CLUB-MUD
Web site: www.glenivy.com

Month 10

How to Start a Support Group
Web site: www.ohionline.osu.ed/ss-fact

James E. Miller. *Effective Support Groups.* Willowgreen Publishing, 1998
Barbara Sher. *Teamworks: Building Support Groups that Guarantee Success.* Warner Books, 1989.

Month 11

Many resources at www.pages.prodigy.net/turnip/childrenandteens.htm
Includes articles and links to support groups for children and for parents

R. Paul St. Amand and Claudia Marek. *What Your Doctor May Not Tell You About Pediatric Fibromyalgia.* Warner Books, 2002.
Devin Starlanyl and Mary Ellen Copeland. *Fibromyalgia and Chronic Myofascial Pain: A Survival Advocate.* New Harbinger Publications, Inc., 2001.
Miryam Erlich Williamson. *Fibromyalgia: A Comprehensive Approach.* Walker, 1996.

Acknowledgments

THERE ARE many debts associated with this book, yet there is still a logical place to start. Dr. R. Paul St. Amand, M.D., who shared his infectious and great love of medicine with me, patiently taught me, and answered all my questions, certainly deserves top billing. He made available to me, and to you, the knowledge he has gleaned from forty-plus years of tirelessly treating fibromyalgics. There is no way I could have ever attempted this book without his generosity.

My husband, Lou, encouraged me to take on this project and shouldered tasks above and beyond the call of duty to allow me to do it, and for that I owe him big time, and also for doing my illustrations. My sons Malcolm and Sean were troupers, and only rarely complained because I was always "too busy," cheerfully for the most part, doing without their mother at baseball games and meals. My father and mother gave me many, many gifts, and the greatest of those was confidence in myself—they taught me to believe I could do anything I turned my heart and mind toward accomplishing.

So many fibromyalgia patients from the office where I work and from online support groups shared their experiences and stories to make this book richer. It is always amazing to me how many rush forward whenever they hear the word "help." I thank them all for using their precious energy to pitch in. The

Administrative Team from fibromyalgiatreatment.com: Gwen Meshorer, Gretchen Evans Parker, Char Melson, Anne Louise, Jan Houp, Cris Croll, and Jayne Cutler, provide an abundance of support, material, and ideas on a daily basis.

Because I continued to work full-time while writing this book, my co-workers Gloria Martinez and my son Malcolm Potter stepped up and helped me get through every day. I don't know how we got it all done, but thanks especially to Gloria, we did.

This book couldn't possibly have been completed without Mari Florence, whose expertise and hands-on work were the bedrock of this task. Carol Mann, my agent, and Matthew Lore and Sue McCloskey from Marlowe & Company also deserve a grateful and heartfelt thanks for their hard work on this project. Last but certainly not least, an acknowledgment is due to Howard Grossman for designing the cover, and to Pauline Neuwirth who did the same for the interior pages.

Index

Solomons, Clive, 86
St. Amand, Paul, 38, 73, 198
Starlanyl, Devin, 34, 106, 192
stimulants, 47–48, 197
stress, 122–37
stretching routines, 152–55
support groups, 3, 78, 84, 289–99
surgery for fibromyalgia, 105
symptoms, 7–9, 162, 170
    central nervous system (CNS), 7, 35–43
    dermal system, 8
    gastrointestinal system, 8
    genitourinary system, 8
    musculoskeletal system, 7, 20–25
syndrome, 10

T

T'ai Chi, 217
teenagers, 313
tender points, 21–23, 27, 105–6, 191
tests, 4
thyroid, 48
topical solutions, 28, 76, 84, 191
    capsaicin, 191
    Emu Oil, 85
    lidocaine cream, 85, 191
    salicylates, 191
    See also creams
Trager, Milton, 218–19
Trager work, 218–19
train travel, 282–83
tranquillizers, 195
travel, 279–88
trigger points, 27, 105–6, 191
TSH-HS, 4

U

ulcerative colitis, 59

V

vacations, 273–78
vegetables, 226
vertigo, 96
vitamins, 204–6
vulvar pain syndrome
    See vulvodynia
vulvar vestibulitis syndrome, 77, 79
vulvodynia, 73, 76, 77–78, 84–86

W

weather, 100
weight, 227
weight loss, 233–38
Whitmore, Kristene, 84
Willems, John, 73, 76, 78, 84, 85, 88
Williamson, Miryam, 255
Wolfe, Dr., 12
work, 135, 241–55
workers' compensation, 253

Y

yeast infections, 74, 76
yoga, 217
Yount, Joanne, 86
Tunis, Dr., 12

Z

Zone diet, 227